Holistic Remedies for Alzheimer's

Natural Strategies to Avoid or Combat
Dementia

By Case Adams, Naturopath

Holistic Remedies for Alzheimer's: Natural Strategies to Avoid or Combat
     Dementia
Copyright © 2016 Case Adams
LOGICAL BOOKS
Wilmington, Delaware
http://www.logicalbooks.org
All rights reserved.
Printed in USA
Front cover illustration: Gerd Altmann

Publishers Cataloging in Publication Data
Adams, Case
     Holistic Remedies for Alzheimer's: Natural Strategies to Avoid or
Combat Dementia
First Edition
1. Medicine. 2. Health.
Bibliography and References; Index

ISBN-13s
Print version: 978-1-936251-50-6
Ebook version: 978-1-936251-51-3

Other Books by the Author:

PURE WATER: The Science of Water, Waves, Water Pollution, Water Treatment, Water Therapy and Water Ecology

THE ANCESTORS DIET: Living and Cultured Foods to Extend Life, Prevent Disease and Lose Weight

THE BRAIN, MIND AND UNCONSCIOUS SELF: Unveiling the Ancient Secrets using Science

THE CONSCIOUS ANATOMY: Healing the Real You

THE LIVING CLEANSE: Detoxification and Cleansing Using Living Foods and Safe Natural Strategies

THE MEANING OF DREAMS: The Science of Why We Dream, How to Interpret Them and How to Steer Them

THE SCIENCE OF LEAKY GUT SYNDROME: Intestinal Permeability and Digestive Health

TOTAL HARMONIC: The Healing Power of Nature's Elements

Table of Contents

Introduction

The first documented case of Alzheimer's disease was discovered by a Bavarian psychiatrist named Dr. Alois Alzheimer. Dr. Alzheimer treated a 51-year old patient who suffered from memory loss and hallucinations. The patient, "Auguste D" was frequently delirious and had extreme short-term memory deficit. She complained of having "lost myself." She was committed to the Frankfurt asylum in 1901 and died five years later. Autopsy revealed a sticky plaque among brain cells and nerve tissue entanglement.

The disease was named after the diagnosis given by Dr. Alzheimer, and this variant of dementia became associated with memory loss and physical damage to the brain apparently relating to a build-up of beta-amyloid plaque among certain regions of the brain.

In the century following this first diagnosis, Alzheimer's disease has become a virtual plague of aging humanity.

In the United States alone, someone new will develop Alzheimer's disease every 67 seconds. By 2050, this number is expected to double to someone developing Alzheimer's every 33 seconds.

Alzheimer's disease is the scourge of our generation—and its increasingly so. This is a disease which insults the very nature of our humanity—our ability to freely draw from and submit to memory the knowledge of the world and access the information we hold dear.

To take this away—to take away this part of our mental capacity—is to remove our ability to connect with each other in ways that provide a sense of family and unity with others around us.

Anyone who has witnessed or experienced a family member with dementia can tell you: It is a nightmare to have a loved one not recognize or remember you.

This is not the only thing dementia steals. It can steal one's entire recent memory. It can steal the memory of what happened yesterday. Or even what happened five minutes ago.

Certainly, there are different forms of dementia—of which Alzheimer's is one—but just imagine such a scenario:

Those around you feel like strangers: Your wife or husband. Your children. Your friends of many years. You wonder why they are coming around to see you. You wonder why they are hugging you and talking so nicely to you. You wonder what they want from you. They seem familiar but you don't know why.

As you speak with each one, they tell you how they know you. You feel embarrassed and ashamed. But you also feel they could be lying to you. They could be pretending to be your friends and family so they could take advantage of you. Should you trust them?

You excuse yourself to go to the bathroom. You walk by the mirror in the bathroom. You wonder who is this person in the mirror? Is this you? You seem to remember seeing a younger version of what you see. But you're not sure.

Then you look around the bathroom sink after going the bathroom. You are not sure what to do now. What are these things sitting around the sink? What is that white bar for? What are the long sticks with bristles for?

Yes, indeed, severe Alzheimer's disease can make a person forget what essential utensils and objects of daily care are and how they are used.

After going to the bathroom, you go out to the living room again. You look around the room and wonder why all these strangers are in your living room? Some come to you and see your confused look and say, "Hey we were just talking, don't you remember?"

Sadly, you don't. You stare into their eyes but recognize no one. Not even your wife and grown up kids.

"These are my kids?" you ask. Yes, says your wife, who you don't recognize. "What are their names?"

Yes, along with forgetting the faces of your loved ones, you could also forget their names. You could even forget that you have a wife or kids or brothers or sisters.

Yes, this is a nightmare, you say. This is truly something that could never happen to me, you say. Yet there is a good chance that if you live in the West, this will happen to you.

According to the 2016 World Health Organization report on AD, over 30 million people have Alzheimer's disease around the world, with over five million new cases each year. About 58 percent of Alzheimer's cases are among Third world or poorer countries, with the rest among richer countries.

According to the 2014 Alzheimer's Disease Facts and Figures study published by the Alzheimer's Association, well over five million Americans have Alzheimer's disease, with rates growing steadily in recent years. And nearly half a million people over the age of 65 developed Alzheimer's disease in the U.S. during 2014.

Alzheimer's is the sixth leading cause of death in the United States. Alzheimer's yields significant burden upon U.S. health care, and this burden is increasing exponentially. It has been predicted that by 2050, Alzheimer's will cost Americans $1.2 trillion a year in health care costs.

Furthermore, Alzheimer's is the only cause of death from the top 10 causes where Western medicine has no cure or manner of prevention.

The research also finds that 11 percent of Americans over the age of 65 currently have Alzheimer's disease. This means one in nine people.

And a third of Americans over the age of 85 have Alzheimer's. Yes, one in three people over 85 have Alzheimer's disease.

According to this data, 38% of Alzheimer's patients are over 85 years old. And 43 percent are between 75 and 84 years old, while 15 percent are between 65 and 74 years old. Only 4 percent of Alzheimer's patients are under 65 years old.

This last group—under 65—has what is referred to as early-onset Alzheimer's disease. Yes four percent seems small enough. Yet we are still talking about 200,000 people who have early-onset Alzheimer's disease.

In terms of gender, currently more U.S. women have Alzheimer's disease than men. Of the 5.1 million people who have Alzheimer's disease in 2015, 3.2 million are women and 1.9 million are men. This means that close to 63 percent are women.

The jury is still out on why. Some studies have indicated this is because women tend to live longer than men.

Yet other studies have shown that the ApoE4 genotype—known to increase ones risk of Alzheimer's—is more prevalent in women.

As we'll discuss more in the book, having a copy of the ApoE4 gene theoretically increases ones risk of Alzheimer's disease. Having two copies of ApoE4 theoretically increases the risk further. It has been estimated that between 20 and 30 percent of the population has a copy of ApoE4, while about two percent have two copies.

Nonetheless, Alzheimer's disease is expected to significantly increase over the next decades. It is estimated that by 2050, the number of people over 65 with Alzheimer's disease will nearly triple to 13.8 million people in the U.S. alone.

In the next ten years, Alzheimer's disease incidence is expected to increase from five million to over seven million in 2025.

Obviously, we are doing something wrong. We are doing something that previous generations did not do. Alzheimer's disease was only discovered in 1906.

Is Alzheimer's strictly a disease of our times? Did it exist prior to 1906? Certainly it did. But certainly not to this extent. Autopsy is not a new invention.

Yes, it may be true that more of our modern-day population is living longer. The number of people in the U.S. over the age of 65 is greater than it has been over the last fifty years. The average life expectancy in the U.S. and Europe has surely ramped up over the past 50 years.

Yet Alzheimer's disease has not been this sort of rampant issue among those over 65 in centuries past—in Eastern or Western countries.

In fact, traditionally, aging has been linked with the ability to transmit knowledge. Those who reached this age and older were often respected as having advanced wisdom.

Living beyond the age of 65 isn't necessarily a rare occurrence in human history. In fact, average lifespan is somewhat of a misnomer. Average lifespan has been traditionally calculated by averaging all births and deaths. In earlier centuries, significantly more babies died during or following childbirth. This statistic has significantly decreased the lifespan numbers of the near past.

As far as the not-so-recent past, many lived to a ripe old age, with little mention of dementia. Most of us have read some of the records in the Book of Genesis, detailing that Methuselah lived 782 years, Noah lived for 500 years and Abraham lived to 175. Other Biblical personalities also lived far longer than humans live now according to the Bible.

These are not the only records showing increased lifespan among earlier humans. The Chinese Encyclopedia of Materia Medica indicates that He Nengci of the Tang dynasty lived 168 years. Chinese medical records further indicate that the Qin dynasty doctor Cuie Wenze lived to 300 years old. Tao master Li Qingyuan lived to 250 years old. Han dynasty ruler Gee Yule lived to 280 years old. Tao monk Hui Zhao lived to 290 years old. Lo Zichange lived to 180 years old.

We also have modern examples of people living long lives. A 1995 India Times article and subsequent reports put Bir Narayan Chaudhary of Nepal's age as 141 years old.

The point is the notion of living past the age of 65 is not new in human history. What is new is that such a significant portion of those living into their advanced years in a state of dementia—mostly with Alzheimer's disease.

This of course says volumes about Alzheimer's disease. The vast increases in incidence says that Alzheimer's disease is not only a modern day disorder. It indicates that there is something about our modern day lives that is increasing the risk of Alzheimer's disease.

This of course presents to us a modern-day mystery. One that requires significant research and a considerable amount of common sense.

These are the elements that are being brought into the picture with this book. There is a considerable amount of research on the Alzheimer's disease disorder today. This includes the basic understandings of the disease: Its symptoms, physiological traits, prognosis and so on. But recent research now offers us insight into associations between lifestyles and risk. These lifestyles include diets, supplements, exercise and other unique features of health.

Yes, some of these have been well-publicized in recent years. But what has often been missing from these portrayals is the common sense behind the associations.

What is this common sense element? It is fitting together all the pieces behind the associations and Alzheimer's disease. These, together with the fact that Alzheimer's disease incidence is growing—just as those associated lifestyles and diets are growing—gives us increasing insight into the ability to prevent Alzheimer's disease as we age.

Then we can add an additional element to this presentation: The scientific findings of use certain natural therapies that may prevent Alzheimer's, slow the progression of Alzheimer's, and perhaps reverse some of its symptoms.

Introducing such therapies could be frowned upon by some in conventional medicine. Does this mean that such therapies come without scientific and clinical testing?

Not necessarily. Yes, it is true that most Alzheimer's disease research funding in recent years has been pointed towards drug therapies for Alzheimer's disease. But we can offer two significant points. First, that all this funding has not offered much of a solution to Alzheimer's disease. There are a few drugs that have been shown to improve some of the symptoms, yes. But little in the way of real treatments.

Yet at the same time, there has been—despite the severe lack of funding—some significant findings among natural therapies for Alzheimer's disease treatment. We will discuss much of this research to date in this book.

This book is aimed towards anyone who wants to know more about the causes of Alzheimer's disease, and what the science shows regarding natural strategies for fighting it. This includes avoiding it or slowing it.

The title mentions dementia in general. This is because, as we will find, many of the potential causes of Alzheimer's are also linked to the other forms of dementia. And most of the natural strategies discussed in this text are also appropriate for other forms of dementia—the primary ones being vascular dementia and Lewy body dementia.

Finally, to clear the air, we must state that this book is not promising to serve to diagnose, prevent or treat any disease. One should seek professional medical advice for that. Furthermore, anyone wishing to utilize any of the information provided here should consult with ones health care professional in advance.

Part I

What is Alzheimer's Disease?

Chapter One

Signs of Alzheimer's Disease

Alzheimer's disease is a mysterious condition. Yes, the mechanisms of Alzheimer's disease has become clearer. But there are still lots of unanswered questions.

First and foremost, Alzheimer's disease is a form of dementia. There are other forms of dementia, and they are related. Their relationship is based on the symptom of cognitive impairment and memory loss. Besides Alzheimer's, forms of dementia include vascular dementia, Lewy body dementia, frontotemporal dementia and alcohol-induced dementia.

In May of 2016, the Centers for Disease Control (Goodman *et al.*) released the results of Medicare recipient care for those over 66 in the U.S. between 2011 and 2013. The research found that 3.1 million patients were treated for dementia. Most of these were diagnosed in terms of subtypes. But among those who were further diagnosed, 45 percent were Alzheimer's patients; 14.5 percent of them had vascular dementia; 5.4 percent had Lewy body dementia; 1 percent had frontotemporal dementia and 0.7 percent had alcohol induced dementia. Other dementia subtypes added up to 0.2 percent of those diagnosed.

Signs of Alzheimer's

The signs of Alzheimer's disease near the top of this list are related to something called mild cognitive impairment or MCI. This means not just memory loss, but the loss of critical thinking, decision making and the ability to converse and live normally with others.

After these, we'll lay out some of the physiological signs and symptoms, which include beta-amyloids and insulin resistance.

Memory Loss

The hallmark sign of Alzheimer's disease is memory loss. Much of this is recent memories, related to what has happened in the recent past. This includes events that just happened, or things that the Alzheimer's patient has just been told.

The event-related memory loss is often termed episodic memory loss, which means forgetting things that have happened in the past. But it also includes forgetting faces and names, as well as forgetting relatives and friends.

It is almost as if the Alzheimer's patient has withdrawn from everyone and everything he or she has done or known in their lifetime. An Alzheimer's patient might remember parts of their childhood, but they will often forget what they did for a career, or who they married, or what college they graduated from. They might also forget many other important milestones in their life, as well as the people who accompanied them during those events.

This sort of memory withdrawal is quite puzzling to doctors, and we'll discuss the more subtle elements of this later on.

Daily tasking memory is also a challenge for a person with Alzheimer's disease. This includes appointments or important dates, or even daily regimens such as eating or taking a daily shower.

What this is not: It is perfectly normal to forget names, dates or events once in awhile. In fact, forgetting someone's name right after meeting them, or even an acquaintance over a period of time is a frequent habit of healthy people. Alzheimer's disease is not the same as information overload, which is what many people suffer from as we attempt to complete all the information challenges required by our households, computers and government agencies. It is perfectly normal to be increasingly forgetful as we age. This is not the same as forgetting the name of our brother or sister, for example.

Losing Things

It is normal to lose something. There are so many things, and places to put things, and we may forget where we put something. This is normal, especially for things we don't often use.

It is another thing to forget where we put things that we regularly use. For example, forgetting where the forks are when we open the silverware drawer on a regular basis. Or forgetting where our car is parked when we park it in the same place day after day.

Confusion

Another sign of Alzheimer's disease is confusing and losing track of dates, times or places. Examples include forgetting what year it is or how old we are. Or thinking it is morning when it is late in the afternoon.

Confusing places is a big one. Traveling to a location and then forgetting why we traveled there is a big sign.

Another is being somewhere and completely forgetting where we are or how we got there. This is a hallmark sign. If this happens more than once in awhile, consider an Alzheimer's disease checkup.

What this is not: Being confused about something complicated or even occasionally about anything is normal. Going into a room and then forgetting why we went into the room is also perfectly normal sometimes. This is different than making a trip across town or to another city and forgetting why we went there (or where we are).

Conversation or Reading Problems

Someone with Alzheimer's disease may have problems conversing with others. They may not be able to understand what the other person says, for example. Or they may not be able to respond correctly. An Alzheimer's patient might be asked a simple question and not be able to answer it.

Forgetting words during a conversation can also be a sign of Alzheimer's, assuming the word loss is overwhelming and multiple words are lost—not just a word here or there.

This can also translate to reading and writing. A drastic inability to read or write simple words and sentences can be a sign of Alzheimer's disease.

What this is not: It is normal to be shy sometimes or even most of the time, and have difficulty communicating with others. Some people simply don't like large crowds, or family events or other gatherings. This doesn't mean they have Alzheimer's disease.

As mentioned above, losing a word here or there while talking is perfectly normal. The English language contains well over one million words (more like about 1,025,109 according to the Global Language Monitor). As we age, we hear more and more words that describe things in so many different ways. It is simply not possible to remember every single word at the precise moment we would like to use that word. We might even think the word was something that we have used before—so why can't we find the word now?

This often relates to our word association—especially for that particular word, topic or situation. We might, for example, be speaking on a subject that we have considered dry and boring in the past—and because of that, have not made enough associations with the words in that subject matter. Then when we speak on that topic, we might forget some of the words because we have not put enough association behind them. Using memory association tools can significantly enhance a healthy person's memory.

Vision Issues

As we age, our vision becomes weaker. We begin to have issues adjusting to light changes, problems reading smaller print and sometimes issues with color. Most of these are a normal part of aging.

A common Alzheimer's disease sign is a stark yet often inconsistent weakening of vision. Not being able to read traffic signs, judge distances or see contrasting images can be a sign of Alzheimer's disease.

Decision-making

A sign of Alzheimer's disease may be an inability to make critical choices or good decisions. For example, if a waiter asks, "do you want water with your dinner" and the person can't seem to answer this simple question quickly and easily, then this could be a sign of Alzheimer's disease.

What this is not: Making decisions can sometimes become difficult if there are consequences to each and the decision requires more consideration. This is normal. But easy decisions are something else entirely.

Mood Changes

Abrupt mood changes may be a sign of Alzheimer's disease. These include becoming hostile or angry with little provocation. Or being in a good mood and then suddenly changing to a bad mood without a triggering event.

This can also include what appears to be a personality change—as a happy-go-lucky mood changes into a sour, angry mood.

What this is not: It is perfectly normal for a person to change moods for a reason. The reason may be readily apparent to an observer, or not. For example, a person might think of a friend who died recently and become sad. This is normal.

Development of Alzheimer's disease

Early or Mild Phase

During the earliest phase of Alzheimer's disease—which may last up to five years—memory is first affected. This is primarily the short- and medium-term memory. Long-term memory typically stays intact during this phase. Speech is typically fluent, however finding the right word may be difficult.

The early Alzheimer's patient may also have difficulty executing complex activities, such as those at work or in their professional life.

These may appear with frustration, depression and even anxiety, as early Alzheimer's disease patients become aware of their mental deterioration. Sometimes apathy, loss of interest or fear arise.

Middle or Moderate Phase

This middle phase can last a couple of years to a decade. The patient may not be able to remember recent thinking or events. And there is difficulty converting thoughts to words.

During conversation, the person won't be able to react intelligently to questioning. There will be misunderstandings of the conversation and difficulty with expression. Repeating words, sentences or even sounds might take place in an attempt to express oneself.

Difficulty with math, reading and writing will occur during this phase. Disorientation may occur, in both unknown and familiar environments, and with time and space. Sometimes, delusion and hallucination may occur.

Late or Severe Phase

This phase typically lasts only a year to three years, as patients often die from a related or unrelated disorder such as an infection or a fall. Difficulty with communication, social interaction and being able to understand place or position becomes severe in this stage.

Memory recall becomes difficult. Sometimes photos can help recall, but sometimes photos are not even helpful. Recognizing friends and family becomes variable—if not completely unrecognizable.

Communications with family and friends becomes severely difficult. Understanding the meaning of what is being said becomes difficult. Tasks that require judgment, reasoning and logic become difficult.

Chapter Two

Mechanisms of Alzheimer's Disease

Yes, the physiological mechanisms of Alzheimer's disease have become clearer. But there are still lots of unanswered questions. Let's work from the most known towards the more mysterious things about the condition. Many consider some of the below issues as causes of Alzheimer's—but we'll discuss, many of these occur without Alzheimer's disease.

The Plaque of Misunderstanding

Perhaps the most readily associated physiological mechanism for Alzheimer's disease relates to the presence of built-up beta-amyloid plaque in the brain, as seen by autopsy or an MRI (magnetic resonance imaging) scan.

The presence of the plaque is apparently the result of beta-amyloid oligomers being present among brain tissues and cerebrospinal fluid. This is the prevailing theory at least.

According to the theory, the accumulation of beta-amyloid oligomer peptides in the brain of Alzheimer's patients produces neurotoxicity, which kills brain cells. This is especially important among the brain cells of the hippocampus and cerebral cortex. These brain cells are critical for storing and transmitting memories and information.

One of the apparent precipitating factors for the development of beta-amyloid plaques is the existence of what are called tau proteins, which likely form as a result of the continuing presence of the beta-amyloid oligomers. These form twisted fibrils called tau tangles.

Oddly enough, as we will explore further, not everyone with significant beta-amyloid plaque deposits or tau tangles has or will have Alzheimer's disease. This is one of many mysterious things about Alzheimer's.

Another mystery is why healthy adults will have significant levels of beta-amyloid proteins in their bloodstream, and many with Alzheimer's will have low levels of beta-amyloids in their bloodstream.

Beta-amyloid plaque continues to be the central hallmark of Alzheimer's disease because it has been found in the dissected brains of Alzheimer's patients. Today, a doctor can see beta-amyloid plaque using MRI using an imaging compound. The question now is, is beta-amyloid plaque the cause for one losing touch with one's family, past and practically everything else in life? Or is the plaque something else? As we'll discover below, it is something else.

The amyloid plaque-Alzheimer's theory was generally accepted through autopsies. But the theory was adjusted in 2002, with the publishing of a cumulative research paper by Hardy and Selkoe.

Their hypothesis presented that beta-amyloid plaque is produced within a pathway related to a particular type of beta-amyloid proteins. These lead to the death of brain cells, according to the hypothesis. The result is cognitive decline and eventually memory loss—as hippocampus and cortical neurons are lost.

The problem has been that the existence of beta-amyloid proteins and plaques and resulting tau tangles in these locations doesn't necessarily mean having Alzheimer's. In fact, at least 30 percent of elderly people who do not have Alzheimer's will still have these amyloid plaques. Still others will also have the neurofibril (tau) tangles—yet won't have or develop Alzheimer's in the future. This problem has perplexed neuroscientists and doctors alike.

For example, University of Pittsburgh School of Medicine researchers (Aizenstein *et al.* 2008) conducted tomography (PET) imaging on 43 elderly people. They found that one in five (21 percent) had significant amyloid plaques.

The researchers also performed cognitive testing on all the subjects. They found no correlation between amyloid plaque and cognitive performance.

Such a result has also been found in other research, such as Engler *et al.* (2006); Kadir *et al.* (2008 and 2011); Scheinin *et al.* (2009) and Jagust *et al.* (2010). Each of these studies found beta-amyloid plaque build-up in one way or another among people did not correlate with Alzheimer's disease.

At the same time, a number of other studies did show the correlation. These have included Jack *et al.* (2009); Grimmer *et al.* (2010); Rinne *et al.* (2010); Koivunen *et al.* (2011); Sojkova *et al.* (2011); Villemagne *et al.* (2011) and Kadir *et al.* (2012).

Pittsburgh Compound B

Testing for beta-amyloid plaque has always been challenging, and one reason is because, as we'll explain, sometimes the amyloid proteins are helpful to brain function. In other words, there can be different sorts of amyloid proteins in the brain.

In recent years, University of Pittsburg researchers discovered a way to test for amyloid plaque buildup within the brain. An agent called the Pittsburgh compound B is injected into the subject. The PiB compound then attaches to fibrous buildups of beta-amyloid plaques within the brain. And apparently, it doesn't attach to the more healthy beta-amyloid buildup.

Illustrating the connection between this fibrous buildup of amyloid-beat, researchers from France's INSERM (Villain *et al.* 2012) tested 32 patients with Alzheimer's disease. They tested 49 people with MCI and 103 healthy people. The researchers found that only one of the Alzheimer's patients were PiB-negative. The rest all had a buildup of this sort of fibrous amyloid-plaque that PiB attaches to.

The researchers also found that four out of five of those who developed MCI (and one who developed Alzheimer's) had a buildup of this sort of plaque.

Yet again, many of the healthy subjects—with no sign of MCI or Alzheimer's—also had the PiB-associated buildup of beta-amyloid plaque. A full 27 of the 97 healthy people who didn't develop Alzheimer's disease during the follow-up period also had the PiB-associated amyloid buildup.

The researchers also measured the accumulation of beta-amyloid plaque after an additional 40 months. They identified each subject as either an "accumulator" or a "non-accumulator," based upon whether their levels of beta-amyloid increased over the period.

Among the healthy people who were considered PiB-negative, 19 were classified as accumulators and 48 were non-accumulators. Among those who were PiB-positive, 16 were accumulators and 16 were non-accumulators. Those who were non-accumulators also tended to be older—averaging 79 years old compared to 75 among the accumulators.

None of these groups showed progression to Alzheimer's—accumulators or non-accumulators, by the way.

Among those with Alzheimer's, the results weren't that different in terms of accumulation of beta-amyloid. Among those who were PiB-positive (32 out of 33), only 17 were accumulators and 12 were non-accumulators. And here, the non-accumulators tended to be younger, at 67 compared to 75 years old.

While some of this disturbs any notion of a certain continuing disease progression—there was a tendency of those who had built up the amyloid plaque to a certain degree to stop accumulating. This was called a *saturable process* by the researchers. That is, there is a certain point to where the plaque accumulation stops after it has built up to a certain point.

But the researchers still found major discrepancies with regard to the build up of beta-amyloid plaque and the progression of Alzheimer's:

> *"Consistent with the regional PiB rate of change, PiB accumulation status was not related to clinical status or disease progression. As discussed earlier, this finding is consistent with the amyloid-*

clinical discrepancy observed in cross-sectional or short-term longi-
tudinal studies."

In their discussion of the research, the scientists hypothesized a 14+ year lag between the accumulation of the plaque and Alzheimer's disease in the future, yet this could not be proven out by the study:

"Nonetheless our estimations suggest that the hypothetical
14.5 years time-lag between the occurrence of detectable amyloid-β
deposition and dementia is far beyond the 20-month follow-up of
this study."

The link between PiB-positive beta-amyloid buildup and Alzheimer's disease was confirmed in another 2012 study (Chételat *et al.* 2012) from Melbourne, Australia. This study tested 74 healthy elderly people. Each subject was tested twice with Pittsburgh compound B PET scans, 18-months apart.

They were also tested each time with MRI (magnetic resonance imaging) scans to determine the rate of atrophy in their brain, if any.

The researchers found that those with the most prevalent PiB-positive scores also had the greatest rates of atrophy in their brains:

"Our findings show that the presence of Beta-amyloid in the brain,
known to occur in about one-third of asymptomatic elderly indi-
viduals, is actually a pathologic state associated with accelerated at-
rophy. They also suggest that therapy aimed to reduce the
neurodegenerative process should be commenced in presymptomatic
individuals with high PiB."

A year later, Australian researchers from Brisbane (Dore *et al.* 2013) tested 93 healthy elderly adults alongside 40 Alzheimer's patients. The researchers also ran MRI and PiB testing, this time at the beginning of the study, at 18 months and at 36 months.

Here again the researchers found that being PiB-positive correlated with Alzheimer's disease and with reduced episodic memory over time. They also found the cortical thickness of the brain was reduced as atrophy increased. The researchers concluded:

"In asymptomatic individuals, Beta-amyloid deposition is associ-
ated with GM atrophy and memory impairment. The earliest signs
of GM atrophy were detected in the hippocampus and the posterior
cingulate and precuneus regions, and with disease progression, atro-
phy became more extensive in the temporal lobes. These findings
support the notion that Beta-amyloid deposition is not a benign

process and that interventions with anti-Beta-amyloid therapy at these early stages have a higher chance to be effective."

We can surmise from this research that the fibroid-buildup of beta-amyloid plaque can be a significant diagnostic tool indicating the advance of Alzheimer's, but also memory impairment in the absence of Alzheimer's disease: More specifically, a buildup of beta-amyloid plaque within the regions of the hippocampus and the frontal cortices of the brain.

Today, beta-amyloid oligomers in the cerebral spinal fluid will also predict or diagnose Alzheimer's for many people.

For example, a 2015 Australian study (Li *et al.*) tested 157 people who had either mild cognitive impairment or Alzheimer's, and compared these with 99 healthy people.

The researchers used PET scans with PiB imaging, and found that the cerebral spinal fluids of the Alzheimer's and MCI patients had beta-amyloid oligomers, with specificities between 85 and 92 percent. This means this sort of non-invasive imaging provides one of the best diagnostic tools in determining ones potential development or current development of Alzheimer's disease.

But there is still enough solid evidence to conclude that many people with atrophy and PiB-positive beta-amyloid oligomers or plaque in these regions do not succumb to Alzheimer's disease. Though accumulating beta-amyloid plaque does correlate with Alzheimer's disease for many, the evidence indicates that the amyloid plaque itself cannot be causative, because so many people who have the plaque do not develop Alzheimer's disease.

In this regard it is critical to understand the difference between correlation and causation. Two things may be present at the same time for a number of reasons. One may cause another, but there might be a common cause for both of them. Or they might be occurring together for another reason.

Beta-amyloid plaque is certainly one of the symptoms of Alzheimer's disease. But this doesn't mean the plaque is causing the Alzheimer's disease.

Rather, what is producing the plaque may also be producing the Alzheimer's disease. Or the plaque may be one of the byproducts of the memory loss.

This doesn't mean that we should ignore the amyloid plaque. Certainly, avoiding the amyloid plaque should still be important. And a case of developing beta-amyloid plaque should be considered a potential diagnostic indicator of a possible developing case of Alzheimer's disease or MCI.

We might compare this situation to being on the battlefield and seeing one's opponent appear waving a white flag. Certainly, the white flag is a good indicator that the opponent is surrendering. But it is still not a certainty. The potential victors should approach with caution, because the enemy may simply be hanging out some underwear. Or they may be waving the white flag to trick their enemy to stop fighting so they can ambush them.

In addition, we can add the many times people wave white flags—or hang their underwear up to try—when they aren't even in a war. Does every time something white is waved mean surrender? Certainly not. In a war, there is a solid relationship between waving the white flag and surrender. But waving a white flag doesn't always mean surrender.

The only certainty of surrender is when the enemy lays down its weapons and stops fighting.

In the same way, beta-amyloid plaque may indicate the potential of a developing case of Alzheimer's, but not in every case. More certainty is indicated by the loss of memory.

This conundrum also indicates something else at play. What is it? What is the real cause of AD?

For this, we must try to understand more about this disease, and more about the brain itself.

The Plaque Defense

The theory that the beta-amyloid plaques seen among Alzheimer's patients is causing Alzheimer's disease has been questioned by many researchers. In fact, many researchers have taken the stance that the plaques are actually the body's defense system against the real culprit: The free-floating beta-amyloid oligomers.

The error of the plaque hypothesis became more evident after multiple drugs aimed at removing the sticky plaques from the brain did not reduce Alzheimer's disease symptoms.

One of these is bapineuzumab—an antibody drug aimed at reducing plaque in the brain. Yes, mice and human studies showed that bapineuzumab successfully removed plaque. But the drug did little to reverse or lessen Alzheimer's disease symptoms. Human studies by drug companies found, in fact, that the drug was no better than placebo. Shortly thereafter, the drug testing was cancelled.

Dr. Scott McGinnis of Harvard Medical School and Brigham and Women's Hospital in Boston has treated Alzheimer's patients and has ran clinical trials of Alzheimer's disease drugs. Dr. McGinnis stated emphatically in 2010:

"The plaque is not the main culprit in terms of toxicity."

Dr. Andrew Dillin of California's Salk Institute in California and the Howard Hughes Medical Institute agreed and further explained:

"If you say Alzheimer's, everyone immediately thinks that it's the plaques that actually cause the disease. That couldn't be further from the truth. The data actually suggest these plaques are a form of protection that the body tries to put on. So this is a sign that your brain was trying to do something very useful and helpful to you, and the remnant was the formation of amyloid plaques."

Let's clarify this. Let's say that you were cutting up a salad and cut your finger. The small cut bleeds for a bit and then begins to scab up. By the next day the cut has a neat brown scab over the wound.

Would you then say that the scab caused the wound? Certainly not. Certainly the knife is the offender that produced the wound. The scab was the body's response to the invasion into the skin by the knife.

The scab is the body's process of helping to protect the wound while the body works to repair the damage.

This is the same process going on in the form of beta-amyloid plaques. The plaques are the body's healing response to the damage produced at least partly by beta-amyloid oligomers.

This was proven out when researchers (Gandy *et al.* 2010) tested mice of different species, some that developed plaques and some that didn't in response to the beta-amyloid proteins. The research indicated that the plaques were definitely not the causative issue, because the mice that didn't get plaques but had the beta-amyloid oligomers got Alzheimer's disease. How could they get Alzheimer's disease without getting the plaques?

This, along with so much of the other research discussed above, proves out that the body forms the plaque in response to being hit with certain types of toxic beta-amyloid oligomers. It is part of the body's healing process.

What are beta-amyloid oligomers?

These are circulating proteins that have become unstable. Their instability comes from what are called Abeta-derived diffusible ligands—or ADDLs. These ADDLs produce a funny thing among brain cells. They produce defects among insulin receptors. This is especially damaging among hippocampus brain cells. They interrupt the ability of these brain cells to operate effectively, because their metabolism is interrupted (Liu *et al.* 2014).

This relationship between ADDLs and insulin receptors also explains why Alzheimer's patients often also have type 2 diabetes, or at least insulin resistance.

Research from the Washington University School of Medicine (Stanley *et al.* 2016) analyzed this correlation closely. They found that Alzheimer's patients typically have elevated insulin levels. They also found that increased beta-amyloid oligomer levels were accompanied by high insulin levels.

There are multiple ways that insulin receptor derangement can produce Alzheimer's disease. First, the brain cell metabolism is reduced due to the lack of energy. When insulin reception is changed, the cell cannot assimilate glucose. Cells use glucose for energy fuel. When cells don't have enough fuel, they slow down, and many die.

Secondly, when insulin reception is blocked, glucose is not taken into the cell. This loading up of unused insulin and glucose within the blood damages the body's blood vessels. When this takes place in the tiny capillaries that feed brain cells, those brain cells starve and die.

Thirdly, type-2 diabetes has been shown to interrupt brain function in itself. This can occur as a result of the brain cells becoming insulin resistant.

Even without beta-amyloid oligomers, diabetes produces issues in the brain. Type-2 diabetes in itself has been linked to cognitive decline (Allen *et al.*, 2004). Type-2 diabetes has also been linked to brain atrophy (Last, *et al.* 2007) as well as reduced brain function (Roberts et al, 2014).

In this last study, 749 people with an average age of 79 years were studied. The researchers found that while the PiB retention ratio was not increased in diabetic people, the diabetic individuals had more than twice the risk of having the abnormal Alzheimer's disease signature for hypometabolism. This means the brain cells among those regions known for Alzheimer's disease were not functioning properly, and their risk for Alzheimer's disease was enhanced.

The researchers stated in their conclusion:

> *"Diabetes and poor glycemic control in nondiabetic individuals may enhance glucose hypometabolism in Alzheimer's disease signature regions. These factors should be investigated in longitudinal studies for their role in detecting onset of symptoms in Alzheimer's disease."*

This illustrates a chicken-and-egg dilemma for researchers. Does the insulin resistance come before the Alzheimer's disease begins to develop?

Or does this insulin resistance come as a result of the progression of the disease.

Paradoxically, both instances have been observed in research. Research from the University of Washington School of Medicine (Craft *et al.* 1998) tested 39 people, including 25 Alzheimer's patients and 14 healthy people. They found the Alzheimer's patients had significantly higher levels of insulin in their plasma, and their CSF-to-plasma insulin levels were significantly lower than the healthy patients. Furthermore, the worse the Alzheimer's disease cases were, the worse their insulin levels were. This also correlated with their amyloid protein levels—higher levels of insulin correlated with higher levels of the beta-amyloid oligomers.

High insulin levels don't always mean the patient is diabetic. Many people have high levels of insulin due to insulin resistance, yet their condition is not considered type-2 diabetes.

Other studies have also correlated insulin resistance to Alzheimer's disease. The most recent comes from the University of Wisconsin School of Medicine (Willette *et al.* 2015). Here, researchers tested 186 people who were "late middle-aged." They utilized the Pittsburgh compound B to conduct positron emission tomography brain scans on each subject. They also tested for the relationship between insulin resistance and blood sugar status on the PiB distribution volume ratio among the frontal, parietal, and temporal brain regions.

Even if the subject had normal blood sugar levels, higher insulin resistance equated with higher PiB levels among the frontal and temporal areas. This, as we discussed above, reflects the current gold standard of increased AD-related beta-amyloid oligomers. The researchers concluded:

> *"This is the first human study to demonstrate that insulin resistance may contribute to amyloid deposition in brain regions affected by Alzheimer's disease."*

So there you have it. The most current evidence of the mechanisms of Alzheimer's disease among the brain's anatomy. Though still, there are certainly people who have type-2 diabetes and insulin resistance but don't have Alzheimer's—just as there are people who have beta-amyloid plaque and even oligomers and no Alzheimer's disease.

But what we do know is that there is some sort of relationship here between the beta-amyloid oligomers, insulin resistance and Alzheimer's disease. There is a progression here.

But as we find in the research, the progression is not irreversible. The presence of the amyloid plaques indicate that the body is trying to repair the damage done by the oligomers. As to whether the insulin resistance can also be turned around—we'll discuss this in depth later.

How do beta-amyloid proteins develop?

Brain plaques that develop in the brain arise as a result of an assembly of fibril material composed of beta-amyloid protein and hyperphosphorylated tau.

These develop in stages, and apparently through separate processes. As the beta-amyloid proteins accumulate, they will develop into larger protein complexes. One of the A-beta protein complexes, called an AB42 because of its string of 42 amino acids, will form what are called oligomers.

In more technical terms, this takes place through a pathological process starting with the appearance of aggregation nuclei, which proceed to form these neurotoxic oligomers.

The odd thing is that A-beta oligomers are also present in many people without Alzheimer's disease. And imaging studies have found that these A-beta oligomers are utilized by the brains of healthy people to build brain connections and even gather memories.

The beta-amyloid protein develops as a result of what is called a amyloid precursor protein, or APP. The APP can develop into amyloid proteins that are helpful to the brain, or potentially damaging to the brain.

In fact, a study from the University of Adelaide (Plummer *et al.* 2016) found that APPs can be used to help treat traumatic brain injury.

But APP can also liberate protein fragments, including the beta-amyloid plaque implicated in Alzheimer's disease.

Recent research has uncovered another protein that may be involved in the process of the APPs. This protein is called the ATP-binding cassette transporter A7 (or ABCA7). The protein is expressed prominently among the microglia cells in the brain—and it can have variants. This means the brain cells' genes may produce a normal version, but also an abnormal version.

Several studies (Li *et al.* 2015; Zhao *et al.* 2015; Sakae *et al.* 2015 and others) have shown that the abnormal expressions of ABCA7 are involved in Alzheimer's disease. Some of these studies have also shown the reason for this is that a healthy version of ABCA7 actually helps protect the brain cells from the beta-amyloid oligomers. The protein actually helps phagotize (which means to break them down) the beta-amyloid proteins.

And conversely, if the ABCA7 gene is a variant—it may not have that capacity to break down the proteins. This results in the damage to the brain cell, and the progression to Alzheimer's disease.

One of the things that ABCA7 is apparently involved in is expressing certain enzymes. Some of these enzymes are suitable for breaking down the amyloid oligomers.

But when the cells express a variant of the ABCA7, the enzymes that normally break down the beta-amyloid proteins turn out to be deranged. This changes the way they break down the beta-amyloid proteins, producing a toxic form of the amyloid proteins—the oligomers involved in damaging brain cells.

This understanding has come only in the past few years, as researchers began connecting the enzymes involved in this fragmentation of beta-amyloid into toxic forms. The first suspects were enzymes called alpha-secretase, beta-secretase and delta-secretase. But then other potential secretases dubbed delta-secretase, mu-secretase and then other forms of beta-secretase also became suspect.

These enzymes create a process called proteolysis—which means the enzymes break down the amyloids in such a way that is helpful for the brain. But when these enzymes are substandard, they will break down the amyloid differently. Their proteolysis turns the amyloid protein into the dangerous oligomers.

Enzyme processes like these will change around the molecules in such a way that will either render the compound inert (metabolically safe) or toxic. The pathway that converts beta-amyloid proteins to the Alzheimer's disease oligomers begins with alpha-secretase. Reaction with beta-secretase continues the pathway and is often followed by the cleavage with gamma-secretase, producing the beta-amyloid oligomers.

Part of the faulty enzyme proteolysis relates to oxidative stress, produced by the removal of the wrong atoms from the molecules on brain cell membranes—something called oxidation. This process can lead to DNA damage which results in the secretase enzyme errors.

As we'll show, this is illustrated by the fact that certain antioxidants and polyphenols have been shown to help protect brain cells from oxidative stress, evidenced by a reduction of amyloid plaque.

The issue is often described as cytotoxicity—which means a toxicity that occurs within the cell. The cell doesn't function properly because of toxicity—which is directly related to oxidation. Why? Because oxidation creates oxidative radicals. Oxidative radicals are missing a hydrogen or similar atom that completes them. In this state they want to steal their missing elements from somewhere else. So they will hurt a cell's composition by stealing elements from it, starting with the cell membrane.

This scenario of free radicals is nothing new. In fact, it has been linked to numerous inflammatory and degenerative diseases, including heart and artery diseases, arthritis and so many others.

Circulatory Issues

Many Alzheimer's patients have also been found to have cardiovascular disease. This may come in the form of atherosclerosis (hardening of the blood vessels) or coronary artery disease (when the blood vessels of the heart become narrowed or blocked).

Vascular dementia and Lewy body dementia are specifically characterized by a narrowing of blood vessels feeding brain tissues. This often develops alpha-synuclein deposits within brain and nerve tissues. This results in the brain cells becoming starved or stressed to the point where they begin to malfunction.

This is also the case with many Alzheimer's patients. But the progression of Alzheimer's disease dementia is typically more dramatic. No matter the type, dementia proceeds with the loss of synapses and the degeneration of brain tissues within the cortices and hippocampus. As this degeneration is progressing, a gradual cognitive decline will become apparent.

Most researchers now agree that oxidative damage and circulatory insufficiencies contribute to these events. This means there are often signs of vascular damage within the blood vessels that should deliver nutrients to brain cells and remove toxins.

Diabetes and Insulin Resistance

Another possible mechanism involved in—or possibly premeditating—Alzheimer's disease is insulin resistance and glucose intolerance (McCrimmon *et al.* 2012 and many others as we'll discuss). These conditions are often seen with type-2 diabetes and pre-diabetes metabolic disorders.

We will dig more into the research on this later. The effect of glucose overload within the bloodstream, related to either glucose intolerance or insulin insensitivity, will leave the blood full of glucose. This leads to a type of oxidative free radicals along with something called advanced glycation end products. These together can damage blood vessels, causing atherosclerosis and narrowing of the arteries. This in turn restricts circulation to the brain.

These radicals can also damage brain cells.

Furthermore, if brain cells are not able to bring in and process enough glucose for energy, they can die. Brain cells are some of the hardest working cells in the body. The brain composes 2 percent of the body's cells but utilizes 20 percent of the body's glucose requirements. So they need lots of energy to keep operating effectively.

As a result of this mechanism, research on both animals and humans has found that insulin resistance and diabetes is often associated with Alzheimer's disease.

The damaging effects of insulin resistance onto brain cells can also promote the diabetic condition. The hypothalamus is involved in the control of insulin and glucose metabolism. When this regions of the brain are damaged from Alzheimer's, this can accelerate the condition of diabetes.

Neuroinflammation

One way or another, free radicals are considered the common denominator when it comes to damage to brain cells and damage to those blood vessels that feed the brain cells. For this reason, neuroinflammation is also associated with other dementias, including vascular dementia and Lewy body dementia.

This is consistent with Schipper's Free Radical-Mitochondrial theory of aging, which results in mitochondrial oxidative phosphorylation. As the brain cell's mitochondria become less efficient, they release more oxidative radicals as they produce energy. These radicals damage the cell membranes and organelles of the neurons and produce inflammation.

Researchers have coined a new word for this, called "inflammaging."

As we discuss Alzheimer's disease further, we'll focus on an important element of the cell that helps shield the cell from the ravaging of free radicals from the inside and outside: The cell membrane. The cell membrane also helps filter incoming fluids, discerning between nutrients and toxins that can damage the mitochondria.

The cell membrane is layered with lipids and phospholipids. The phospholipids provide structure and ionic potential that gives structure and flexibility to the cell. They are also critical to nerve cell electrical conduction and surface receptors. A healthy phospholipid membrane will retain healthier mitochondria in part because it's insulin receptors will remain intact.

The problem is that phospholipids among brain cells tend to break down and get weaker with age. Whether this is specific to certain diets has yet to be completely established. However, we will, through the means of different research, establish the relationship between diet at the strength of the cell membrane.

Oxidative stress is caused by a combination of poor lifestyle choices and a diet that produces increased levels of oxidative radicals and lower levels of antioxidants.

Researchers from the Beijing Hospital of Traditional Chinese Medicine and the Capital Medical University in China (Shi *et al.* 2012) analyzed urinary biomarkers of oxidative stress among 46 patients with vascular dementia, 24 patients with vascular disease without dementia, and 26 people without symptoms of either.

They found that patients with dementia had significantly higher levels of a urinary biomarker called 8-hydroxydeoxyguanosine (or 8-OHdG). 8-OHdG is associated with significantly high levels of oxidative stress. These levels were significantly higher than both of the other groups of patients.

Another study, this one from Qingdao University's School of Medicine, analyzed multiple studies and two large genome studies and concluded that Alzheimer's disease patients have significantly higher levels of clusterin, also known as apolipoprotein J. Clusterin has been found to bind to beta-amyloid proteins, and has the ability to reduce fibril formation.

It is now thought that in an attempt to resist the formation of the Abeta proteins and fibrils, the body produces clusterin as a defense measure against oxidative stress. This has been confirmed in studies showing that clusterin lowers cell death and levels of oxidative stress. .

New research is increasingly finding that not only are many cognitive disorders such as Alzheimer's and other forms of dementia related to inflammation among brain tissues, but classic mental diseases such as schizophrenia and depression may also be connected to brain inflammation.

Microglia and Neuroinflammation

A study from Japan's Kyushu University Medical School and Saga University (Monji 2012) helped us understand that many mental disorders are produced by inflammation involving the microglia cells of the brain.

The microglia are immune cells categorized as macrophages, but they are focused upon the health of the central nervous system—particularly the brain and spine. Microglia roam the neurons of these areas in search for toxins, intruders and possible infections.

Particularly at issue in cognitive issues such as dementia and Alzheimer's disease is the build up of amyloid plaque among brain cells. The microglia are the immune cells that are supposed to help prevent and clean up plaque build up among brain cells.

Neuroinflammation is the result of damage among brain cells. Healthy microglia populations are focused upon preventing inflammation among neurons, in turn preventing damage to brain cells.

However, when brain cells are damaged, microglia work harder to repair the damage by producing a variety of inflammatory factors. The damage to neurons, evidenced by these inflammatory factors, hamper the brain's function.

When the microglia populations are damaged or otherwise altered, the brain and central nervous system become increasingly susceptible to mental disorders such as Alzheimer's and other forms of dementia. This is because the microglia not only do not do their job: They actually contribute to brain cell damage.

Like other types of macrophages, the microglia are formed within the bone marrow. Once they migrate to the brain, they differentiate into particular responsibilities and different regions. Some microglia are focused on infections, others are focused upon toxins or damaged cells. Others stimulate the repair of brain tissues.

The build-up of plaque among brain cells stimulates the microglia as they work to try to remove the damage. Damage from oxidative stress and glycation byproducts have been linked to this build up of plaque among brain cells and the damage of microglia in the process.

Research by Dr. Akira Monji and associates connected dementia and cognitive issues to these increases in microglia inflammatory factors such as nitric oxide and cytokines. When the microglia have rapidly expanded in the face of damage to brain cells, they produce these inflammatory factors. Dr. Monji's research has shown that the brain tissues of schizophrenia, depression and dementia patients have increased levels of these microglia inflammatory factors.

Furthermore, the research has found that one of the central mechanisms of psychiatric drugs is that they reduce levels of these inflammatory factors—temporarily.

Like most pharmaceuticals, this temporary reduction of inflammatory factors does little to prevent or reduce the cause of the inflammation. Furthermore, by blocking inflammatory factors, the drugs interfere with the damage repair that is taking place, driven by the microglia immune cells. This is often the scenario for drugs that are focused upon the symptoms rather than the causes of a condition.

What Causes Neuroinflammation?

The cause of neuroinflammation, as shown in numerous dementia studies, again relates to oxidative damage. Oxidation is produced through an imbalance between toxins that form oxidative radicals and those antioxidants that neutralize those radicals. When the system is not balanced, oxidation takes place. This takes place not only among tissues among the cardiovascular system, but also among brain tissues.

Should the brain tissues become overloaded with lipid peroxidation, microglia can become damaged just as other cells can be damaged.

The bridge to these relationships has been provided by various research finding that neuroinflammation is one of the key factors affecting mental disorders of many types.

Numerous studies have shown that antioxidants neutralize oxidative radicals that produce inflammation. The very term "antioxidant" is founded upon research showing that particular phytochemicals directly neutralize the oxidative effects of radicals formed by toxins.

For example, in a large French study (Kesse-Guyot *et al.* 2012) published in the *Journal of Nutrition*, researchers found that a healthy diet with greater antioxidant intake was associated with reduced risk of cognitive decline after the researchers removed factors relating to exercise, alcohol intake, calories, gender, age, education and obesity.

This is of course is supported by other research finding that smoking and lack of exercise both increase the rate of cognitive decline, as illustrated in a study by some of the same INSERM researchers (Singh-Manoux *et al.* 2012) that linked obesity with cognitive decline. All these factors are related to oxidative stress.

What this all means is that cognitive disorders are no longer conditions that necessarily fall within the domain of psychiatrists and treatments such as lobotomy, electric shock and psychotropic drugs that have produced a myriad of adverse mental and physical effects.

As we will show, many cognitive disorders are in fact produced by poor diets and poor lifestyles, and thus are to a great degree preventable.

This research also brings mental disorders within the realm of natural health and nutrition. What is now known is that a person with a healthy diet containing plenty of antioxidants, together with an active lifestyle, has a significantly reduced risk of having dementia.

Furthermore, as we will prove in this text, a person with a healthier, antioxidant-rich diet will also stand a better chance of remaining alert into their elderly years.

Chapter Three

Risk Factors for Alzheimer's Disease

There are many different associations with Alzheimer's disease. We can draw upon many studies that illustrate these associations between Alzheimer's disease—which include certain lifestyle and diet choices, but also related conditions.

It must be made clear that associations are different than causes. Something may be related to a condition by something once removed. There may be a direct relationship—perhaps something that causes both. Or it may be the association is once-removed to a direct relationship. Whatever the relationship between Alzheimer's disease and the risk factor, it is worth considering as we continue to unlock the mysteries of this condition.

Before we start, we should clarify that a long-standing assumption about trauma—blows to the brain—was recently disproven. A large study from the University of Washington (Crane *et al.* 2016) found that traumatic brain injury is not related to a higher risk of Alzheimer's disease.

The researchers followed 7,130 people and found that traumatic brain injury did increased the risk of Parkinson's disease, but did not increase the risk of Alzheimer's disease.

With that in mind, let's look at risk factors that have been clearly linked to Alzheimer's:

Age

This goes without saying for most, but needs to be clarified. As explained earlier, only a small portion of Alzheimer's patients are diagnosed prior to turning 65. Thus, we find the age of 65 to be one of the most obvious and certain risk factors.

To restate what was discussed in the introduction, 11 percent of Americans over the age of 65 currently have Alzheimer's disease. This means one in nine people over 65 years old. When more advanced age is considered, a third of Americans over the age of 85 have Alzheimer's disease.

In terms of the entire population of Alzheimer's patients, 38 percent of Alzheimer's patients are over 85 years old. Another 43 percent are between 75 and 84 years old, and 15 percent are between 65 and 74 years old. Only 4 percent of Alzheimer's patients are under 65 years old.

Certainly age is not the only factor, since three-quarters of Americans over 85 don't have Alzheimer's disease. This means a one in four chance, but it also means there are other relationships between Alzheimer's disease outside of age. Otherwise, everyone who turns 86 would have it.

Genetics

How strong is the genetic factor in Alzheimer's? This is debatable, but worthy of consideration. A series of studies from the University of Southern California on over 12,000 Swedish twins established there was a 45 percent concordance between the twins and Alzheimer's disease. This means that two people who share the same genetics will not share Alzheimer's disease in more than half the time.

Concordance means that having a particular genetic trait for a condition will always subject the person to that condition.

Put more precisely, somewhere between 40 to 65 percent of people with Alzheimer's disease have the ApoE4 gene. But not everyone with the ApoE4 gene will contract Alzheimer's disease.

Let's put this another way. Having a genetic variant of the ApoE4 does not always result in Alzheimer's disease, but having one E4 allele can increase the risk of Alzheimer's disease by three times and having two E4 alleles can increase the risk of Alzheimer's disease by 12 times.

And at the same time, there are many with Alzheimer's disease that don't have the ApoE4 gene.

Conversely, many people who have the ApoE4 gene will never develop Alzheimer's disease.

So is that really a genetic factor? In addition to this gene, other genes have been seen prominent in those with Alzheimer's disease. But the same facts about these ApoE4 also apply to these other genes.

Let's consider an example. Let's say that someone finds that many people with Alzheimer's disease also have gray hair. Should we then conclude that gray hair is a risk factor?

Not so fast. Of course, the reason many of those with Alzheimer's disease have gray hair is because gray hair is more prominent among elderly people.

That seems obvious, but one might take a similar course with genes. While many assume that we are all born with all our genes, that just isn't the case. Many genes develop over our lifetimes, according to our lifestyles, diets, environments and so on. The body responds to environmental factors with genetic changes.

This is often referred to as epigenetics. But the reality is, many of those epigenetic changes will indeed be passed onto the next generation. And if those epigenetic changes are related to doing things that can cause Alzheimer's, then there is your connection. Because diets and other lifestyle factors also have a link to Alzheimer's.

Some may simply call these genetic changes mutations. But in reality, the body is constantly re-adjusting its genes so that the cells are able to adapt. This science of epigenetics—our changing genetic structure based upon our environment and consumption—defines how our lifestyle, diet and environment choices shape our future and future generations.

The other issue to consider about ApoE4 is that this part of our genes is involved in how the body transports fats, cholesterol, vitamins and others through the blood and lymphatic system. Furthermore, issues with these mechanisms—of cholesterol and fats—can relate directly to blood vessel disorders such as atherosclerosis.

Atherosclerosis is also linked with Alzheimer's disease as well as other dementias, as we'll discuss. This is because decreased circulation within the brain can relate directly to the brain cell damage that results in Alzheimer's disease.

Furthermore, atherosclerosis is specifically linked to diet. In other words, one may have a certain particular genetic mutation for transporting fats and cholesterol poorly. But ones diet will still exasperate those mechanisms, creating a greater risk of not only Alzheimer's, but heart attacks, strokes and other disorders.

Yet Alzheimer's is not always the result of the ApoE4 gene variant, though it is often seen among those with vascular damage—damage to the tiny blood vessels in the brain. As we've discussed with other Alzheimer's disease research, diet is one of the greatest determinants for Alzheimer's. And vascular damage is also seen without the E4 gene variant.

So, just as gray hair shouldn't be considered a direct cause of Alzheimer's, we shouldn't jump to the conclusion that there is necessarily an independent genetic cause for Alzheimer's disease.

Obesity and Heart Disease

With this in mind, we continue gingerly forward in our discussion of risk factors for Alzheimer's disease. We'll carefully use the words "linked" or "associated" from here on out to carefully differentiate between cause and a possible indirect association.

As expected, several studies, including a large 2012 French and Finnish INSERM study, has linked cognitive decline to increased obesity, diabetes and heart disease.

The study, led by Dr. Mika Kivimaki and associates from the French government's investigative body, INSERM, with support from the U.S. National Institutes of Medicine, studied 6,401 adults between 39 and 63 years old. They found that people who were obese and suffered from metabolic disorder (cardiovascular disease and/or diabetes) had more than a 22% greater cognitive decline than those who were of normal weight with no metabolic disorder.

This study has been confirmed by others that have related cognitive decline to cardiovascular disease, sedentary lifestyles, obesity and increased levels of toxins.

Alcohol Consumption

There is a dementia subtype called alcohol-induced dementia. Among subtypes from 3.1 U.S. Medicare patients, 0.7 percent of the dementia patients were diagnosed with alcohol-induced dementia.

A 2015 study from Norway (Langballe) followed 40,435 people who were born between 1905 and 1946. They each completed a questionnaire that assessed their alcohol consumption. The research found that consuming alcohol five or more times every two weeks was associated with a 40 percent increased risk of dementia compared to those who drank between 1 and 4 drinks every two weeks. Yet abstinence did not decrease the risk of Alzheimer's disease compared to moderate and infrequent group.

A 2016 study, from Sweden and the University of Southern California (Handing *et al.*), investigated 12,328 people part of the Swedish Twin Registry. They found that moderate to heavy drinking increased the risk of dementia by 57 percent, and sped up the development of dementia by nearly five years. They concluded that averaging more than 12 grams of alcohol per day increased dementia risk. Drinking spirits had the most association with dementia.

A 2016 study (Boissoneault *et al.*) on 51 people between 55 and 70 years old and 70 people between 25 and 35 years old found that working memory and cognitive power is significantly more affected by alcohol in an older person. The study found that alcohol affected working memory greater among the older people with the same amount of alcohol.

Smoking

Another French study, based upon the Whitehall II cohort study (Sabia *et al.* 2013) connected smoking and dementia. The researchers calculated data from 5,099 men and 2,137 women, with an average age of 56 years old when they were first tested for cognition.

They were given a battery of tests for memory, vocabulary and executive function. They also calculated a summary score they called a global cognitive score.

The researchers found that those who never smoked had the best cognition and lowest levels of cognitive impairment.

This compares with the current men smokers, who experienced the most cognitive decline during the testing period of ten years. In contrast, those who had quit smoking more than 10 years earlier showed no increased cognitive impairment.

Attention Deficit/Hyperactivity Disorder

Adult attention deficit and hyperactivity disorder (AD/HD) may be related to, or possibly may increase the risk of Alzheimer's disease. A definite answer is not apparent at this time, but there are a few caveats. Let's discuss some of these.

First, let's discuss some of the statistics on AD/HD.

Attention deficit and hyperactivity disorder (AD/HD) incidence is growing, particularly among Western industrialized societies. Research has found that about 5% of children between 9 and 17 have been diagnosed with AD/HD, while possibly 2-4% of adults have it. Some research has estimated that up to 10% of the U.S. population may be affected by AD/HD.

Boys have more AD/HD diagnoses than girls, at a rate of nearly 5 to 1. Some have suggested this is the result of girls having different symptoms than boys.

We should point out that this sort of association may simply mean that the same factors that produce a higher risk of Alzheimer's disease also produce a higher risk of AD/HD. Those may be related with the body's metabolism or they may be related with issues among brain cells.

It is also important to note that older adults with AD/HD may be misdiagnosed as having Alzheimer's disease or some other form of dementia. This is because some of the clinical symptoms of the two diseases are similar. These include memory impairment and short-term forgetfulness. There may also be functional impairment, which means not being able to function on a day-to-day basis very well. Those with AD/HD may have all of these signs.

As a result, clinicians and researchers have reported the existence of many older people with AD/HD being diagnosed with dementia.

Some other research has linked AD/HD with a later diagnosis of dementia. This included a study from Argentina (Golimstok *et al.* 2011) that linked AD/HD earlier in life with a later development of Lewy body dementia. However, later researchers have considered that perhaps this study result had to do with misdiagnosing AD/HD with this type of dementia.

So we'll leave this risk factor in the realm of unknowns for now.

Periodontal Disease

Gingivitis and periodontal disease in general have been linked with a greater risk of Alzheimer's disease.

A study presented at the first Alzheimer's Association International Conference on Prevention of Dementia, from the University of Southern California and Sweden's Karolinska Institute, analyzed data from over

12,000 twins as part of the Swedish Twin Registry. The twins filled out questionnaires that included information on their dental history and conditions. Forty years later, their medical histories were analyzed with this data. They found 109 instances of one twin being diagnosed with dementia while the other hadn't. Those twins diagnosed with Alzheimer's had four times the likelihood of having periodontal disease in middle age when compared to their twin.

The researchers, including Dr. Margaret Gatz, psychology professor at USC, attributed this effect as part of the "inflammatory burden" relating to Alzheimer's disease. Inflammation can be produced by bacteria as well as oxidative stress. Both have been linked with Alzheimer's disease as we'll be discussing throughout this book.

Lack of Sunshine

International research (Russ *et al.* 2016, Grant 2016 and others) has established that Alzheimer's disease incidence—and dementia in general—is more prevalent in regions that are furthest away from the equator. This relates directly to the availability of sunshine, and indirectly to the production of natural vitamin D.

Other studies have shown that people with Alzheimer's tend to have low circulating levels of vitamin D.

Less Education

Dr. Gatz' research with Swedish twins revealed another risk factor, which other studies have also found: Those who are less educated have about double the risk of dementia and Alzheimer's disease compared to those who have completed a higher degree in education.

The education in itself may not be the actual factor, however. Dr. Gatz detailed that this and other lifestyle factors may actually reflect levels of inflammation during ones younger years.

Let's look at this practically. It may be that a person who is seeking a higher degree will be less likely to party during their younger years.

I would personally beg to differ in that universities are often centers for party life. My suggestion here would be that when one seeks a higher degree, they begin to utilize greater levels of their brain's memory centers. This greater use of the hippocampus and other memory neurons activate those cells in ways that those with less education may not.

Furthermore, assuming that someone with a higher degree goes on to work as a professional, this use of the deeper memory centers of the brain would certainly continue. A professional degree will typically require continued learning in that area of expertise. Further to this point, many professional licenses actually require continued education (CE) units each year. This means such a professional will continue being a student on an ongoing basis.

Sleep Disturbance

A number of studies have now linked Alzheimer's disease with sleep deprivation or disturbance—especially REM-state sleep. For example, a study from Johns Hopkins School of Medicine (Spira *et al.* 2014) tested 13 adults, including eight who were healthy and five who had mild cognitive impairment. The researchers found those with sleep disturbance related to apnea who had less oxygen saturation had a greater likelihood of developing the beta-amyloid deposits in the brain—one of the hallmarks of Alzheimer's disease as we have discussed.

This and many other studies have shown that cognitive impairment in many forms is significantly associated with sleep disturbance.

Poor Diet

Alzheimer's disease has been significantly linked to certain diets and certain classes of foods, as we will discuss shortly in depth. The largest interaction revolves around the Western diet.

As we'll discuss, the research illustrates not only that certain diets can increase the risk of Alzheimer's: But some diets and foods in particular have been shown to reduce the risk of Alzheimer's disease.

Diabetes and Insulin Resistance

Alzheimer's has been linked to both diabetes and insulin resistance. This was confirmed by a study from Japan's Kyushu University Medical School (Ohara *et al.* 2011), which found that dementia and Alzheimer's disease are associated with type 2 diabetes.

The researchers, from the Graduate School of Medical Sciences' Environmental Medicine Department, followed 1,017 adults over the age of 60 years old for fifteen years. The elderly adults lived in an adult community and were dementia-free at the beginning of the study.

The adults were given oral glucose tolerance tests periodically. At the end of the fifteen years, those adults whose glucose tolerance testing confirmed a diagnosis of diabetes by the end of the study were more than twice as likely to have Alzheimer's disease, and had 74% increased incidence of vascular dementia.

Dementia and Alzheimer's disease risk also significantly increased among those whose two-hour post-load glucose levels were over the 7.8 mmol/Liter levels, and the highest risk was found among those with two-hour post-load glucose levels over 11 mmol/Liter.

The study was published in the medical journal *Neurology*, and has been coined the Hisayama Study.

The researchers concluded:

> *"Our findings suggest that diabetes is a significant risk factor for all-cause dementia, Alzheimer's disease, and probably vascular dementia."*

Why is insulin resistance and diabetes a risk factor? Insulin helps glucose into neuron cells. When neurons become resistant to insulin, glucose doesn't get into the cells, starving them of their energy source.

This also leaves unused glucose floating around the bloodstream. This produces oxidative radicals and advanced glycation endproducts. These together damage blood vessels and damage cells.

This means they can also damage brain cells.

These glucose-related reactive oxygen species produces oxidative stress. Oxidative stress is an imbalance between reactive oxygen species production and the body's antioxidant defense system.

Oxidative Stress

Speaking of oxidative stress, research has repeatedly proved that Alzheimer's disease and dementia are linked with lifestyle factors and exposures that lead to an increase in oxidative stress. We've discussed some of the mechanisms earlier.

Oxidative stress is produced with increased levels of toxin exposure, either within the diet, water or air, combined with lower levels of antioxidants and increased levels of lifestyle stressors. Toxins more easily become oxidized and become radicals, damaging cells, blood vessels and tissues.

Chemical Exposures

In 2013, toxicology chemist Harold Zeliger, Ph.D. published findings that irrefutably linked exposures to certain toxic chemicals to neurological diseases such as Alzheimer's disease, amyotrophic lateral sclerosis (ALS), attention deficit/hyperactivity disorder (AD/HD), autism and other forms of neuropathy.

Dr. Zeliger, a certified forensic examiner, conducted a review of 140 toxicology studies to arrive at his conclusions.

Dr. Zeliger found that chemical exposures to lipophilic (fat-soluble) chemicals such as polychlorinated bisphenols (PCBs), organochlorine pesticides, dioxins, polybrominated biphenyl ethers (PBDEs) and perfluorooctanoic acid esters—in many household and industrial products—were specifically linked to dementia and other neurological disorders.

Other research, as we'll discuss below, has linked Alzheimer's disease to fine particle air pollution and ozone, as well as pesticide exposure.

Aluminum or Lead Toxicity

A link between Alzheimer's disease and aluminum toxicity has been the subject of many studies over the past 50 years. Yet a certain link has yet to be confirmed or agreed upon.

In the 1960s and earlier, several autopsies found higher levels of aluminum within the brains of Alzheimer's patients. Some of these were not controlled or randomized, so they have been later dismissed. However, a few still showed a link. For example, one study (Trapp et al. 1978) found that Alzheimer's patients had an average of 1.4 times the aluminum levels compared to controls.

Yet another study (Markesbery et al. 1981) studied 74 Alzheimer's patients post-mortem along with 137 healthy control subjects. They found no increase in aluminum in the brain compared to the controls. They did, however, find that aluminum levels tended to increase with age among both the Alzheimer's and healthy subjects.

Still, the suspicion has continued. In a study of bone content from Canada's McMaster University (Mohseni et al. 2016), researchers tested bone samples from 30 people—half of which had Alzheimer's. Because aluminum tends to build up in the bones, the researchers tested their bone content for aluminum and aluminum-calcium ratios. The researchers found that while the Alzheimer's patients tended to have more than five times the amount of aluminum in their bones, the relationship was all about age. The older the subject—healthy or not—the more aluminum they tended to have in their bones. So again, they found no link between aluminum and Alzheimer's.

But then we have another interesting study to add to the equation. Researchers from France's INSERM (Rondeau et al. 2000) studied 3,777 people in lived in different areas of France. They also tested 2,698 people as a control group. The researchers found that those people who lived in areas where the aluminum levels were higher had double the incidence of Alzheimer's disease compared to those whose water did not have high levels of aluminum.

Where does this leave us? Many studies have shown there is a mechanism between nerve and brain cell damage and aluminum toxicity. The topic is still somewhat debatable, but we can certainly accept that there may well be an association between aluminum toxicity and Alzheimer's.

The association between Alzheimer's disease and lead is also circumspect, but deserves some mention as well. Lead toxicity has been linked with other neurological issues, especially in children. Findings that lead exposures is linked with reduced IQ scores and increased attention deficit issues was found in a study from South Korea's Seoul National University College of Medicine (Hong *et al.* 2015). In 2013, University of Southern Mississippi researchers (Goodlad *et al.* 2013) found a similar link in a study of 10,232 children.

While lead toxicity is known to cause neurological damage, the link between Alzheimer's and lead has yet to be clearly established.

Part II: Strategies to Prevent or Slow Alzheimer's Disease

Chapter Four

Vitamins and Nutrients for AD

Some vitamins and nutrient supplements have been shown to improve cognition and memory, and even stave off Alzheimer's disease. There are even some scientific reports showing that certain nutrient supplements may slightly improve memory and cognition for those with Alzheimer's.

As we have discussed, there is considerable evidence that one of the major hallmarks of Alzheimer's disease is extraordinary levels of inflammation. That is, that Alzheimer's patients have been seen having higher-than-normal inflammation levels. This indicates the potential of lower levels of anti-inflammatory nutrients in the diet.

Researchers from Canada's University of Sherbrooke (Khalil *et al.* 2012) did blood work on 20 healthy people and 39 Alzheimer's patients. They found that the circulation of HDL-cholesterol and Apolipoprotein A1 were impaired, indicating that the Alzheimer's patients had greater levels of oxidative stress. The end result was that the anti-inflammatory effects of HDL were significantly lower in Alzheimer's patients.

Is it as simple as replacing anti-inflammatory nutrients with supplements? Sorry, but it isn't.

One of the ongoing messages we'll see in the below summary of research over the past two decades is that many isolated nutrients will not deliver the same potency as the foods they are found in. Then again, often many foods just won't have the nutrient content enough to have the effects found in this research. So supplements often provide a good strategy—depending on the particular nutrient.

Vitamin E and AD

In 2014, researchers from Yale and other universities around the U.S. (Dysken *et al.*) tested vitamin E and compared its effects with the Alzheimer's drug memantine on Alzheimer's disease. The research tested memantine against vitamin E for Alzheimer's.

What is memantine?

This expensive pharmaceutical is branded as Mimetix by Abbott, Ebixa, Abixa by Lundbeck, and Namenda by Forest Pharmaceuticals. It is prescribed for existing Alzheimer's patients—with mild to moderate forms of the condition. It is also often prescribed for some other forms of dementia.

Memantine is a acetylcholinesterase inhibitor. It is also a dopaminergic receptor agonist—as it binds with this receptor. It is also a noncompetitive antagonist with the binding of 5HT receptors and acetylcholine receptors.

Okay, I'm not expecting you to understand all that. What is important is that this chemical has complex responses within the body—it is a complex pharmaceutical that significantly affects the nervous system. And while it has shown some benefit in some situations, it also comes with various adverse effects, including anxiety, headaches, insomnia, dizziness, drowsiness, vomiting and even hallucinations.

Yes, that was hallucinations. And insomnia and anxiety. In a drug that is supposed to help with dementia.

Consider the contrast between this drug and vitamin E—notably one form of vitamin E, alpha-tocopherol. This is a nutrient that is prevalent in a number of natural foods. These include sunflower seeds, almonds, beets, pumpkin, peanuts, peppers, avocado and many other foods. It has no known adverse effects—only positive side effects.

Could such a basic vitamin beat out the billion-dollar pharmaceutical, memantine? You betcha.

First of all, this is research published in the most respected U.S. medical journal—the *Journal of the American Medical Association—JAMA*. The research was conducted by a large team of researchers—at 14 Veteran's Administration research centers in Minneapolis, New York, Madison, Albuquerque, Cleveland, Washington, DC, Philadelphia, Miami, Baltimore, Charleston, Ann Arbor, Boston, Seattle, Iowa City, and elsewhere. Researchers from medical schools of the University of Maryland, the University of Washington, the University of Iowa, the University of South Carolina and Yale University's School of Public Health were involved in the research.

The research was randomized, double-blinded and placebo-controlled. It began in 2007 and concluded in 2012, and was published in 2014.

The research involved 613 patients with mild to moderate Alzheimer's disease. They were veterans treated at the 14 VA centers mentioned above.

The patients were divided into four groups: 152 patients were given 2000 IU per day of alpha tocopherol; 155 were prescribed 20 milligrams per day of memantine; 154 patients were given both of these together, and 152 were given a placebo. This placebo group provided the control group with which to compare the treatments of the other three groups.

The results of the study were measured by the Alzheimer's Disease Cooperative Study/Activities of Daily Living (ADCS-ADL) Inventory test. The ADCS-ADL Inventory test has a range of scores, from 0 to 78—with 78 being the highest and best score. This bases its measure on functioning levels of dementia—the ability to function on a day-to-day basis.

The researchers also otherwise measured the patients' cognition, nervous and mood-related symptoms, their ability to function and the levels of caregivers they required during the five-year period. One of the more prominent alternative tests they used was the MMSE test—the widely used Mini–Mental State Examination—along with the Alzheimer Disease Assessment Scale–Cognitive Subscale (ADAS-cog).

After an average of nearly two-and-a-half years of treatment, a total of 561 patients completed the study with appropriate analytical results. (Some died during the study and some had to drop out for different reasons). Completed were 140 vitamin E patients, 142 memantine-treated patients, 139 who took both and 140 who were given the placebo.

To summarize, the research found that the vitamin E-treated group had Alzheimer's progression from between nearly 1 point up to 5.4 points *lower* than the placebo group declines. The average difference in reduced scores was 3.15 points. This means the vitamin E group's decline in functioning—their Alzheimer's condition—worsened less than the placebo group's decline by 3.15 points.

This difference was significant. The difference was calculated to be equivalent to a delay of nearly 20% of Alzheimer's disease progression. This was also converted to be about six months of reduced progression over the total four year trial period.

The researchers also found that the vitamin E-alone group scored better for caregiver time—meaning the vitamin E group required significantly less caregiver time than the other groups.

These positive effects of the vitamin E occurred throughout the group, but better among those with more advanced stages of the condition.

Meanwhile, the memantine treatment group also slowed a slight delay in their Alzheimer's disease progression. However, the difference between the placebo group and the memantine treatment group's Alzheimer's progression was a meager 1.98 points—which the researchers qualified was too low to be considered a significant difference:

"There were no significant differences in the groups receiving memantine alone or memantine plus alpha tocopherol."

This means that not only was the memantine not effective for delaying the progression of Alzheimer's; when the Vitamin E was mixed with memantine, the significant positive effect of Vitamin E was lost:

> *"When compared with placebo, the alpha tocopherol alone group showed significant benefit, but paradoxically, the combination of alpha tocopherol and memantine had less effect than either alpha*

tocopherol alone or memantine alone. Although it is possible that memantine could have interfered with the effectiveness of alpha tocopherol, it is difficult to postulate a plausible mechanism. To our knowledge, no studies have examined whether memantine interferes with alpha tocopherol's antioxidant effects."

In contrast, the researchers were clear that Vitamin E had a clear positive effect:

"These findings suggest benefit of alpha tocopherol in mild to moderate Alzheimer's disease by slowing functional decline and decreasing caregiver burden."

Many of the patients who were tested were older. So there were deaths during the trial period. But the Vitamin E group suffered significantly fewer deaths during the study.

Statistically, the Vitamin E group had a nominal death rate of 7.3%—over 25% lower than the death rate of 9.4% among the placebo group. Meanwhile, the memantine group had a whopping 11.3% mortality rate during the trial—over 50 percent higher than the Vitamin E group.

In addition, adverse effects were significantly greater in the memantine group. The memantine suffered 31 adverse events among 23 patients, while the combination groups suffered 44 events among 31 patients. The placebo group had 13 events among 11 patients.

Previous research confirms vitamin E's effectiveness in reducing Alzheimer's disease progression. In 1997, researchers from the Columbia University's College of Physicians and Surgeons (Sano *et al.*) studied 341 moderately severe Alzheimer's patients for two years. In this study, the Mini-Mental State Examination was used to test the patients. The group that was treated with alpha-tocopherol had significantly less progression of Alzheimer's compared to the placebo group—by a score of 670 to 440 days.

In this study, the pharmaceutical drug selegiline was tested as well. And it did result in a slower progression similar to that of the Vitamin E group. However, further study on Selegiline has proven it to not be such a hot Alzheimer's drug. In a large 2003 Cochrane Database review from Oxford University, medical researchers concluded:

"Despite its initial promise, i.e. the potential neuroprotective properties, and its role in the treatment of Parkinson's disease sufferers, selegiline for Alzheimer's disease has proved disappointing. Although there is no evidence of a significant adverse event profile, there is also no evidence of a clinically meaningful benefit for Alzheimer's disease sufferers. This is true irrespective of the outcome measure evaluated, i.e. cognition, emotional state, activities of daily

*living, and global assessment, whether in the short, or longer term
(up to 69 weeks), where this has been assessed. There would seem
to be no justification, therefore, to use it in the treatment of people
with Alzheimer's disease, nor for any further studies of its efficacy
in Alzheimer's disease."*

Yet we do not find this sort of disappointment among the Vitamin E
research and among other studies of natural remedies for slowing the
progression of Alzheimer's disease.

Importance of Other Vitamin E Forms

It must be understood that the alpha-tocopherol version of vitamin
E is only one dimension of this critical brain vitamin. Nature provides
eight different molecules categorized as vitamin E. Four are tocopherols—alpha-tocopherol, beta-tocopherol, gamma-tocopherol, and
delta-tocopherol. Of these, alpha-tocopherol is the more prevalent within
the body—easily stored and used.

But there are also four important tocotrienol forms of vitamin E—
alpha-tocotrienol, beta-tocotrienol, gamma-tocotrienol, and delta-
tocotrienol.

Research from Sweden's Karolinska Institute (Mangialasche *et al.*
2013) has shown that Alzheimer's disease and cognition decline is linked
not just to tocopherol levels—but also to tocotrienols.

The researchers studied 81 Alzheimer's patients, 86 patients with
mild cognitive impairment, and 86 matched volunteers who where cognitively healthy.

The researchers found that plasma levels of both tocotrienols and
tocopherols corresponded with levels of cognitive decline: Those with
Alzheimer's disease had the lowest levels of both.

Furthermore, MRI scans were compared with blood levels of
gamma-tocotrienols and alpha-tocotrienols—along with gamma-
tocopherols. The researchers found that lower levels of these different
forms of Vitamin E were associated with greater levels of cognitive decline.

Another study from the Karolinska Institute and Stockholm University (Mangialasche *et al.* 2013) followed 140 advanced-age people without
cognitive issues at the beginning of eight years. They measured their
blood levels of vitamin E together with the advancement of cognitive
decline.

They tested for all eight vitamin E molecules as mentioned above.

The researchers found that over the eight-year period, cognitive decline was less among those who had higher blood levels of gamma-

tocopherol and beta-tocotrienol. Those with higher levels of total to-cotrienols also had significantly less cognitive decline.

In their conclusion they summarized their findings:

"Elevated levels of tocopherol and tocotrienol forms are associated with reduced risk of cognitive impairment in older adults."

Multiple studies have also found that tocotrienols are significantly beneficial to cardiovascular health.

While these can be supplemented, a mix of different forms of Vitamin E can be found with a diverse diet containing whole grain foods, whole rice, coconut and palm foods. This combination will provide both tocotrienols and tocopherols.

B Vitamins

Researchers from the University of Oxford (Douaud *et al.* 2013) determined that B vitamin supplementation can slow and possibly reverse the progression of Alzheimer's symptoms, along with cognitive impairment.

The researchers—from Oxford's Nuffield Department of Clinical Neurosciences—conducted a clinical trial with 156 elderly patients who had mild cognitive impairment and a high risk of dementia and Alzheimer's disease. The researchers randomized the patients and for two years, gave one group a daily supplement with 800 micrograms of folic acid, 20 milligrams of vitamin B6, and 500 micrograms of vitamin B12. They gave a placebo supplement to the control group.

Before the trial and during the testing period, the researchers utilized magnetic resonance imaging (MRI) to measure the patients' atrophy levels of grey matter in their brains. Atrophying grey matter is a sign of the progression of Alzheimer's disease and other forms of dementia. Atrophy in the grey matter is shown as the amount of grey matter shrinks in the imaging tests.

While grey matter regions did shrink among both groups, the researchers found that those given the B vitamin supplements had about seven times less grey matter shrinkage than did the placebo group.

The researchers also found that those whose grey matter shrunk fastest had higher levels of homocysteine, and those with higher homocysteine levels received the greatest benefit from the B vitamin supplements. They summarized the effects thus:

"B vitamins lower homocysteine, which directly leads to a decrease in grey matter atrophy, thereby slowing cognitive decline."

The researchers also conducted neuropsychological testing on the patients to correlate their grey matter losses with neuropsychological function. Their testing concluded that the B vitamins not only helped reduce grey matter losses, but also reduced the drop in neuropsychological scores among the supplement group.

In their conclusion the researchers stated:

> *"Our results show that B-vitamin supplementation can slow the atrophy of specific brain regions that are a key component of the Alzheimer disease process and that are associated with cognitive decline."*

Other studies have linked B vitamins and high homocysteine levels with cognitive decline, Alzheimer's disease and dementia.

For example, in a study from Korea's Ewha Womans University (Kim *et al.* 2013), 321 elderly people were studied and tested for cognitive function, together with their levels of vitamin B12, folate and homocysteine.

After using multiple regression analysis, low folate levels were associated with low scores on naming tests, and low levels of vitamin B12 in the blood were related to low scores on word list memory. High homocysteine levels were also associated with low scores on word memory and construction recall testing.

The researchers stated in their conclusion:

> *"These results suggest that plasma folate, vitamin B12, homocysteine and tissue factor pathway inhibitor are associated with cognitive function in cognitively impaired (Alzheimer's disease and Mild cognitive impairment) elderly and that the association was stronger in patients with Alzheimer's disease."*

Increased homocysteine relate directly to higher levels of inflammation and greater oxidative stress. Higher homocysteine levels have also been linked with cardiovascular disease—more specifically the progression of atherosclerosis or the hardening of the arteries. Thus, high homocysteine levels have been found among those who have suffered from strokes and heart attacks.

Elevated homocysteine levels are anything higher than 10-15 μmol/L depending upon the age and health of the patient. The Oxford researchers classified their high homocysteine patients as those with levels of 11 μmol or more.

Homocysteine and its two partners methionine and cysteine are involved in the metabolic detoxification process called methylation. This transfers methyl groups from one molecule to another. When a methyl group is transferred to a oxidative toxin, it speeds its discharge from the body. Higher levels of homocysteine are typically accompanied by higher levels of oxidative radicals and toxins in the liver and blood stream.

If not neutralized, these toxins cause oxidative damage to blood vessels and cells—including brain and nerve cells.

It should also be noted that folate—nature's form—is a better form of the B9 vitamin than folic acid. Excessive folic acid supplementation has been linked with increased cancer risk. A 2009 study showed folic acid fortification increased colon cancer risk.

Food sources of folate include parsley, turnip and mustard greens, collard greens, romaine lettuce, spinach, asparagus, broccoli, cauliflower and beets. Lentils and brewer's yeast are also good sources. In supplements, the 5-methyltetrahydrofolate (5-MTHF) nutrient offers an option to synthesized folic acid.

Despite its reputation for cognitive improvement, vitamin B12 by itself doesn't seem to help dementia that much. A study from Yale (van Dyck *et al.* 2009) gave 28 dementia patients with low blood B12 a vitamin B12 supplement for four months. They compared findings with patients who were matched but didn't have low B12 levels.

The researchers didn't find much cognitive improvement or lessened dementia as a result of taking the B12.

The vitamin B supplementation plan doesn't appear to help everyone either. A study published in 2008 in the *Journal of the American Medical Association* (Aisen *et al.*) conducted a large multicenter study on B vitamins and Alzheimer's disease. The researchers tested 302 Alzheimer's patients with a placebo or daily high-dose folate (5 mg), vitamin B6 (25 mg), and vitamin B12 (1 mg) for 18 months. Of the whole population, 202 were given the supplement and 138 were given the placebo.

The B supplement did help the treatment group reduce their homocysteine levels. The treatment group's levels averaged -2.42 while the placebo group had -0.86. However, the vitamin supplementation had no obvious benefits to cognition:

> *"it had no beneficial effect on the primary cognitive measure, rate of change in ADAS-cog score during 18 months."*

There was a small effect, however, with the ADAS score, which changed 0.372 points per month for the placebo group versus 0.401 points per month for vitamin treatment group.

In 1996, researchers from Japan's Hiroshima University School of Medicine (Mimori *et al.*) tested patients using fursultiamine (TTFD), a derivative of thiamine. They supplemented the patients with 100 mg per day and found the patients' emotional, mental and intellectual functions improved. Yet only the mildly impaired patients showed cognitive improvement.

In another study, of Taiwanese Alzheimer's patients, researchers (Sun *et al.* 2007) gave vitamin B6, B12 and folic acid to 89 Alzheimer's patients for six months. Again, the researchers found their homocysteine levels were reduced by the supplementation, yet there was no noticeable change in their cognitive health. They concluded:

> *"In this population of patients with mild to moderate Alzheimer's disease in Taiwan, a multivitamin supplement containing vitamins B(6) and B(12) and folic acid for 26 weeks decreased homocysteine concentrations. No statistically significant beneficial effects on cognition or ADL function were found between multivitamin and placebo at 26 weeks."*

But vitamin B may be important in conjunction with other treatments. For example, researchers from Australia's University of Dundee (Connelly *et al.* 2008) treated 57 patients with "probable" Alzheimer's disease.

The researchers gave either a placebo or 1 mg of folic acid per day together with cholinesterase inhibitors (ChI) for six months. Scores in the Mini-Mental State Examination (MMSE) did not change significantly. But there was a significant difference in Activities of Daily Living and Social Behavior scores between the two groups. Here is what they concluded:

> *"This pilot double blind study suggests that response to cholinesterase inhibitors in patients with Alzheimer's disease may be improved by the use of folic acid."*

Researchers from the University of Western Australia (Flicker *et al.* 2008) tested 299 older men. For two years, they gave them either a placebo or 2 mg of folate, 25 mg of B6 and 400 micrograms of B12.

The researchers found that after the two years, the increase of the A-beta protein 1-40 was 4.9% (7.0 pg/ml) in the supplement group and (4.9%), and 18.5% (26.8 pg/ml) in the placebo group. The researchers wrote:

> *"We conclude that B vitamins may decrease the plasma level of A beta 40 and have a role in the prevention of Alzheimer's disease."*

Researchers from the University of Oxford (Douaud *et al.* 2013) gave MRI scans to 156 Alzheimer patients at the beginning of a two-year study. Then 80 were given a high-dose vitamin B supplementation program, and 76 were given a placebo. The vitamins given to the supplement group were: 0.8 milligrams folic acid, 20 milligrams of vitamin B-6, and 0.5 milligrams of vitamin B-12.

After two years, the researchers gave all the subjects MRI scans again. They found that those taking the B vitamins had less brain shrinkage than the supplemented group.

The average gray matter loss among the placebo group after two years was 3.7 percent. The average gray matter loss in the supplemented group after two years was only 0.5 percent.

That is a significant difference.

Researchers from the University of Oxford (de Jager *et al.* 2012) tested 266 people with mild cognitive impairment. Half were given 0.8 mg of folic acid, 0.5 mg of vitamin B12 and 20 mg vitamin B6; and the other half were given a placebo for two years.

The researchers found that the average blood levels of homocysteine were 30% lower in those given the B vitamins, compared to the placebo group. They also found that the B vitamins stabilized their executive functions. Furthermore, the B-vitamin treatment improved global cognition levels for the patients' who had higher homocysteine levels. They also had higher episodic memory and higher semantic memory scores.

They concluded:

> *"In this small intervention trial, B vitamins appear to slow cognitive and clinical decline in people with MCI, in particular in those with elevated homocysteine. Further trials are needed to see if this treatment will slow or prevent conversion from with mild cognitive impairment to dementia."*

A similar result was found by some of the same researchers from Oxford (Smith *et al.* 2010) two years earlier. This study tested 271 people over 70 with MCI and gave half of them 800 mcg of folic acid, 500 mcg of vitamin B12 and 20 mg vitamin B6 per day. The other half were given a placebo. And 187 of the patients also were given MRIs to test their brain's rate of atrophy.

After two years of supplementation or placebo, the researchers found that the B vitamin group's brain atrophy was 53% less than the placebo group. However, this change was only found among those people who had homocysteine levels that were greater than 13 micromoles per liter.

Those with greater brain atrophy also had more cognitive decline.

A study from the University of Western Australia (Ford *et al.* 2010) studied 299 men who were 75 or older. For two years, they gave half 2 milligrams of folic acid, 25 milligrams vitamin B6 and 500 micrograms B12. The other half were given a placebo for the two years.

The researchers found no difference between the two groups in the Alzheimer's Disease Assessment Scale (ADAS-cog) after two years. However, they did find a decrease in cognitive impairment risk when they followed up after eight years. This was considered insignificant and they concluded that the B vitamins didn't make a difference.

B Vitamins and Methylation

Why are B vitamins so important to preventing and slowing the progression of AD?

Our bodies conduct an interesting process called *methylation*. To simplify a very complex biological process, this is a process where methyl groups replace hydrogen atoms on larger molecules. The critical biological methylation process is called DNA methylation. In this process, methyl donors convert the DNA component cytosine to 5-methylcytosine using a special enzyme called methyltransferase. This CpG-to-Me-CpG is an important gene expression, which is related to adapting to various stress-factors.

Should there be a lack of methyl groups available to construct this exchange, the likelihood for nervous disorders increase substantially.

Another type of methylation is called protein methylation, which will modify proteins for biological processes. Lysine and arginine are usually the amino acid portions of the proteins where methylation often occurs.

Methylation is a critical mechanism. It is a key process for energy production and detoxification. Through methylation, the body can produce co-enzyme Q. It is the key mechanism for the repair of tissues and neutralizing toxic elements.

Methylation is also critical to neurotransmitter production, stimulating the production of dopamine, melatonin, norepinephrine and others. Methyl transfer also enables the body to produce SAM-e and DMG—critical to our moods and our energy levels.

Homocysteine processing is also dependent upon methyl transfer. High homocysteine levels have been linked with cardiovascular disease. Methyl transfer is what the body uses to neutralize homocysteine levels.

B vitamins are known methyl donors. For this reason, B12 and folate are critical for health, as are choline and S-adenosyl methionine (SAM)—which is derived from the amino acid methionine. Methionine is one of only two sulfur amino acids the body uses for protein synthesis (cysteine is the other, which can be converted by methionine and is the precursor for the all-important detoxificant glutathione).

Methionine is a powerful chelating agent, which through the trans-sulfuration pathway assists in the production of carnation, cysteine, and taurine. It is also an important component of fatty acid synthesis. Methionine is critical for phosphatidylcholine production as well—critical for brain cell function.

A lack of methyl groups in the diet causes a state of *hypomethylation*. This can produce imbalances among our DNA, stimulating possible mutation as the cells attempt to adjust to the lack of methyl donors. The resulting genetic adjustment to too few methyl groups can result in the production of damaged alpha-secretases and related enzymes, which are unable to properly break down the beta-amyloid proteins—resulting in the beta-amyloid oligomers that damage our brain cells.

For this reason, it is important to have a wide selection of foods in the diet containing B vitamins and methionine. Foods like whole grains, lentils, sesame seeds, garlic, onions, sunflower seeds, Brazil nuts, spinach, peppers and dairy foods are great sources of methionine.

Outside of supplements, nutritional yeast and fermented foods such as yogurt and kefir are great sources for producing B vitamins and other methyl group donors.

The planet also undergoes a process of methylation, by the way. This is conducted through various bacteria within the seabed, converting toxic elements like lead, arsenic and mercury into their innocuous methyl forms such as dimethyl mercury and trimethyl arsine. This process speeds up ocean detoxification while rebalancing the environment to the extent possible—just as methylation does in the body. The methylation process basically converts toxins into useable or harmless molecules.

Vitamin C and E

Researchers from Ulm University in Germany (von Arnim *et al.* 2012) tested blood levels of the antioxidants vitamin C, vitamin E, beta-carotene, lycopene, and coenzyme Q10 among 74 people with mild dementia. They compared these levels in the blood with 158 healthy people of the same age and gender as the dementia patients.

The researchers found that blood levels of vitamin C and beta-carotene were significantly lower in the dementia patients. This was found even after the researchers adjusted for their school education, supplementation, smoking habits, body weight, and alcohol consumption—all of which affect ones antioxidant levels.

At the same time, the researchers didn't find any differences for vitamin E, lycopene or coenzyme Q10.

The researchers concluded that deficiency in vitamin C and beta-carotene were linked to dementia.

Research from (Kontush *et al.* 2001) Germany's University Hospital Eppendorf tested whether vitamin C and E supplementation could increase the antioxidant status among Alzheimer's patients. As other research has found, the researchers tested 20 Alzheimer's patients and found the antioxidant levels in their cerebrospinal fluid (CSF) was low. They proceeded to give half the patients vitamin C (1,000 mg) and E supplements (400 IU) or just vitamin E (400 IU).

After a month, the patients in the C and E group showed significantly increased antioxidant potential in the CSF. But the vitamin E-alone patients did not change anything.

However, some research has not found evidence that vitamin E and C supplementation treats existing Alzheimer's disease. Research from Duke University (Fillenbaum *et al.* 2005) tested 616 people with either delayed dementia or Alzheimer's disease. The researchers analyzed their vitamin use over a period of 13 years. They found those who took vitamin E, C or both did not have any difference in terms of their progression of the disease.

The problem with this study is the lack of quality control over the form and dose of the nutrients. Not all forms of nutrients are the same. Plus the results were based on patient reports, leading to subjective bias.

These nutrients definitely reach the brain. A 2003 study (Quinn *et al.*) found that both vitamin E and C supplementation increased levels of these antioxidants among the central nervous system.

Omega-3s

Turns out that omega-3s support the function of B vitamins.

A study from the UK's University of Oxford (Jernerén *et al.* 2015) followed 185 people with mild cognitive impairment. They were 70 years old or older. The researchers gave all the subjects MRI brain scans at the beginning of the study and at the end of the two years. They also tested the blood of all subjects for omega-3s (eicosapentaenoic acid (EPA) and docosahexaenoic acid (DHA)).

They gave half the group a daily dose of 0.8 milligrams folic acid, 20 milligrams of vitamin B-6, and 0.5 milligrams of vitamin B-12. The other half were given a placebo.

The brain scans two years later indicated those who took the vitamin B supplements had a 40% decrease in atrophy compared to the placebo group: But this only occurred among those who had higher levels of EPA and DHA. Those higher levels were greater than 590 micromoles per liter.

Those people who had taken the vitamin B supplements but had lower levels of EPA and DHA in their bloodstreams did not have less brain atrophy compared to the placebo group.

In other words, higher levels of circulating DHA and EPA assist the benefits of vitamin Bs on our brains.

How can we do this? There are three basic choices: Taking DHA supplements, as DHA easily converts to EPA in the body. Eating foods that have DHA—namely algae or fish. Or eating ALA (alpha linolenic acid) foods, such as flaxseeds, chia seeds, walnuts and others. These foods will be converted to DHA and EPA in the body.

While certainly fish is an alternative, the problem lies with mercury. Mercury levels are increasing among fish and seafoods around the world. While some say that the conversion of ALA to DHA is not efficient, the liver produces a neat enzyme called delta-saturase, which does this very efficiently, at a rate of 15 percent or more in healthy people. See the section on omega-3s in my book, *"The Ancestors Diet."*

Beta-carotene

Researchers from Spain's University of Alcala de Henares in Madrid (Jiménez *et al.* 1999) studied 38 Alzheimer's patients along with 42 healthy patients. The researchers found that blood levels of beta-carotene and vitamin A were much lower in the Alzheimer's patients.

This doesn't mean that beta-carotene supplements will necessarily improve an Alzheimer's disease condition, or prevent Alzheimer's disease. But it does indicate an action step for ones diet. Beta-carotene is found prominently in carrots and leafy greens.

Alpha Lipoic Acid

Researchers from Hannover, German (Hager *et al.* 2007) tested nine patients with Alzheimer's disease. They gave all the patients 600 mg of alpha-lipoic acid for one year. They tested the patients before and after the year. The supplementation program increased cognitive function according to the Mini-Mental State Exam (MMSE) and the Alzheimer's Disease Assessment Score Cognitive Subscale, ADAS-cog.

The researchers then increased the group to 43 patients, and extended the study to 48 months. Among the patients with mild dementia, their dementia progressed more slowly. Of those with moderate dementia, their disease progressed twice as slow.

What about citicoline?

In studies on rats, citicoline has been shown to benefit rats with Alzheimer's. However, human studies have not been so conclusive. For this reason, citicoline is not recommended for Alzheimer's.

This said, one study (Cotroneo *et al.* 2014) tested citicoline on 349 elderly people with mild vascular cognitive impairment. The patients were given 1,000 milligrams of citicoline per day. Functional cognition was tested with the Activities of Daily Living (ADL) and Instrumental Activities of Daily Living (IADL) tests. And their moods were tested with the Geriatric Depression Scale (GDS).

The patients were tested after three months and nine months. The research found that MMSE scores of the patients were better in the supplemented group compared to the control group. The other tests didn't show much difference. The researchers explained their hypothesis on how citicoline works:

> *"Citicoline activates biosynthesis of phospholipids in neuronal membranes, increases brain metabolism as well as norepinephrine and dopamine levels in the central nervous system, and has neuro-protective effects during hypoxia and ischemia. Therefore, citicoline may be recommended for patients with mild vascular cognitive impairment."*

We should note that while some Alzheimer's patients may also have vascular cognitive impairment, this is a quite different disorder from Alzheimer's.

Phospholipids

Remember our discussion of the health of the cell membrane. The cell membrane can secure and trap free radicals before they enter the cell and damage the cell's DNA.

Three phospholipids in particular have thus been shown in clinical studies to help with cognitive decline: Phosphatidylserine (PS), glycerophosphocholine (GPC) and citicholine. Let's quickly review a small sampling of the research:

In a multi-center placebo-controlled Italian study, researchers (Cenacchi *et al.*, 1993) gave 300 milligrams of phosphatidylserine per day for 6 months to 494 cognition-impaired elderly patients. The phosphatidylserine group showed significant improvements in behavior and cognition compared to the placebo group.

Stanford University and Vanderbilt University researchers (Crook *et al.* 1991) gave 149 age-associated memory-impaired patients 300 milligrams of phosphatidylserine or placebo per day for twelve weeks. The phosphatidylserine group improved in learning and memory performance assessments by 30% over the placebo group. The improvements among the phosphatidylserine group were significantly greater among those with the most cognitive impairment.

Due to this and related research, the U.S. Food and Drug Administration has approved two health claims for phosphatidylserine:

(1) "Phosphatidylserine may reduce the risk of dementia in the elderly."

(2) "Phosphatidylserine may reduce the risk of cognitive dysfunction in the elderly."

These are quite generous claims for natural supplements.

Glycerophosphocholine has also shown positive results in research. In one multi-center study, 2,044 patients who suffered from cognitive damage following a recent stroke were given 1000-1200 mg per day of glycerophosphocholine for six months. The glycerophosphocholine group had significantly more improvements in memory, and a reduction in cognitive decline compared with the placebo group (Barbagallo *et al.*, 1994).

Another choline that has showed clinical benefits for cognition is citicoline (cytidine diphosphate choline, or CDP-choline). In a study of 4,191 cases of acute ischemic stroke, citicholine supplementation for six weeks was found to significantly improve "neurological outcomes" of the patients.

In a study of brain activity using magnetic resonance imaging technology found that brain frontal lobe activity increased significantly after six weeks of citicoline supplementation (Silveri *et al.* 2008).

While these studies are peer-reviewed and in good-standing among the medical community, they are typically missing from the mass media's discussion about Alzheimer's disease and dementia. Why is that? Because much of commercial media is financed and subsidized by the pharmaceutical industry. Have you watched the commercials of any of the network news shows lately? A good percentage of them are about pharmaceuticals.

These choline and phosphatidylserine products are not pharmaceuticals. They are derived from natural products such as soybeans. They are not patentable, in other words. Without a patent, pharmaceutical companies are typically not interested.

Mixed Supplements and Multivitamins

Multivitamins in commercial standardized nutrient levels may provide little or no protection or improvement for Alzheimer's, unless there is a deficiency. This has been illustrated in the research. A 14-year study (Grodstein *et al.* 2013) of 5,947 male physicians who were 65 or older found that taking multivitamins did not have any benefits to cognitive health. The researchers stated:

> *"In male physicians aged 65 years or older, long-term use of a daily multivitamin did not provide cognitive benefits."*

Many may find these results questionable. But one must also consider that doctors are typically well-fed. Most have at least a cursory understanding of nutrition and tend to eat better than the general population.

The basic benefits of vitamins, as shown in many studies, is to cure nutritional deficiencies. In study after study on particular vitamins this fact becomes apparent: When ones needs for vitamins are met, vitamins don't have a lot of therapeutic value if they are over-supplemented. In fact, over-supplementation can cause its own problems in some cases.

The researchers also felt this way as they commented on the study:

"Doses of vitamins may be too low or the population may be too well-nourished to benefit from a multivitamin."

It should also be noted that part of the funding for this study came from DSM—a large supplement company.

Then again, there are multiple-nutrient supplements that are formulated specifically for memory or cognitive issues. Are these any better? The research says yes.

Researchers from Italy's University of Genoa (Pardini *et al.* 2015) gave 125 milliliters per day of a multi-nutrient product called Souvenaid™ or a placebo to 26 people with early frontotemporal dementia for 12 weeks. After the period, the groups were switched. This is called a cross-over study. The researchers tested the subjects before and after the treatment and found that taking the supplement significantly reduced their behavioral symptoms of Alzheimer's. But the effect stopped after the supplementation period stopped. And no other differences were seen among the patients for executive function.

Here is what Souvenaid contains:
Eicosapentaenoic acid, 300 mg
Docosahexaenoic acid, 1200 mg
Phospholipids, 106 mg
Choline, 400 mg
Uridine monophosphate, 625 mg
Vitamin E (alpha-tocopherol equivalents), 40 mg
Selenium, 60 μg
Vitamin B12, 3 μg
Vitamin B6, 1 mg
Folic acid, 400 μg
Vitamin C, 80 mg

Another study (Olde Rikkert *et al.* 2015)—from Spain and Holland—found that Souvenaid increased exploratory memory among Alzheimer's patients after a 48-week trial.

A 2014 study from Amsterdam's VU University Medical Center (de Waal *et al.*) also showed favorable results with Souvenaid. The researchers tested 179 people with Alzheimer's for 24 weeks with the supplement or a placebo.

The researchers compared the network connectivity and global network integration of the brains of the patients, before and after the trial.

The research found no increases in memory. But they found the supplement helps protect brain networks from continuing to slide. While the placebo group's network scans found continued deterioration, the supplemented group had significantly less deterioration.

A study from the University of Maryland (Remington *et al.* 2015) gave a combination of folate, alpha-tocopherol, B12, S-adenosyl methionine, N-acetyl cysteine and acetyl-L-carnitine for three or six months. Others took a placebo. The research found that the combination improved cognitive performance, and mood and behavior for those taking the supplements.

Researchers from the University of Massachusetts tested 12 people with moderate to late-stage Alzheimer's disease. They gave half a placebo. The other half were given a formulation of folate, vitamin B12, alpha-tocopherol (vitamin E), S-adenosyl methionine, N-acetyl cysteine and acetyl-L-carnitine. The researchers found those given the nutrient formula, *"demonstrated a clinically significant delay in decline in the Dementia Rating Scale and clock-drawing test as compared to those receiving placebo."*

The researchers also stated:

> *"Institutional caregivers reported approximately 30% improvement in the Neuropsychiatric Inventory and maintenance of performance in the Alzheimer's Disease Cooperative Study-Activities of Daily Living for more than 9 months."*

Another study from UOM (Chan *et al.* 2008) had similar findings. This study gave a formula with folate, vitamin B6, alpha-tocopherol, S-adenosyl methionine, N-acetyl cysteine, and acetyl-L-carnitine to 14 people with early-stage Alzheimer's disease. This study lasted for 12 months and some continued for another 16 months. Again the research found the nutrient formulation improved scores in the Neuropsychiatric Inventory (NPI) and the Alzheimer's Disease Cooperative Study-Activities of Daily Living (ADL). Their caregivers also reported that these improvements were sustained over the next 16 months.

A 2010 study (Chan *et al.*) from the University of Massachusetts tested a formulation consisting of folic acid, B12, Vitamin E, S-adenosylmethionine, N-acetyl cysteine and acetyl-L-carnitine. They gave half the Alzheimer's patients a placebo. Those 74 years old and younger showed some improvement after six months. Those over 74 did not show any improvement.

As discussed earlier, nutrient antioxidants are typically low among those with Alzheimer's disease and mild cognitive impairment. Researchers from Italy's University of Perugia (Rinaldi *et al.* 2003) tested blood levels of vitamin C, vitamin A, vitamin E and carotenoids (including lutein, zeaxanthin, beta-cryptoxanthin, lycopene, alpha- and beta-carotene) among 25 MCI patients, 63 Alzheimer's patients and 53 healthy control patients. They found these antioxidants were lower in the MCI and Alzheimer's patients compared to the controls. But they weren't worse in the

Alzheimer's patients. They were about the same between the MCI and the Alzheimer's patients.

Research from the Memorial University of Newfoundland (Chandra 2001) tested 86 patients over the age of 65. For one year, they gave half the subjects a multivitamin-mineral supplement. The other half took a placebo. The supplemented group significantly improved in every cognitive test except for long-term memory recall. While the subjects did not have Alzheimer's, the researchers felt the supplement program might delay any onset of the disease. They wrote:

> *"Cognitive functions improved after oral supplementation with modest amounts of vitamins and trace elements. This has considerable clinical and public health significance. We recommend that such a supplement be provided to all elderly subjects because it should significantly improve cognition and thus quality of life and the ability to perform activities of daily living. Such a nutritional approach may delay the onset of Alzheimer's disease."*

Another study from UOM (Chan *et al.* 2008) had similar findings. This study gave a formula with folate, vitamin B6, alpha-tocopherol, S-adenosyl methionine, N-acetyl cysteine, and acetyl-L-carnitine to 14 people with early-stage Alzheimer's disease. This study lasted for 12 months and some continued for another 16 months. Again the research found the nutrient formulation improved scores in the Neuropsychiatric Inventory (NPI) and the Alzheimer's Disease Cooperative Study-Activities of Daily Living (ADL). Their caregivers also reported that these improvements were sustained over the next 16 months.

Other research confirms the benefits for supplementation for those over the age of 72—assuming they are not deficient in nutrient intake. Research (Chew *et al.* 2015) published in the *Journal of the American Medical Association* found that taking omega-3 fatty acids, lutein/zeaxanthin, or vitamins C, E, beta carotene or zinc did nothing to reduce cognitive decline among over 3,500 people at an average age of 72. The researchers gave them either a placebo or 1,000 milligrams of omega-3 and/or 10 milligrams of lutein, 2 milligrams of zeaxanthin. Others took these plus different combinations of the other nutrients.

The researchers followed up with the subjects for between two and five years. Cognitive improvements were no greater than the placebos among those tested.

Are supplements better than a good diet?

While the research above is convincing, it is still up for debate whether supplements will do better than a good nutrition-rich diet. A good diet in general improves the prospects for those with cognitive decline.

Researchers from France (Kesse-Guyot *et al.* 2011) tested 2,135 people with the French National Nutrition and Health Program. They used the Guideline Scores (PNNS-GS) to measure their diets over a period of 13 years.

The researchers found those who had better adherence to the Guidelines over the period had 41% better reflecting verbal memory.

That is a significant change—one that matches or beats much of the research above on supplements.

At question is a person's access to healthy whole foods—and of course ones determination to adhere to a healthy diet.

Researchers from the Beijing Hospital of Traditional Chinese Medicine and the Capital Medical University in China (Shi *et al.* 2012) analyzed urinary biomarkers of oxidative stress among 46 patients with vascular dementia, 24 patients with vascular disease without dementia, and 26 people without symptoms of either.

They found that patients with dementia had significantly higher levels of a urinary biomarker called 8-hydroxydeoxyguanosine (or 8-OHdG). 8-OHdG is associated with significantly high levels of oxidative stress. These levels were significantly higher than both of the other groups of patients.

Another study, this one from Qingdao University's School of Medicine (Wu *et al.* 2012), analyzed multiple studies and two large genome studies and concluded that Alzheimer's patients have significantly higher levels of clusterin, also known as apolipoprotein J. Clusterin has been found to bind to beta-amyloid (Abeta) proteins, and has the ability to reduce fibril formation.

It is now thought that in an attempt to resist the formation of the Abeta proteins and fibrils, the body produces clusterin as a defense measure against oxidative stress. This has been confirmed in studies showing that clusterin lowers cell death and levels of oxidative stress.

Oxidative stress is produced with increased levels of toxin exposure, either within the diet, water or air, combined with lower levels of antioxidants and increased levels of lifestyle stressors. Toxins become oxidized and become radicals, which can damage our arteries and tissues.

Researchers from Columbia's University of Pontificia Javeriana (Albarracin *et al.* 2012) studied the connection between antioxidant intake and Alzheimer's disease in a variety of studies. They found that an increased consumption of "polyphenol-rich" foods significantly lowered the risk of Alzheimer's disease. Plant-based foods provide polyphenols.

The researchers confirmed their findings:

"It has been demonstrated, in various cell culture and animal models, that these [polyphenol] metabolites are able to protect neuronal cells by attenuating oxidative stress and damage."

Chapter Five

The Anti-Alzheimer's Diet

As promised, let's expose the relationship between Alzheimer's disease and diet. As you will find within the research outlined below, Alzheimer's disease is related to reduced fruits and vegetables and other types of foods that reduce oxidative stress.

Systemic Inflammation

Alzheimer's disease is a form of systemic inflammation that impacts regions and cells of the brain. Systemic inflammation indicates the immune system is overburdened. The extent or combination of the elements mentioned simply overwhelms the immune system. Typically, the immune system can resolve most of these problems when it is presented with a small amount or a few of them at a time. But when an avalanche of them becomes too great, the immune system goes on alert, resulting in systemic inflammation.

Systemic inflammation is the immune system's version of all-out war. The immune system begins to launch the nukes. These can include fever, vomiting, diarrhea, swelling and pain.

The rest of this chapter will more specifically discuss lifestyle choices that produce or worsen systemic inflammation within the body. In other words, these are all *contributing causes*. This means that just one of these factors may not in itself cause systemic inflammation. But any one of these, in addition to others, can overwhelm the immune system—producing systemic inflammation.

Factors of Systemic Inflammation

While toxin overload is the primary condition, the following list summarizes conditions that collectively contribute to systemic inflammation:

1) *Toxemia:* An overload of toxins that produce radicals.
2) *Infections:* Infection with microorganisms that produce mutagenicity: viruses, bacteria, yeasts and parasites.
3) *Antioxidant enzyme deficiencies:* An undersupply of antioxidizing enzymes that stabilize radicals, including glutathione peroxidase, glutathione reductase, catalase and superoxide dismutase.
4) *Dietary antioxidant deficiencies:* An undersupply of antioxidants from our foods to help stabilize radicals.
5) *Barriers to detoxification:* Lifestyle or physiological factors that block our body's ability to rid waste products and toxins.

65

Detoxification requires exercise, fresh air, sweating, sunshine and so on.

6) **_Poor dietary choices:_** A poor diet burdens the body with toxins, unstable fatty acids, refined sugars and overly processed foods.

7) **_Immunosuppression:_** A burdened or defective immune system.

Aging and Free Radicals

As we've discussed, oxidative stress caused by free radicals is specifically linked to Alzheimer's disease. This is because brain cells become damaged by these free radicals. The resulting oxidation produces damaged saturase enzymes which produce destructive amyloid oligomers.

Over the past few decades, researchers have tried to figure out what causes aging and more disease as we age. Studies have investigated the body's biological clock—linked to RNA and the methylation of DNA—also referred to as epigenetic aging.

But a more tangible approach to aging and disease is the understanding that disease and the aging of the cell is linked to free radicals and oxidative stress. This is more tangible because we can chemically determine levels of oxidative stress in an individual.

In addition, research over the last few years has concluded that oxidative stress—damage to the body's tissues and cells from free radicals—increases with age.

But this has neither been confirmed nor quantified with regard to how much oxidative stress increases over the years.

Technology and recent research now affords scientists the ability to quantify the level of oxidative stress within an individual's body. And this quantification can be done at a particular period of time, with comparisons made.

In the first study of its kind, researchers from Italy's University of Bologna (Valgimigli et al. 2014) conducted a study of 247 healthy people who were between two days old and 104 years old. The researchers utilized a technique called electron paramagnetic resonance to test the blood of each of the people for their level of oxidative stress.

The test is similar to a nuclear magnetic resonance (NMR) scan but it also measures unstable molecules—considered oxidative and described as free radicals.

As expected, the researchers found that oxidative stress levels increase from childhood into the elderly years. But they also found that the rate of oxidative stress increases by an average of 1.1 percent per year. They also found there was little difference in this oxidative stress progression between men and women.

Some of the techniques and philosophy were born from a study (Filosa *et al.* 2005) that utilized electron paramagnetic resonance to study the oxidative stress levels of patients with sickle cell related thalassemia— a recessive blood disorder. The researchers tested 38 of the patients and compared their results with healthy control subjects that were matched— same age and so on.

The researchers found that the electron paramagnetic resonance results coincided with levels of oxidative stress determined from the blood of the patients.

They called the electron paramagnetic resonance testing a *radical probe*.

The radical probe is referring to counts of free radicals, which are present in all of our bodies to one degree or another. Other research has confirmed that free radical levels tend to be higher in disease—related to oxidative stress.

Free radicals are often produced from toxins, but can also be products of nature as well. In nature, however, free radicals are typically balanced by antioxidants.

Multiple studies over the years have shown that our synthetic chemical society has become more harmful in general because of the increases in free radicals produced by consuming these chemicals.

This doesn't mean that nature doesn't produce free radicals. It does. Free radicals are a natural part of metabolism. As long as we don't get overloaded with them by consuming synthetic toxins.

What these researchers determined is that high levels of free radicals are proportionate to higher levels of oxidative stress because free radicals need electrons. As they steal electrons from cells and tissues, those remaining molecules will often combine one way or another with oxygen— producing an oxidation reaction.

And because such an free radical-caused oxidation reaction will in effect rip away molecules from tissues and cells, the result is disease and aging.

But now we know—from the University of Bologna study discussed above—that levels of free radicals increase over the years. We also know that they increase in a fairly uniform and predictable manner.

If we assume the rate of free radical intake is constant, this means the body is slowing down its ability to neutralize free radicals over time. This relates directly to the liver's production of glutathione, superoxide dismutase and others, as well as the ability of our immune system and probiotic system to neutralize free radicals as we age.

While this in itself does not explain how we age—because we don't know why these mechanisms are slowed down with aging—understanding this allows a new understanding of how we can reduce our proclivity to disease as we age.

This of course gives us a means to help slow the process of cell and tissue damage as we age—by decreasing our exposure to toxins as our bodies get older.

The Role of Antioxidants

This leaves the potential means for combating degenerative disease: increase the consumption of antioxidants.

Antioxidants are foods, nutrients and phytocompounds we can consume that will naturally neutralize free radicals. Even if our liver and immune system is slowing down as we age, we can increase our intake of antioxidants to help defer degenerative disease. If we are increasing our antioxidant consumption by at least by 1% per year to keep up with our free radical increases, we stand a chance to seriously defer degenerative diseases, which include cancers, Alzheimer's and others.

This doesn't mean we can live forever in these bodies. Aging is part of nature's way of telling us this lifetime is only a part of our journey. But perhaps we can keep our body and brain a little healthier—and more useful—during this lifetime.

This and other studies give us a mature view of how our dietary habits today will effect our future mental health. Diets that produce high levels of oxidative free radicals have been shown to produce a higher risk of not just cardiovascular disease, but also dementia, because what damages the heart and blood vessels can also damage brain and nerve cells. And when it comes to blood flow, brain cells will suffer first when arteries become damaged.

Lipid Peroxidation

An important form of oxidative stress in Alzheimer's disease is something called lipid peroxidation. Lipids are quite simply, fats—fatty acids. Lipid peroxidation means the lipids or fats become oxidized and unstable. They are missing an atomic part—often just a hydrogen ion. This means that like any other type of free radical, they need electrons to make themselves complete, or stable.

The special issue of lipid free radicals is that lipids make up the cell membranes. When these molecules are being robbed of electrons, the 'robbery' results in an unstable cell membrane.

Fatty acids that make up the membranes of cells are the likely candidates for peroxidation. Remember, the name "lipid" refers to a fatty acid. Fatty acids include saturated fats, polyunsaturates, monounsaturates, and so on (see fatty acid discussions later on).

Let's take a closer look at the process of lipid peroxidation.

The first step takes place with the entry of an oxidized lipid. This occurs frequently when low-density lipoproteins (LDL) accumulate in the blood. LDL is easily oxidized, forming free radical lipids.

Other radicals can also promote lipid peroxidation, such as high levels of free glucose in the blood; chemical or drug metabolites; and many other synthetics.

When these reactive oxygen species come into cell membrane proximity, they damage cell membranes by robbing the lipid cell membranes.

Several types of lipids make up the cell membrane. Fatty acids will combine with other molecules to make phospholipids, cholesterols and glycolipids. Saturates and polyunsaturates are typical, but there are several species of polyunsaturates. These range from long chain versions to short versions. They also include the cis- configuration and the trans- configuration. Cell membranes that utilize predominantly cis- versions with long chains are the most durable. Those cell membranes with trans- configurations can be highly unstable, and irregularly porous. This is one reason why trans fats are unhealthy. The other reason is that trans fats easily become peroxidized.

Cell membranes with more long chain fatty acids are more stable and are less subject to peroxidation. Shorter chains that provide more double bonds are less stable, because these are more easily broken. Also, monounsaturated fatty acids such as GLA are more stable.

Once the fatty acid is degraded by an oxygen species, it becomes a fatty acid radical. The fatty acid will usually become oxidized, making it a peroxyl-fatty acid radical. This radical will react with other fatty acids, forming a cyclic process involving radicals called cyclic peroxides.

This becomes a chain reaction that results in the cell membrane becoming completely destroyed and dysfunctional. This forces the cell to signal to the immune system that it is under attack and about to become malignant. The T-cell immune response will often initiate the cell's self-destruct switch: TNF—tumor necrosis factor. Alternatively, the cell may be directly destroyed by cytotoxic T-cells. The combined process stimulates inflammation. As these cells are killed or self-destruct, they are purged from the system—provoking increased mucous formation.

While this peroxidation and cell destruction is taking place, the immune system is not simply standing by. The body enters a state called *systemic inflammation.* As we discussed earlier, during systemic inflammation, the immune system launches an ongoing supply of eosinophils, neutrophils and mast cells, which release granulocytes that inflame the airways.

In other words, due to this ongoing peroxidation, the immune system is on a hair-trigger. Imagine a person at work who is stressed from being buried in work and a myriad of problems. You walk into their office and they immediately react: "And what do *you* want?" they demand.

If they were not overloaded with work, problems and deadlines, your coming into their office would probably be met without such a frantic response. But since they were overloaded, they reacted (hyper reacted is a better word) more defensively than needed, *because they thought you were going to add to their workload.*

In other words, inflammation is simply a defense measure by an immune system that is overwhelmed.

Typical associations with inflammation include artery damage and plaque build-up, obesity, diabetes, a sedentary lifestyle, and a diet high in saturated fats and/or fried foods. High blood pressure and fast or irregular heart rate, especially in persons over 40 years old, are also strong markers.

Along with these associations come higher levels of total cholesterol, low-density lipoprotein (LDL) and very low-density lipoprotein (VLDL) cholesterol, and total triglycerides are also key markers. The link between small LDL particle size and atherosclerosis is a key factor, and the oxidation of LDL particles is the match that lights the fuse. These involve hyperperoxides, as they readily form oxidative radicals. The cascade towards LDL oxidation also seems to be accelerated by lipooxygenases like 15-LOX-2 along with cyclooxygenases (COX). The process as a whole is lipid peroxidation.

In addition to launching systemic inflammation due to widespread cell damage, the body also produces processes that attempt to halt the peroxidation cycle. One of these components is the glutathione peroxidase enzyme discussed earlier, formed by the body using selenium as a substrate. Depending upon the rate of lipid peroxidation, however, this could be like trying to blow out a forest fire. There is simply too much fire spreading too quickly.

The critical component in this mystery is glutathione peroxidase—an enzyme produced in the liver. Glutathione peroxidase is the leading enzyme responsible for the breakdown and removal of lipid hydroperoxides. Lipid hydroperoxides are oxidized fats that damage cell membranes. As they do this, they create pores in the cell. The resulting damage eventually kills most cells.

Lipid hydroperoxides are one of the most damaging molecules within the body. They are responsible for many deadly metabolic diseases, including heart disease, artery disease, Alzheimer's disease and many others.

When lipid hydroperoxides accumulate in the body, they can also damage the cells of the airways, causing irritation and inflammation. The damage from lipid hydroperoxides stimulates an inflammatory response. Researchers have called the start signal from the cell that initiates this inflammatory response *lipid peroxidation/LOOH-mediated stress signaling.* In other words, the cells are stressed by lipid peroxidation, and this initiates a distress signal to the immune system.

By virtue of removing lipid hydroperoxides, glutathione peroxidase— not to be confused with glutathione reductase—regulates pro-inflammatory arachidonic acid metabolism. In other words, glutathione regulates the release and populations of those pro-inflammatory mediators, the leukotrienes. Leukotriene activity is directly associated with the damage created by lipid hydroperoxides. Thus, when lipid hydroperoxide levels are reduced by glutathione peroxidase, leukotriene density is reduced.

Selenium is required for glutathione peroxidase production. Should the body be overloaded with lipid hydroperoxides, more glutathione is required to clear out the damage. As more glutathione is produced, more selenium is utilized, which runs selenium levels down.

This issue was illustrated by research from Britain's South Manchester University Hospital (Hassan 2008). The researchers studied 13 aspirin-induced asthmatics and a healthy matched control group. They found that the asthmatics maintained higher levels of selenium in the bloodstream— especially among blood platelets. This high selenium content in the bloodstream correlated with higher glutathione peroxidase activity. The research illustrated how selenium is used up faster in by those with inflammation through this glutathione peroxidase process.

Reactive Lipid Oxygen Species

The initiation process of the lipid peroxidation is started by a reactive oxygen species. This reactive species is a free radical—an unstable molecule or ion that forms during a chemical reaction. In other words, the molecule or ion needs another atom, ion or molecule to stabilize it. Once it is stable, it is not reactive.

While a free radical is unstable, it can damage any number of elements it meets. These include the cells, organs and tissues of the body.

Nature produces many, many free radicals. However, nature typically accompanies radicals with the molecules, atoms or ions that stabilize the radical. In the atmosphere, for example, radicals become stabilized by ozone and other elements. In plants, radicals become stabilized by antioxidants from nutrients derived from the sun, soil and oxygen. In the body, radicals are stabilized by antioxidizing enzymes, nutrients and other elements. These include glutathione peroxidase, as we have been discussing.

Confirming this, the research from South Manchester University Hospital mentioned earlier concluded with a comment that the increased glutathione peroxidase activity related to radical oxidation: *"administration of aspirin to these patients increases the generation of immediate oxygen products..."*

Another anti-oxidation process within the body utilizes the *superoxide dismutase* (SOD) enzyme. The SOD enzyme is typically available within the cytoplasm of most cells. Here SOD is complexed by either copper and zinc, or manganese—similar to the way selenium is complexed with the glutathione peroxidase enzyme. Several types of SOD enzymes reside within the body—some in the mitochondria and some in the intercellular tissue fluids. SOD neutralizes superoxides before they can damage the inside and outside of the cell—assuming the body is healthy, with substantial amounts of SOD. The immune system produces superoxides as part of its strategy to attack microorganisms and toxins.

Another broad anti-oxidation process utilizes *catalase*. Here the body provides an enzyme bound by iron to neutralize peroxides to oxygen and water. It is a standard component of many metabolic reactions within the body.

Yet another enzyme utilized for radical reduction is *glutathione reductase*. This enzyme works with NADP in the cell to stabilize hydrogen peroxide oxidized radicals before they can damage the cell.

Notice that all of these antioxidizing enzymes require minerals. We have seen either selenium, copper, zinc, manganese or iron as necessary to keep these enzymes in good supply. Many other minerals and trace elements are used by other antioxidant and detoxifying enzyme processes. These minerals, and many of the enzymes themselves, are supplied by various foods and supplements, as we'll discuss further.

Another tool that the healthy body utilizes to stabilize radicals are the antioxidants supplied by plant foods. Plants produce antioxidants to protect their own cells from radical damage. Thus, their plant material contains a host of these oxidation stabilizers, which our bodies use to neutralize radicals.

The antioxidant capacity of a food is often measured with an ORAC (oxygen radical absorbance capacity) assay. This test specifically measures the ability of the food to neutralize quantities of peroxyl radicals. By measuring this capacity to reduce the number of peroxyl radicals in a solution, that food is judged for its antioxidant capacity. The theory behind this is that if a molecule has *unpaired electron* then those electrons must become paired somehow, so they in effect "steal" electrons or donate their unpaired electrons to another molecule. In effect, this donating or stealing process is thought to be what damages biological tissues.

Investigation on antioxidant capacity reveals assays besides ORAC assays. There is the Total Radical Trapping Antioxidant Parameter assay (TRAP), the Crocin Bleaching assay, Folin-Ciocalteu Reagent assay (RCR), the Trolox Equivalence Antioxidant Capacity assay (TEAC), Ferric Ion Reducing Antioxidant Power (FRAP) and a Total Antioxidant Potential assay, which uses copper as an oxidant. While some of these assays apparently measure the ability of some molecules to transfer hydrogen atoms, others are thought to measure electron transfer only. While ORAC is considered one of the more reliable measurements of antioxidant capacity, it is rendering only a narrow window of what happens within a (living) biological system (Huang *et al.* 2005).

In reality, radicals are not bad guys in themselves. The biological system produces radicals through normal metabolic activities, and they are necessary for many physiological functions. As energy is produced through the Krebs cycle, oxygen is a necessary part of the process, and oxidative radicals are part of the byproduct. Superoxide can both accept electron moments or donate electrons. Even though superoxide is considered a radical, it is a necessary species for other metabolic functions. It is part of the feedback-response regulating mechanism within cells. Superoxide reacts either independently or through catalytic conversion with superoxide disumutase to form the biological version of the natural antibiotic, hydrogen peroxide along with oxygen. This 'free radical' superoxide is thus an important component working within the body's immune functions.

Interestingly, research indicates the body's own production of melatonin neutralizes reactive singlet oxygen. While not providing the classic antioxidant identity, melatonin production appears to substantially reduce reactive oxygen species and other harmful radicals such as the *peroxynitrite anion*—caused by the consumption of nitrites.

Tryptophan—another molecule naturally produced in the body—also appears to stimulate radical neutralization. In fact, both tryptophan and melatonin not only neutralize radicals, but they also provide protective mechanisms, preventing cells from being damaged. They assist in the production of various enzymes. They will even enter cells and line cell membranes. These wonderful biochemicals protect the body against oxidative radical and other types of free radical damage (Reiter *et al.* 1999; Tax *et al.* 2000).

Now should the body not properly manufacture these protective bio-chemicals, radical species such as singlet oxygen can invade cell membranes, disfiguring and genetically damaging the cell. This is especially true if the lipid quality of the cell membrane is not structurally sound (i.e. through the eating of trans fats, etc.). The radicals themselves can damage the cell membrane. This will allow other radicals to pour into the cytoplasm and damage proteins, organelles and more importantly, the cells' DNA.

Should radicals get into cells and damage the DNA within the nuclei, dangerous mutations of the cells can develop. While cells have a tremendous capacity to repair genetic damage, a large population of radicals can overwhelm this capacity. This is the mechanism most thought to instigate metastasizing and invasive cancers.

Should a radical encounter the electromagnetic structure of a stable molecule such as triplet oxygen, there will be a change in the biochemical aspects and characteristics of that molecule. As the body's personal defense systems recognize that capacity for damage, various detox biochemicals are drawn in to neutralize it.

What's this have to do with Diet?

We have discovered in our research on antioxidants that tremendous neutralizing biochemicals are produced through the process of the conversion of chlorophyll. While this process is underway, plants produce various phytochemicals such as sterols, anthocyanidins and others.

In the case of devitalized foods, over-processed and/or foods blended with chemicals, these foods are often chemically imbalanced. The bonds that tie together the various minerals, vitamins and amino complexes—have become serrated. The resulting molecular structure is homogenized. The bonds have been robbed of much of their capacity though processing (notably heat, freezing and reheating). Electromagnetic waveforms interact with the bonds of the nutrient factors, creating instability. The instability breaks apart many of the cofactors, releasing ions and breaking bonds. A fractured and minimized array of nutrients is now available.

When we cook at home we can prevent much of this nutrient release by cooking with the lid on at lower temperatures. Studies out of Britain's University of Warwick (2007) and the American Chemical Society (2007) illustrate that while boiling and frying reduces the nutritional content of vegetables, steaming vegetables will not only retain nutrient content, but may even—as in the case of anti-carcinogenic glucosinolates—be increased with steaming. Whatever heat remains in the food can also assist in a recombant molecular bonding, retaining some of the energy released with the breaking of bonds.

This is especially the case when food is lightly cooked in water. The water will absorb many of the nutrients as they are released from the food. This occurs in slow-cooked soups. Hot soup more nutritious than after it is cooled down (careful, do not burn the tongue) as well.

In overly processed food, both the heat and the nutrients are gone by the time it reaches the shelf of the store. Only a fraction of the covalent nutrient bonds will remain in the food. The complex high-energy bonds are broken. Many of the fat- and water-soluble nutrients that were once part of the whole food will have either evaporated or broken up into denatured fractions. The complex oscillating bonding binding the various nutrients to their carbon chain skeletons (often polysaccharides or glycerides) have been separated.

What we slowly discovered from the refining of cane, beets and wheat will also be what we learn about the rest of nature's nutrients: We cannot separate the nutrient from its surrounding matter and achieve the same effects. This goes for the concept of antioxidants and free radicals. Nature produces antioxidants like polyphenols and sterols within a molecular field of components derived from living organisms. These bond the nutrients to elements such as fiber, carbohydrates, glycosides, minerals, phytosterols, fatty acids, lignans, and even special polysaccharides like beta-glucans. All of these components and many others we have yet to discover come together within plants. Once we denature them, free radical species are created.

Antioxidant Diets and AD

These points are not simply theory. There is hard evidence that substantiates the connection between the consumption of antioxidants (or the lack thereof) and Alzheimer's disease:

Researchers from Columbia's University of Pontificia Javeriana (Albarracin *et al.* 2012) studied the connection between antioxidant intake and Alzheimer's disease in a variety of studies. They found that an increased consumption of "polyphenol-rich" foods significantly lowered the risk of Alzheimer's disease. Plant-based foods provide polyphenols.

The researchers confirmed their findings:

> *"It has been demonstrated, in various cell culture and animal models, that these [polyphenol] metabolites are able to protect neuronal cells by attenuating oxidative stress and damage."*

A fifteen year study of elderly persons, Japanese researchers (Ozawa *et al.* 2013) confirmed that ones diet can dramatically reduce our chances of Alzheimer's disease and dementia.

The researchers, from Japan's Kyushu University Graduate School of Medical Sciences, followed 1,006 people who were between 60 and 80 years old. They tracked their diets, and tracked whether they contracted vascular dementia and/or Alzheimer's disease during that period.

The researchers grouped the diets among the subjects into seven general categories. These included Western diet patterns, traditional Japanese diets and more or less vegetable intake, more or less soy intake, more or less rice intake, more or less dairy intake and more or less algae (seaweed) intake—part of the traditional Japanese diet.

Among the total population, after an average of fifteen years, 144 people developed Alzheimer's disease and 88 developed vascular dementia—the second-leading type of dementia after Alzheimer's disease. (Research has estimated that 20-30% of dementia cases are vascular, and vascular dementia can also produce Alzheimer's symptoms.)

The researchers found that those whose diets had the highest intakes of vegetables, soybeans, algae, milk and dairy products, and low in rice had a 65% reduced incidence of Alzheimer's disease, 66% less incidence of any dementia, and 45% less incidence of vascular dementia.

It should be pointed out that white polished rice is the primary rice being eaten among the Japanese today. We discuss the problems with white rice and why brown rice is healthier for a myriad of reasons in my book, *"The Ancestor's Diet."*

Other research has found that diets rich in fruits and vegetables—notably the Mediterranean Diet—decrease the risk of Alzheimer's disease and other forms of dementia. In a study from Australia's Edith Cowan University (Gardener *et al.* 2013), it was found that diets that most closely adhere to the Mediterranean Diet reduce the risk of Alzheimer's disease and mild cognitive impairment. This study followed 970 people—including 149 with Alzheimer's and 98 with mild cognitive impairment (MCI).

In research funded by the National Institutes of Health, Columbia University Medical Center researchers found that a diet with higher consumption of vegetables, fruits, grains and legumes, with lower saturated fat levels and higher monounsaturated fats reduced the risk of brain damage.

The diets of 712 New Yorkers were divided into three groups. They were followed up with brain scans an average of six years later. The scans indicated that 238 people had brain damage of some sort.

The group following more closely to a Mediterranean diet (primarily vegetarian and fish diet with little or no meat) had a 36% lower risk of brain damage. The group that had a closer Med-diet had 21% lower risk of brain damage than the group that ate the typical (red meat with low plant-based foods) Western diet.

In another study, Columbia University (Gu *et al.* 2010) researchers followed 2,148 elderly persons for four years, giving them dementia testing every 18 months. This research found that a diet high in nuts, fruits, cruciferous vegetables, leafy green vegetables, nuts, tomatoes and fish—and had a lower intake of red meat and high-fat dairy products—were 38% less likely to develop Alzheimer's disease by the fourth year. None of the elderly subjects had symptoms of Alzheimer's or dementia at the beginning of the study and they were all over 64 years old.

In another study from the Columbia University researchers (Scarmeas *et al.* 2009), 1,880 elderly people without dementia at the beginning of the study were followed for over five years. At the end of the study, 282 people contracted Alzheimer's disease. The researchers found that adhering to a Med diet decreased the risk of Alzheimer's by 40%.

In a study (Scarmeas *et al.* 2006) on 2,258 elderly New Yorkers, those who adhered more closely (highest third) to the Mediterranean diet had a 40% reduced risk of developing Alzheimer's disease within four years.

In another study (Scarmeas *et al.* 2006) that compared 194 Alzheimer's patients with 1,790 healthy elderly persons, it was found that those adhering more closely (highest tertile) with the Mediterranean diet had a 68% reduced risk of Alzheimer's compared to those with the lowest adherence—the highest consumption of the Western diet.

Another study by the same researchers (Scarmeas *et al.* 2007) found that a higher adherence to the Med diet reduced the risk of dying for Alzheimer's disease patients as well.

Researchers from Spain's University of Navarra (Martínez-Lapiscina *et al.* 2013) conducted a series of studies that have determined that a Mediterranean diet supplemented with either nuts or extra virgin olive oil results in a reduced risk of mild cognitive impairment (MCI)—and thus Alzheimer's disease. Another study found that the Med diet with olive oil decreased the risk of MCI even further.

In the major study, 522 elderly adults participated. They had an average age of 75 years. They were split into three groups and followed for six and a half years. One group consumed a standard (Western) low-fat diet, another group consumed a Mediterranean diet supplemented with mixed nuts, and the third group consumed a Mediterranean diet supplemented with virgin olive oil.

The supplemented nuts group consumed 30 grams of mixed nuts per day in addition to their diets, and the supplemented olive oil group consumed one liter of extra virgin olive oil per week.

The subjects were evaluated using the Mini-Mental State Examination and Clock Drawing Test. The Mini-mental exam is a 30-point test used by doctors to check patients for dementia and cognitive impairment. The Clock Drawing Test uses clock drawings to test the patient's ability to accurately convert, copy and understand—another test for dementia and cognitive impairment.

After nearly seven years, the researchers found those who ate the Mediterranean Diet with the olive oil had 62% better scores on the Mini-Mental exam than did the control group. This group also had an average of 51% better scores on the Clock Drawing Test. The group consuming the Mediterranean Diet supplemented with nuts had 57% better scores than the conventional diet on the Mini-Mental exam, and 33% better scores on the Clock Drawing Test.

A 2015 review by researchers from Australia's Swinburne University of Technology (Hardman *et al.* 2016) analyzed 18 studies that followed the diets of aging adults. They found that the Med Diet significantly reduced the incidence of Alzheimer's, along with other forms of dementia . Here is what the researchers stated:

> *"Eighteen articles meeting our inclusion criteria were subjected to systematic review. These revealed that higher adherence to a Med-Diet is associated with slower rates of cognitive decline, reduced conversion to Alzheimer's disease, and improvements in cognitive function. The specific cognitive domains that were found to benefit with improved Mediterranean Diet Score were memory (delayed recognition, long-term, and working memory), executive function, and visual constructs."*

Further in their discussion, the researchers stated:

> *"The more specific cognitive domains that improved with Med Diet were memory, delayed recognition, executive function, long-term working memory, and visual constructs. These are mainly tests of fluid intelligence that decline with age. Interestingly, benefits to cognition afforded by the Med Diet were not exclusively in older individuals. The two studies included that were in younger adults both found improvements in cognition using computerized assessments."*

The researchers also summarized the contents of the Med Diet:

> *"The key components of a Med Diet are abundant consumption of plant foods, such as leafy greens, fresh fruit and vegetables, cere-*

als, beans, seeds, nuts, and legumes. The Med Diet is also low in dairy, has minimal red meats, and uses olive oil as its major source of fat."

In 2013, Researchers from the University of Athens School of Medicine (Psaltopoulou *et al.* 2013) conducted a review of research that studied the connection between the Med diet and the risk of stroke, depression, cognitive impairment, and Parkinson's disease. They found 22 well-designed studies that followed many thousands of patients. Their meta-analysis of these studies found that the Mediterranean diet reduced the risk of stroke by 29%, reduced the risk of depression by 32%, and reduced the risk of cognitive impairment by 40%.

In one of these, researchers from Australia's Edith Cowan University (Féart *et al.* 2011) studied nearly 1,000 people—including some with mild cognitive decline and Alzheimer's. They found those who had diets closest to a Mediterranean Diet had the least incidence of cognitive decline and Alzheimer's disease. Many other studies have confirmed these results over the past few years.

The question also arises is what are the factors of the Mediterranean diet and why does this diet help reduce cognitive decline? As stated recently by researchers from the University of Malta (Solfrizzi *et al.* 2011)—the Med Diet:

"is rich in the antioxidants Vitamins C and E, polyunsaturated fatty acids and polyphenolic compounds."

What do these elements have in common with the Mediterranean diet? Yes, the Med Diet certainly does contain many of these nutrients. But the Med Diet, as pointed out by the University of Malta scientists—contains numerous nutrients that synergize with each other. And because the Med Diet is rich in plant-based foods, the Med Diet contains polyphenols.

These polyphenols are plant components that include flavonoids, proanthocyanidins, sterols and many other types of special compounds. These compounds work synergistically within plant-based foods to provide a host of benefits, which include brain cell health, artery health, heart health, liver and kidney health and many others. The combination of these plant-based foods provide the ultimate in cognitive decline prevention, because along with other benefits they reduce damage produced by free radicals—which are ultimately at the core of cognitive decline according to most research.

What about meat consumption? The research above is very clear, that a reduced consumption of red meat lowers the risk of Alzheimer's disease. But other research has been even more concise in this aspect.

Research (Grant 2016) on the prevalence of Alzheimer's in ten different countries—the United States, Brazil, Chile, Cuba, Egypt, India, Mongolia, Nigeria, Republic of Korea and Sri Lanka—analyzed diets 5, 10, and 15 years prior to Alzheimer's diagnoses. The research found that eating meat and other animal products (with the exception of milk) five years before diagnosis was found to be the most relevant correlation with Alzheimer's incidence. The research concluded:

> *"Thus, reducing meat consumption could significantly reduce the risk of Alzheimer's disease as well as of several cancers, diabetes mellitus type 2, stroke, and, likely, chronic kidney disease."*

The brain does not sit in a laboratory jar isolated from the rest of the body. The brain operates as part of the rest of the whole body. The health of the rest of that body—including the arteries, heart, liver, kidneys, bloodstream and so on—directly affects the health of our brain cells.

A primarily plant-based diet and regular exercise are the key elements in keeping the whole body healthy. This is proven not only in cognitive research, but in cancer research, heart disease research, liver and kidney research and elsewhere. Turns out, those plant-based foods the Western diet relegates to a small portion at the edge of the plate are the very medicines our body needs to keep itself healthy.

After reviewing some of the same research, Dr. Gad Marshall, a Harvard Alzheimer's researcher and Assistant Professor of Medicine at Harvard concluded that ones diet can delay and even prevent cognitive decline and Alzheimer's. According to Dr. Marshall:

> *"My strongest recommendations are a Mediterranean-style diet and regular physical exercise," he says. "There's good evidence from multiple studies showing that these lifestyle modifications can prevent cognitive decline and dementia and also slow down existing cognitive decline."*

These two factors have been proven to reduce memory and cognitive decline without question. The evidence comes from numerous studies and reviews from eminent researchers around the world.

Other research has had similar findings: Vassallo *et al.* 2012; Wyka *et al.* 2012; Devanand *et al.* 2012; Solfrizzi *et al.* 2011; Solfrizzi *et al.* 2011 among others.

The bottom line is that nature works in synergy, just as the body does. The brain does not sit in a laboratory jar isolated from the rest of the body. The brain operates as part of the rest of the whole body. The health of the rest of that body—including the arteries, heart, liver, kidneys, bloodstream and so on—directly affects the health of our brain cells.

Obesity and Alzheimer's

According to the latest statistics from the Centers of Disease Control, about 36% of American adults are obese and 69% are overweight. This means that the majority of Americans are either overweight or obese.

The United States is first in the world in obesity. This is followed by Mexico, where 30% of adults are obese, and New Zealand, where 27% of adults are obese. Australia is fourth with 25% of adults, followed by the UK, where 25% is also obese. Canada is the sixth most obese country, with 24% of adults. Ireland is seventh, with 23% obesity among adults, and Chile is eighth with 22%. Iceland is ninth with 20% obesity among adults.

Other countries with higher percentages include Hungary, Greece, Germany, Finland and Poland.

The countries that are the least obese include Japan, Korea, China, India, Indonesia, Italy and others. China, for example, has 2.9% obesity, and India has about 5% obesity. Korea and Japan are close to China's rate. Italy is about 7% obesity.

What is a consequence of the most obese countries versus the countries with less obesity? First, these are countries with the highest rates of Alzheimer's disease. These countries with higher rates of obesity are also the countries that consume the Western diet to the greatest degree.

The Western diet is composed primarily of red meats, fried poultry and seafood, processed starchy foods, and sugary foods and sodas. Could this possibly be a coincidence that the countries that consume more of a Western diet have greater levels of obesity? Nada. Numerous universities and governmental agencies have been studying the relationship between obesity and diet for many years, and have concluded that the Western diet is by far the most fattening diet.

For example, research from China has shown that as more people begin to eat the Western diet, obesity rates have been rising (Wang and Zhai 2013).

Most of us realize that diet and obesity are related. But do we know that toxicity and obesity are related? As we discussed earlier, many toxins—especially many dangerous ones—are fat soluble. This means that they will build up among our fat cells. This also means that the more and larger fat cells we have, the more build up of toxicity we can have.

Obesity is also associated with a disorder now called *metabolic syndrome*. According to the American Heart Association, metabolic syndrome is related to the following conditions:

- Blood sugar issues (diabetes, insulin resistance, hypoglycemia)
- Obesity (most specifically abdominal obesity)

- Cholesterol issues (high LDL, low HDL, high triglycerides)
- High blood pressure
- Chronic inflammation markers (including homocysteine, C-reactive protein, high white blood cell count, high eosinophils)
- Atherosclerosis (damage and hardening to the arteries—indicated by fibrinogen, circulation problems and so on.)

As we discussed earlier, these conditions are also linked with greater risk of Alzheimer's disease.

Metabolic syndrome is characterized by cholesterol problems, high blood pressure, diabetes or hypoglycemia, chronic inflammation, cardiovascular disease, high CRP levels, and heart disease. All of these issues add up to the same issue: systemic inflammation. Furthermore, each of these conditions have the same underlying issues as we have discussed: Poor dietary choices, high levels of reactive oxygen species, increased infections, an overburdened immune system, lack of exercise and other poor lifestyle choices.

It is thus not an accident that the relative intake of our fats is specific to our levels of toxicity. This has been studied by a number of researchers, who have concluded that obesity and inflammation are irreparably tied.

It is a well-known fact that obese people have higher rates of cardiovascular disease, diabetes, kidney disorders, liver diseases, arthritis, asthma, hay fever, dementia, intestinal disorders and many, many other conditions. Just about every medical condition is worsened by obesity, and we need no scientific reference for this fact, simply because the research is so widely known.

In a recent study from Boston University's School of Medicine, led by cardiologist and medical professor Noyan Gokce, MD, fat tissues from 109 obese and lean people provided clear evidence. Tissue from none of the lean patients illustrated any signs of inflammation. In comparison, fat tissues from the obese patients showed "significant" signs of inflammation.

In addition, the lean patients showed "no sign" of poor vascular function while the obese patients showed significantly poor vascular function. This of course relates to inflammation, as we've discussed. When the blood vessel walls become damaged by free radicals and lipid peroxides. This results in scarring and artery deposit build-up, which inhibits healthy circulation and releases clots that block other arteries.

The research also illustrated that the obese persons exhibited varying degrees of inflammation, indicating that a toxic environment and intake of toxins is also associated with higher levels of inflammation. Obesity simply allows for a better 'net' to capture more filters within the fat cells.

So other than consuming fewer calories, can a change in our diet really make a difference?

The evidence says yes. Researchers from Northwestern University's Feinberg School of Medicine (Shay *et al.* 2012) followed 1,794 adult Americans from eight different population samples. Of course, they found that lower calorie intake related directly to lower levels of Body Mass Index (BMI).

But they also found that calories equal, those who ate more fresh fruit, pasta and rice had lower BMIs. Lower BMI was also associated with less meat intake and lower saturated fat consumption, while higher dietary fiber (read plant-based foods) were associated with lower levels of BMI.

The researchers concluded:

> *"The consumption of foods higher in nutrient-dense carbohydrate and lower in animal protein and saturated fat is associated with lower total energy intakes, more favorable micronutrient intakes, and lower BMI."*

In a study from the School of Public Health of the UK's Imperial College (Romaguera *et al.* 2011) followed 48,631 men and women from five different European countries for an average of five and a half years. They found that those eating more meat, processed breads, margarine and soft drinks had a significantly greater risk of becoming obese. They concluded:

> *"A dietary pattern high in fruit and dairy and low in white bread, processed meat, margarine, and soft drinks may help to prevent abdominal fat accumulation."*

Another study found that a mostly-vegan diet plan with daily green-foods and apple cider vinegar supplementation in addition to a daily supplement can result in significant weight loss and reductions of "bad" cholesterol in just three weeks.

The researchers (Balliett *et al.* 2013) gave 49 adult men and women a three week diet containing mostly vegan meals. The meals totaled 1200-1400 calories for the women and 1600-1800 calories for the men.

The men and women were also given, once daily, nutritional supplements. The daily supplement contained a greenfood drink with alfalfa, wheatgrass and apple cider vinegar. In addition, the group was given a nutritional supplement with enzymes and vitamins.

During the second week, the adult subjects—with an average age of 31—were given a daily cleanse supplement. This supplement contained magnesium, chia, flaxseed, lemon, camu camu, cat's claw, bentonite clay, turmeric, pau d'arco, chanca piedra, stevia, zeolite clay, slippery elm, garlic, ginger, peppermint, aloe, citrus bioflavonoids, and fulvic acid. The cleanse supplement was given before every meal during the second week.

During the third week, the researchers gave the subjects supplements with probiotics and prebiotics instead of the cleanse supplement.

The average weight loss after 21 days was nearly nine pounds per person—equating to a 2-3% drop in weight per person.

And the average drop in total cholesterol was 30 mg/dL while the drop in low-density lipoprotein (LDL)—the "bad" cholesterol—was 21 mg/dL. Their average LDL levels prior to the three-week diet was 103 mg/dL, dropping to an average of 83 mg/dL, while total cholesterol went from an average of 185 mg/dL to 155 mg/dL. These are significant drops in both total and LDL cholesterol by any standard, let alone from only three weeks of a diet with natural supplements.

Triglycerides also decreased dramatically. Average triglyceride levels went from 93 mg/dL to 83 mg/dL during the three weeks.

In addition, testosterone levels among the women in the group went up significantly, from an average of 400 n/dL (nanograms per deciliter) to over 511 n/dL.

Average blood pressure went down as well. Average systolic blood pressure went from 116 to 112 mmHg during the three weeks, while diastolic pressure went from 76 to 71 mmHg.

In a large review of studies from the University of Naples (Esposito *et al.* 2011), researchers found that among the 19 studies that fit their quality standards, the Mediterranean diet resulted in significant weight loss, especially in studies lasting longer than six months.

Diabetes, Insulin Resistance and Alzheimer's

We discussed how type-2 diabetes and in particular, insulin resistance has been linked to the progression of Alzheimer's disease. The reality is, these conditions have been growing just as Alzheimer's disease has been growing. Let's take a closer look.

Research from Japan's Kyushu University Medical School (Ohara *et al.* 2011) found that dementia and Alzheimer's disease are associated with type 2 diabetes.

Researchers from the Graduate School of Medical Sciences' Environmental Medicine Department, followed 1,017 adults over the age of 60 years old for fifteen years. The elderly adults lived in an adult community and were dementia-free at the beginning of the study.

The adults were given oral glucose tolerance tests periodically. At the end of the fifteen years, those the adults whose glucose tolerance testing confirmed a diagnosis of diabetes by the end of the study were more than twice as likely to have Alzheimer's disease, and 74% increased incidence of vascular dementia.

Dementia and Alzheimer's disease risk also significantly increased among those whose two-hour post-load glucose levels were over the 7.8 mmol/Liter levels, and the highest risk was found among those with two-hour post-load glucose levels over 11 mmol/Liter.

The study was published in the medical journal *Neurology*, and has been coined the Hisayama Study.

The researchers concluded:

> *"Our findings suggest that diabetes is a significant risk factor for all-cause dementia, Alzheimer's disease, and probably vascular dementia."*

Diabetes rates around the world are at epidemic levels, according to Harvard researchers. Almost 350 million adults have diabetes worldwide, and over 25 million U.S. adults or 11% of U.S. adults have diabetes—most of which is type 2.

Are type-2 diabetes and insulin resistance really linked to our diets?

Researchers from Harvard (Pan *et al.* 2013) followed 26,357 men for 20 years, 48,709 women for 20 years and 74,077 women for 16 years, and compared their diets with incidence of type 2 diabetes.

In a pooled multivariate analysis, the researchers found that increasing red meat consumption for at least four years increased the risk of diabetes significantly during that period.

Their data found that an average increase in ½ serving of red meat per day resulted in a 48% increased incidence of type two diabetes.

This increase in meat consumption also resulted in weight gain risk by 30%.

Meanwhile reducing red meat consumption for a four year period resulted in a 14% lower risk of diabetes. The researchers concluded that:

> *"Increasing red meat consumption over time is associated with an elevated subsequent risk of T2DM, and the association is partly mediated by body weight. Our results add further evidence that limiting red meat consumption over time confers benefits for T2DM prevention."*

Researchers at the Harvard School of Public Health found in a huge study that eating red meat regularly increases the incidence of type 2 diabetes. Furthermore, they found that replacing red meat in the diet with non-meat proteins significantly lowers incidence of type 2 diabetes.

The research was led by An Pan, PhD and Frank Hu, PhD, a professor of nutrition and epidemiology at Harvard's School of Public Health.

The researchers followed 37,083 men for 20 years, 79,570 women for 28 years, and 87,504 women 14 years. In addition, they performed a meta-analysis review by combining their data with previous studies, to arrive at a massive total of 442,101 human subjects. Of this population, 28,228 developed type 2 diabetes during the period of study.

The study eliminated trends related to lifestyle and other dietary risk facts, as well as age and body mass index (BMI). In the final analysis, a average of 50 grams of processed meat per day increased diabetes incidence by 51%, while a 100 gram serving of unprocessed red meat per day increased diabetes incidence by 19%.

Dr. Hu explained the results in a press release by Harvard:

> *"Clearly, the results from this study have huge public health implications given the rising type 2 diabetes epidemic and increasing consumption of red meats worldwide. The good news is that such troubling risk factors can be offset by swapping red meat for a healthier protein."*

The Harvard press release also stated this was the largest study of its kind to link red meat with diabetes—confirming the findings of other smaller studies. The study was supported by the National Institutes of Health's National Institute of Diabetes and Digestive and Kidney Diseases, along with the National Heart, Lung, and Blood Institute.

The Harvard researchers suggested that processed red meats such as bacon, sausage, hot dogs, and deli meats, as well as unprocessed red meats should be "minimized" or "reduced." They recommended replacement with healthier protein sources.

Healthier proteins, according to the researchers, include nuts, grains, beans and low-fat dairy.

The study also found that even substituting one serving of grains per day instead of meat protein lowered diabetes incidence by 23%. Substituting one serving with nuts reduced incidence by 21%, and low-fat dairy resulted in a 17% reduction.

This study confirms another Harvard study done in 2010 (Micha *et al.*), which found that meat consumption increased the risk of diabetes along with coronary heart disease and strokes. This study analyzed 20 clinical studies that met their quality review, which included 1,218,380 total human subjects. Among other findings, they found that red meat increased incidence of coronary heart disease by 42%.

Dr. Pan stated in a follow-up interview:

> *"Our study clearly shows that eating both unprocessed and processed red meat—particularly processed—is associated with an increased risk of type 2 diabetes,"*

He also suggested that it was unfair to lump other healthier sources of protein together with the unhealthier red meats.

Other research has found that type 2 diabetes is associated with a lack of exercise, obesity and diet.

In one, researchers from Simmons College in Boston (Fung *et al.* 2004) followed 69,554 women between 38 and 63 yeas old for ten years. They found that for every single serving increase in red meat resulted in a 26% increased risk of diabetes. The risk increased to 38-43% for processed meats, 73% for bacon, and 49% for hot dogs.

In a study of 42,504 men by researchers from the Harvard School of Public Health (Van Dam *et al.* 2002), it was found that the frequent consumption of processed meat was associated with a 46% higher risk of type 2 diabetes.

Another study from Harvard (Schulze *et al.* 2003) that followed over 91,000 women between 26 and 46 years old found that eating processed meat for more than five times a week increased the risk of type 2 diabetes by 91%.

Dutch researchers van Woudenbergh *et al.* 2012) analyzed 4,366 participants who did not have diabetes initially. After more than 12 years, the researchers reviewed the diets and the incidence of diabetes among the study group.

The research determined that eating 50 grams more processed meat per day increased the incidence of type 2 diabetes by 87%. Eating 50 grams more meat in general increased the incidence of type 2 diabetes by 42%, and 18% after adjusting for BMI levels.

The researchers also looked into the connection between C-reactive protein levels and diabetes, since other research has recently linked meat consumption with increased levels of CRP. Higher CRP levels are associated with heart attacks and cardiovascular disease.

While the research confirmed the link between meat consumption and CRP, they found that increased CRP seems to be unrelated to diabetes when considering meat consumption. In other words, they are independent associations with meat consumption.

Other studies have linked type 2 diabetes with diet.

In a study from the Britain's University of Bristol (Andrews *et al.* 2011) studied 593 type 2 diabetes patients, and found that while the control group (no diet or exercise regimen) worsened over a six month period, those who underwent diet therapy had 28% increased glycemic control, and those who underwent diet and exercise therapy had 31% increased glycemic control after six months.

A study from Italy (Panunzio *et al.* 2011) shows that the Mediterranean diet significantly improves metabolism, glycemia, insulin levels, C-reactive protein levels and body mass index.

All of these factors present the issues related to metabolic syndrome. Metabolic syndrome is symptomized by cardiovascular disease, being overweight and a tendency for type 2 diabetes.

The study followed 80 volunteers who were between 51 and 59 years old. They were randomly split into two groups, and one group ate the Mediterranean diet and the other ate a Western diet. Before and after six months, the subjects underwent extensive testing.

After 25 weeks on the diet, the Mediterranean diet subjects had an average of 12.4% lower body mass index, 8.3% less weight, 9.2% lower fasting glycemia and 32% lower fasting insulin. The Med diet group also had 34% lower levels of C-reactive protein.

C-reactive protein is a marker for inflammation. High CRP levels indicate systemic inflammation, often accompanying the hardening of the arteries, also called atherosclerosis, coronary artery disease and a higher risk of heart disease and stroke in general—and Alzheimer's as we've discussed.

Lower fasting glycemia levels means lower levels of blood sugar, related to a lower risk of diabetes.

Lower fasting insulin levels are also a marker that is associated with a reduced risk of diabetes.

The diets of the Med diet group proved consistent with these in this study. The Med diet group showed 39% higher levels of fruit, 30% higher levels of vegetables, 18% higher cheese and 38% higher levels of fiber.

Diet and Attention Deficit

We discussed earlier that Alzheimer's disease has been linked to Attention Deficit and Hyperactivity Disorder (AD/HD) in adults. We also pointed out that the reason may be that Alzheimer's disease and AD/HD have mutual causes.

Diet may be at least one of the links that associate these two conditions.

For example, research from the University of Western Australia (Howard *et al.* 2011) found that AD/HD in children is linked to diet, and more specifically, to the Western diet.

The study reviewed the dietary patterns of 1,799 children. The children's diets were followed for fourteen years. The researchers divided the children into two basic groups based on their diet habits: A "Healthy" group and a "Western" group.

Of the 1,799 children, 115 were diagnosed with AD/HD.

Those children who ate a Western diet were more than twice as likely to have AD/HD—2.21 times more likely, to be exact.

Dr. Wendy Oddy, a professor at the University of Western Australia, was the lead author of the study. Dr. Oddy commented about the study for Perth's Telethon Institute for Child Health Research, which participated in the study:

"We found a diet high in the Western pattern of foods was associated with more than double the risk of having an AD/HD diagnosis compared with a diet low in the Western pattern, after adjusting for numerous other social and family influences."

In this study, the "Western pattern" was defined as the higher intake of red meats, fried foods, fast foods, sweets and processed foods. The "Healthy pattern" diet pattern was defined as a diet high in whole grains, fresh fruit, vegetables and fish.

The AD/HD group also were more likely to eat certain foods.

"When we looked at specific foods, having an AD/HD diagnosis was associated with a diet high in takeaway foods, processed meats, red meat, high fat dairy products and confectionary," Dr Oddy said.

For those who doubt the connection between diet and AD/HD, there are other studies to consider.

For example, the AD/HD Research Center in Enhoven, Netherlands (Pelsser *et al.* 2011) studied 100 children aged 4-8, who were randomly assigned to either a control group or an elimination diet group. The control group was instructed to eat a healthy diet, while the elimination group eliminated particular foods according to food challenge tests. This study found that many children's AD/HD was indeed induced by certain foods.

While the above studies have focused upon children with AD/HD, many children with AD/HD become adults with AD/HD—which has been linked with Alzheimer's disease as discussed.

The Anti-arachidonic Acid Diet

Alzheimer's disease is an inflammatory disease. And numerous studies have connected inflammatory diseases to the conversion processes of arachidonic acid—a fatty acid.

The critical enzymes used for this conversion to prostaglandins, thromboxanes, and leukotrienes are cyclooxygenase (COX) and lipoxygenase (LOX). A significant amount of research over the past decade has confirmed that a disproportionate amount of arachidonic acid in the diet will produce increased levels of inflammation (Calder 2008 and many others) due to an oversupply of these messengers.

In fact, research headed up by Dr. Darshan Kelley from the Western Human Research Center in California illustrated that diets high in arachidonic acid stimulated four times more inflammatory cells than diets low in arachidonic acid content. And this problem actually increases with age. In other words, the same amount of arachidonic acid-forming foods will cause higher levels of arachidonic acid the older we get (Chilton 2006).

This also relates to many other health-related problems as people age. For example, higher arachidonic acid levels in the bloodstream correlate with greater platelet aggregation. This creates a higher risk of blood clots. Higher levels of arachidonic acid can also cause difficulties with glucose utilization, lung efficiency, intestinal health and so many other disorders related to inflammation.

According to the USDA's Standard 13 and 16 databases, animal meats and fish produce the highest amounts of arachidonic acid in the body. Diary, fruits and vegetables produce little or no arachidonic acid. Grains, beans and nuts produce none or very small amounts. Processed bakery goods produce a moderate amount of arachidonic acid.

Hundreds of studies have now confirmed that an increase in long-chain fatty acids such as DHA, EPA, ALA and GLA in the diet slows down inflammation in the body. How do they do that? Because these fats convert to other compounds—such as phospholipids used for cell membranes—leaving less fat available to convert to prostaglandins, leukotrienes and thromboxanes.

Plant-based antioxidants have been shown to significantly reduce the severity of a number of disorders, including dementia, arthritis, atherosclerosis, heart disease, liver disease, diabetes and others. This is because they support the immune system's process of removing toxins before they do any further damage. This was illustrated in a study (McAlindon *et al.* 1996) at the Boston University School of Medicine.

The study revealed that people consuming more than 200 milligrams a day of vitamin C were one-third less likely to experience a worsening of their osteoarthritis. Dr. Timothy McAlidon, a professor at the University suggested that the reduction in free radicals by the antioxidant vitamin C was the likely mechanism.

Alzheimer's and Gut Bacteria

In 2013, a team of leading medical researchers (Scher *et al.*) found that inflammatory conditions also tend to follow intestinal dysbiosis and the overgrowth of pathogenic gut microbes.

The researchers—from the New York University School of Medicine, Cornell Medical College, Italy's University of Trento, Harvard School of Public Health, Spain's University of Valencia, Oxford and the Howard

Hughes Medical Institute—found that the overgrowth of a bacteria called *Prevotella copri* within the gut was linked with inflammatory conditions such as rheumatoid arthritis.

The researchers used DNA analysis of the microbiome (the gut's total bacteria load) together with specific analyses to relate the overgrowth of this particular bacteria.

But the growth of the bacteria didn't happen in isolation. In a predominance of the cases, the bacteria overgrowth was related to the loss of colonies of healthy probiotic colonies—an event called dysbiosis.

The researchers based their findings upon DNA sequencing of 114 stool samples from patients with rheumatoid arthritis and healthy control subjects. This indicated the total DNA of the gut's microbiome: The general species make up of intestinal bacteria. The researchers then took 44 of the samples and analyzed them with more detail to isolate the particular species of bacteria at the root of the dysbiosis.

Using further analysis of the genetic composition of the patients' microbiome together with the patients' own DNA, it was established that rheumatoid arthritis is linked with the overgrowth of this *Prevotella copri* bacteria combined with dysbiosis.

While the Prevotella enterotype is related to plant-based diets, the condition of dysbiosis is related to the Western diet. This is because the Western diet has a reduced compatibility with healthy probiotic bacteria within the gut.

A healthy microbiota consists of a balance of many organisms. An overgrowth of any of these species leads to dysbiosis and the risk of inflammation.

This pro-inflammatory condition relates to several variables, as we'll discuss further. With regard to intestinal bacteria, the Western diet maintains a lack of prebiotic conditions. That is, a lack of complex prebiotics as we will describe in detail. Plant-based prebiotics feed our healthier species of intestinal bacteria.

Meanwhile, the Western diet promotes the growth of pathogenic organisms. As these pathogenic organisms gain in colony strength and territory, they begin to push aside the probiotic organisms that support intestinal health.

Healthy probiotic organisms also support the immune system and thus are anti-inflammatory in nature.

Contrasting this, pathogenic organisms facilitated by the Western diet produce an array of waste products, which can find access to the blood stream, where they can promote inflammatory responses.

These waste materials from pathogenic organisms are typically called endotoxins. Why? Because as they find their way into the bloodstream, they become toxins within the body—which is why they are described with the word *"endo."*

Once in the bloodstream, these endotoxins produce inflammation as the immune system works to remove them. These endotoxins and their metabolites can affect our brain cells because they damage cell membranes.

Recently, significant research has established a link between gut bacteria and Alzheimer's disease. Not only Alzheimer's, but other cognitive disorders. Is this true?

Researchers from Louisiana State University (Bhattacharjee and Lukiw 2013) reviewed the data and found a number of relationships. Most notably, the production of particular types of microbiome-derived RNA, including small non-coding RNA (sncRNA) and micro RNA (miRNA) has been discovered at heightened levels among Alzheimer's patients. These miRNA appear to evolve from pathogenic bacteria in the gut have been linked with Alzheimer's inflammatory factors.

For example, research from the Russian Academy of Medical Sciences (Alexandrov *et al.* 2012) also found this link. The researchers tested human cerebrospinal fluid from Alzheimer's patients and healthy people post-mortem. They found that Alzheimer's patients had increased levels of pro-inflammatory miRNA-9, miRNA-125b, miRNA-146a and miRNA-155 in their brain tissues and fluids. These miRNA were associated with higher levels of beta-amyloid-40 proteins—which are associated with Alzheimer's.

A number of other studies (Meyer *et al.* 2007 and others) have found that eating yogurt reduces levels of pro-inflammatory cytokines within the bloodstream.

To these points we can add that at least three animal studies have shown that a particular probiotic can reduce memory issues and cognitive impairment. The studies (Yoo *et al.* 2015; Jeong *et al.* 2015; Woo *et al.* 2014; Jung *et al.* 2012) utilized Lactobacillus plantarum—or more specifically, Lactobacillus pentosus var. plantarum. All three studies showed the mice and rats' memory impairment was halted by the probiotic supplementation program. While these are animals, not people, the studies may provide at least an indication that probiotic supplementation may be useful as an anti-Alzheimer's strategy.

What this all means is that having a healty microbiome can help prevent the pro-inflammatory miRNAs. This means eating a variety of cultured and fermented foods, such as yogurt, kefir, sauerkraut and others. Supplementing with probiotics can also be a helpful strategy.

Learn more in my book, *"Probiotics—Protection Against Infection."*

The Nutty Diet

New research is matching diet with cognition. Two Harvard University studies have now concluded that a Mediterranean Diet and a diet high in nuts will decrease cognitive decline among elderly persons.

In the first, Harvard University researchers (Samieri *et al.* 2013) followed 16,058 women over the age of 70 years old for six years. Their diets were followed for more than 13 years, as part of the Nurses' Health Study.

For six of those years, the researchers conducted phone interviews with each four times a year. These tested their cognitive status using the Telephone Interview for Cognitive Status (TICS) test. This tests cognition skills using memory recall, fluency and attention span tests.

The researchers found that those women who ate closest to a Mediterranean diet had significantly better cognitive scores as the women grew older. The differences in their cognitive scores calculated to about one to 1.5 years of aging—meaning the Med diet slowed their aging decline in cognition.

Another study by different researchers from Harvard University and Brigham and Women's Hospital (O'Brien *et al.* 2013) confirmed that eating more nuts every day will increase cognitive skills among women.

Using the same Nurses study as a foundation, the researchers followed 16,010 women 70 years old or older. In this study, 15,467 completed the final cognitive interview. And the TICS cognitive skills testing was utilized.

The researchers found those women who consumed at least five servings of nuts per week had higher cognitive scores compared to those who did not consume nuts. (Most nut serving sizes are about one ounce— about a small handful). The average difference in scores was 0.08 units, which is equivalent to two years of cognition decline during the aging process.

They could not correlate cognitive decline with long-term nut consumption, but the association was clear, as concluded by the researchers:

> *"Higher nut intake may be related to better overall cognition at older ages, and could be an easily-modifiable public health intervention."*

The Problems with Processed Foods

Let's now connect how processed foods contribute to Alzheimer's disease. Food processing consists of one or a combination of the following actions on food:

- chopping or pulverizing
- heating to high temperatures

- distilling or extracting its constituents
- otherwise isolating some parts by straining off or filtering
- clarifying or otherwise refining

Most consider food processing a good thing, because we humans like to focus on one or two characteristics or nutrients within a food. The idea is that we want the essence of the food, and don't want to fool around with the rest. In most cases—in terms of commercial food—it is a value proposition, because all the energy and work required to produce the final food product must equal or be greater than the increase in the processed food's financial value. Therefore, the more concentrated or isolated the attractive portion is, the more financial value is added.

Typically, this increase in financial value is due to the food being sweeter, smoother or simply easier to eat or mix with other foods. In the case of oils or flours, the food extract is used for baking purposes, for example. In the case of sugar—which is extracted and isolated from cane and beets—it is added to nearly every processed food recipe.

Ironically, what is left behind in this extraction is the food's real value. The healthy fiber and nutrients are stripped away in most cases. Plant fiber is a necessary element of our diet, because it renders sterols that aid digestion and reduce LDL cholesterol. Many nutrients are also attached to and protected by the plant's fibers. Once the fiber is stripped away, the remaining nutrients are easily damaged by sunlight, air, and the heat of processing.

What is being missed in the value proposition of food processing is that nature's whole foods have their greatest value—nutritionally—prior to processing. When a food is broken down, the molecular bonds that attach nutrients to the food's fibers and complex polysaccharides are lost. As these bonds are lost, the remaining components can become unstable in the body. When these components—such as refined sugar and simple polysaccharides (starches)—become unstable, they can form free radicals in the body. They thus add to our body's toxic burden because they can damage our cells.

In other words, whole foods provide the nutrients our bodies need in the combinations our bodies recognize. Nutrients are bonded within a matrix of structure and fiber, rendering their benefits as our bodies require them.

In some cases, we might need to physically peel a food to get to the edible part. In other cases, such as in the case of beans and grains, we may need to heat or cook them to soften the fibers to enable chewing and digestion. In the case of wheats, we can mill the whole grain (including the bran) to deliver the spectrum of fibrous nutrients. In other words, the closer we match the way our ancestors ate foods, the more our bodies will recognize them, and the better our bodies will utilize them.

Because many of our processed foods have been in our diet for many decades, it is difficult to prove that our modern diet of overly-processed foods produces greater levels of systemic inflammation. This doesn't mean that it is impossible, however.

To test this hypothesis, French researchers (Fremont *et al.* 2010) studied the effects of processed flax. Foods containing processed flax are a new addition to our diet—although our ancestors certainly ate raw or cooked whole flax. So they studied the introduction of modern processed flax into the French diet. In a study of 1,317 patients with allergies, they found that those who were allergic to flax could be identified by their sensitivity to extruded, heated flax, rather than raw flax seed. This of course indicates that the increase in flax allergies among the French is due to the increase in *processed flax* rather than the increased availability of flax.

Certainly, over time, as flax allergies proceed, there will be more crossover allergies to raw flax. But now, while flax exposure is fairly recent, allergies to processed flax but not raw flax indicate that it is the extrusion processing that causes the identification of flax protein as an allergen.

What does processing do to create more inflammatory sensitivity? Our digestive enzymes and probiotics have evolved to break down (or not) certain types of molecules. Imbalanced or denatured molecules can be considered foreign.

We can also see how processing increases diseases when we compare the disease statistics of developing countries with those of developed countries.

For example, like many developing countries, India has more heart disease in recent decades because of increased consumption of processed and fried foods. In the same way, the Chinese thrived for thousands of years on a rice-based diet. But when modern processing machines introduced degermed white rice, malnutrition diseases began to occur. This is because the degerming and bleaching process results in the loss of important lignans, B vitamins, E vitamins and others.

Processed and refined foods damage intestinal health and promote free radicals. They are nutrient-poor. They burden and starve our probiotics. Frying foods also produces a carcinogen called acrylamide (Ehling *et al.* 2005).

Glycation and AD

In general, food manufacturing glycation is produced when sugars and protein-rich foods are combined and heated to extremely high temperatures. This is a typical process used for the manufacture of many commercial packaged foods on the grocery shelves today. During the process, sugars bind to protein molecules. This produces a glycated protein-sugar complex and glycation end products, both of which have been implicated in cardiovascular disease, diabetes, some cancers, peripheral neuropathy and Alzheimer's disease (Miranda and Outeiro 2010).

With regard to Alzheimer's disease, one of the end products of the glycation reaction is deranged amyloid protein. Deranged amyloid proteins have been found among the brain tissues and cerebrospinal fluids of Alzheimer's patients as we have discussed. Glycation is implicated in the deranged amyloid plaque buildup found in Alzheimer's.

Glycation also takes place within the body. This occurs especially with diets with greater consumption of refined sugars and cooked or caramelized high-protein foods.

Refined Sugar

The Western diet is also laden with refined sugars. Today, nearly every pre-cooked recipe found in mass market grocery stores contains refined sugar. Many brands now try to white-wash the massive sugar content of their products by calling their sugar content "all natural." This is a deception, because nature in the form of fiber has been unnaturally stripped away from their refined sugars. This is hardly a "natural" proposition.

Research has linked refined sugars to dementia, diabetes, obesity, kidney diseases, Candida and many other conditions. This is hardly news to those who have investigated natural health literature.

Nature attaches sugars to complex fibers, polysaccharides and nutrients in such a way that prevents them from easily attaching to proteins. Sugars that are cooked and stripped of these complexes are assimilated too quickly, and drive the pancreas to produce and even overproduce insulin. This has the effect of stressing the pancreas and producing insulin resistance.

Remember that insulin resistance has been linked directly to Alzheimer's.

Refined sugars also stress the liver that feeds the pancreas, and stresses the detoxification processes that must metabolize the insulin, glucose and glycogen byproducts. All of this slows down the body's immunity and detoxification processes.

Refined sugars also feed pathogenic microorganisms. While our probiotics feed on oligosaccharides such as FOS, GOS and others, pathogenic microorganisms tend to feed on refined sugars. This is the case for *Candida albicans,* a virtual sugar fiend.

Refined sugars also become immediate unnatural glycation candidates within the body.

As our digestive system combines refined sugars with proteins, many of the glycated proteins are identified as foreign by IgA or IgE antibodies in immune-burdened physiologies. Why are they considered foreign? Because glycated proteins and their AGE end products damage blood vessels, tissues and brain cells. In this case, the immune system is launching an inflammatory attack in an effort to protect us from our own diet!

There is no surprise that glycation among foods and in the body is connected with systemic inflammation. It is also no accident that the increased consumption of overly-processed foods and manufacturing processes that pulverize and strip foods of their fiber; and blend denatured proteins and sugars using high-heat processes has increased as our rates of inflammatory diseases have increased over the past century.

In fact, this connection between inflammatory diseases and processed foods has been observed clinically by natural physicians over the years. They may not have understood the precise mechanics, however. Many of these reputable health experts have categorized the effect of processed foods as one of acidifying the bloodstream. The concept was that denatured and over-processed foods produced more acids in the body.

This thesis did not go over too well among scientific circles, because the acidification mechanism was not scientifically confirmed, and there was no concrete mechanism.

Well this can now change, as we are providing the science showing both the mechanism and the evidence that glycation end products do produce acidification in terms of peroxidation radicals that damage cells and tissues.

We should note that a healthy form of natural glycation also takes place in the body to produce certain nutrient combinations. Unlike the radical-forming glycation formed by food manufacturing and refined sugar intake, this type of glycation is driven by the body's natural enzyme processes, resulting in molecules and end products the body uses and recognizes. When glycation is driven by the body's own enzyme processes, it is termed *glycosylation,* however.

Alkaline Nutrition

This discussion of diet should also include the reflective effects of the proper acid-alkaline balance among the blood, urine and intercellular tissue regions. The reference to acidic or alkaline body fluids and tissues has been made by numerous natural health experts over the years. Is there any scientific validity to this?

Many nutritionists condemn an acidic metabolism and loosely call appropriate metabolism as a *state of alkalinity*. Strictly speaking, however, an alkaline environment is not healthy. The blood, interstitial fluids, lymph and urine should be *slightly acidic* to maintain the appropriate mineral ion balance. Let's dig into the science.

Acidity or alkalinity is measured using a logarithmic scale called pH. The term pH is derived from the French word *pouvoir hydrogene*, which means 'hydrogen power' or 'hydrogen potential.' pH is quantified by an inverse log base-10 scale. It measures the proton-donor level of a solution by comparing it to a theoretical quantity of hydrogen ions (H+) or H_3O+.

The scale is pH 1 to pH 14, which converts to a range of 10^{-1} (1) to 10^{-14} (.00000000000001) moles of hydrogen ions. This means that a pH of 14 maintains fewer hydrogen ions. It is thus *less acidic* and *more alkaline* (or basic).

The pH scale has been set up around the fact that water's pH is log-7 or simply pH 7—due to water's natural mineral content. Because pure water forms the basis for so many of life's activities, and because water neutralizes and dilutes so many reactions, water was established as the standard reference point or neutral point between what is considered an acid or a base solution. In other words, a substance having greater hydrogen ion potential (but lower pH) than water will be considered acidic, while a substance with less H+ potential (higher pH) than water is considered a base (alkaline).

Now the solution with a certain pH may not specifically maintain that many hydrogen ions. But it has the same *potential* as if it contained those hydrogen ions. That is why pH is hydrogen power or hydrogen potential.

In human blood, a pH level in the range of about 6.4 is considered healthy because this state is slightly more acidic than water, enabling the bodily fluids to maintain and transport minerals. It enables the *potential* for minerals to be carried by the blood, in other words. Minerals are critical to every cell, every organ, every tissue and every enzyme process occurring within the body. Better put, a 6.4 pH offers the appropriate *currency* of the body's fluids: This discourages acidosis and toxemia, maintaining a slight mineralized status.

Acidosis is produced with greater levels of carbonic acids, lactic acids, and/or uric acids among the joints and tissues. These acids are readily oxidizing, which produces free radicals. However, an overly alkaline state can precipitate waste products from cells, which also floods the system with radicals. For this reason, *toxemia* results from either an overly acidic blood-tissue content or an overly alkaline blood-tissue content. In other words, pH *balance* is the key.

Ions from minerals like potassium, calcium, magnesium and others are usually positively oriented—with alkaline potential. But to be carried through a solution, the solution must have the pH potential to carry them.

Besides being critical to enzymatic reactions, these minerals bond with lipids and proteins to form the structures of our cells, organs and tissues—including our airways, nerves and mucosal membranes.

Natural health experts over the past century have observed among their patients and in clinical research that an overly acidic environment within the body is created by a diet abundant in refined sugars, processed foods, chemical toxins and amino acid-heavy animal foods. More recently, research has connected this acidic state to toxemia. The toxemia state is a state of free radical proliferation, which damages cells and tissues. It is also a state that produces systemic inflammation, because the immune system is over-worked as it tries to remove the cell and tissue damage.

As mentioned earlier, animals accumulate toxins within their fat tissues. They are bioaccumulators. Thus, animals exposed to the typical environmental toxins of smog and chemical pollutants in their waters and air—along with pesticides and herbicides from their foods—will accumulate those toxins within their fat cells and livers. And those who eat those animals will inherit (and further accumulate) these accumulated toxins. In addition, animals secrete significant waste matter as they are being slaughtered.

Plants are not bioaccumulators. While they can accumulate some pesticides and herbicide chemicals within their leaves and roots, they do not readily absorb or hold these for long periods within their cells. This is because many environmental toxins are, as mentioned, fat soluble. Because plants have little or no fat, they can more easily systemically rid their tissues of many of these toxins over time.

Further, as the research has shown, a diet heavy in complex proteins—which contain far more amino acids than our bodies require—increases the risk and severity of inflammation. Amino acids are the building blocks of protein. A complex protein can have tens of thousands of amino acids. While proteins and aminos are healthy, a diet too rich in them will produce deposits in our joints and tissues, burdening our immune system.

As we discussed in the last chapter, research also reveals that diets rich in red meats discourage the colonization of our probiotics, and encourage the growth of pathogenic microorganisms that release endotoxins that clog our metabolism and overload our immune system. Diets rich in red meats also produce byproducts such as phytanic acid and beta-glucuronidase that can damage our intestinal cells and mucosal membranes within the intestines. Greater levels of cooked saturated fats also raise cholesterol levels, especially lipid peroxidation-prone low-density lipoproteins (LDL).

The complexities of digesting complex proteins produce increased levels of beta-glucuronidase, nitroreductase, azoreductase, steroid 7-alpha-dehydroxylase, ammonia, urease, cholylglycine hydrolase, phytanic acid and others. These toxic enzymes deter our probiotics and produce systemic inflammation. Not surprisingly, they've been linked to colon cancer.

By contrast, plant-based foods contain many antioxidants, anti-carcinogens and other nutrients that strengthen the immune system and balance the body's pH. Plant-based foods also discourage inflammatory responses. Plant-based foods feed our probiotics with complex polysaccharides called prebiotics. They are also a source of fiber (there is little fiber in red meat)—critical for intestinal health.

The Mediterranean diet does not completely eliminate meat, but it is focused on more plant-based foods, healthier oils and less red meat. However we configure our diet, there are choices we can make at every meal. The research shows that the greater our diet trends toward the Mediterranean diet, the lower our toxic load will be and the stronger our immunity will be. This will allow us to better combat and eventually lower systemic inflammation.

This also not a condemnation of dairy. Milk is a great food, assuming it contains what nature intended: probiotics. Real milk is inseparable from probiotics, and when probiotics are killed off by pasteurization, milk becomes a dubious food.

Nature's food packages as delivered by living organisms are better than the stripped down, refined and purified versions we produce. This seems just too complicated for us. We cannot seem to understand this. Why cannot we just isolate those constituents contained in the healthy food versions and just add them into our unhealthy foods and make them healthy? Perhaps it might help to consider that scientists have found more than 400 medicinal compounds in ginger and more than 27 medicinal constituents in garlic along with hundreds of other phytochemicals.

In addition, research has established that a tomato can contain up to 10,000 phytocompounds.

When these and other raw foods are over-processed, the medicinal elements of the foods become lost due to overheating, glycation and other chemical processes that result from the application of mechanical processes to whole foods.

In some cases, it is best to heat or process certain foods. This is the case for many grains, where the husk or shaff needs to be separated from the seed. Then the cooking of grains, as well as beans, is a good idea in order to soften up the fibers so they can be more readily digested. Cooking is also a good idea for foods in the nightshade family—of which tomatoes are included. Tomatoes are good fresh or cooked, however.

The bottom line in these types of processing is they should be done minimally. Minimal processing means to apply heat or other separation in a judicious manner—without destroying the food's nutrients or separating the fibers from the food.

Chapter Six

Superfood Strategies for AD

We've laid out the evidence showing that antioxidant-rich diets significantly reduce our risk of developing Alzheimer's disease. Such diets may also actually prevent Alzheimer's disease from developing. This is because antioxidants neutralize oxidative radicals and allow our body to minimize brain cell damage.

As we've discussed, oxidative radicals particularly damaging to brain cells—and involved in the production of beta-amyloid oligomers—are the lipid peroxidation radicals. These can harm cell membranes and effectively disrupt the production of enzymes. When brain cell DNA is damaged, it produces enzymes that cannot properly break down beta-amyloid proteins. The incorrectly-broken down beta-amyloid proteins become oligomers that in turn ruin brain cells.

In this section, we will introduce some very special types of antioxidants. These are superfoods, which are rich in phenols—or phenolic acids—along with other compounds. Phenols and similar antioxidant compounds in these superfoods exert a significantly stronger protective effect upon the body by preventing or reducing outbreaks of lipid radicals.

Superfood Antioxidants

As we've discussed, a plethora of research has confirmed that damage from free radicals is implicated in Alzheimer's disease. Free radicals from toxins damage cells, cell membranes, organs, blood vessel walls and airways—producing systemic inflammation—as the immune system responds to an overload of tissue damage.

Free radicals are produced by synthetic chemicals, pathogens, trans fats, fried foods, red meats, radiation, pollution and various intruders that destabilize within the body. Free radicals are molecules or ions that require stabilization. They reach stabilization by 'stealing' atoms from the cells or tissues of our body. This in turn destabilizes those cells and tissues—producing damage.

Antioxidants serve to stabilize free radicals before our cells and tissues are robbed—by donating their own atoms. A diet with plenty of fruits and vegetables supplies numerous antioxidants. Although antioxidants cannot be considered treatments for any disease, many studies have proved that increased antioxidant intake supports immune function and detoxification. These effects allow the immune system to respond with greater tolerance.

Antioxidant constituents in plant-based foods are known to significantly repeal free radicals, strengthen the immune system and help detoxify the system. These include *lecithin* and *octacosanol* from whole grains; *polyphenols* and *sterols* from vegetables; *lycopene* from tomatoes and watermelons; *quercetin* and *sulfur/allicin* from garlic, onions and peppers; *pectin* and *rutin* from apples and other fruits; *phytocyanidin flavonoids* such as *apigenin* and *luteolin* from various greenfoods; and *anthocyanins* from various fruits and oats.

Some sea-based botanicals like kelp also contain antioxidants as well. Consider a special polysaccharide compound from kelp called *fucoidan*. Fucoidan has been shown in animal studies to significantly reduce inflammation (Cardoso *et al.* 2009; Kuznetsova *et al.* 2004).

Procyanidins are found in apples, currants, cinnamon, bilberry and many other foods. The extract of *Vitis vinifera* seed (grapeseed) is one of the highest sources of bound antioxidant *proanthocyanidins* and *leucocyanidines* called *procyanidolic oligomers* or PCOs. Pycnogenol® also contains significant levels of these PCOs. Blueberries, parsley, green tea, black currant, some legumes and onions also contain PCOs and similar proanthocyanidins.

Research has demonstrated that PCOs have protective and strengthening effects on tissues by increasing enzyme conjugation (Seo *et al.* 2001). PCOs have also been shown to increase vascular wall strength (Robert *et al.* 2000).

Oxygenated carotenoids such as *lutein* and *astaxanthin* also have been shown to exhibit strong antioxidant activity. Astaxanthin is derived from the microalgae *Haematococcus pluvialis*, and lutein is available from a number of foods, including spirulina.

Most of these phytonutrients specifically modulate the immune system. For example, the flavonoids *kaempferol* and *flavone* have been shown to block mast cell proliferation by over 80% (Alexandrakis *et al.* 2003). Sources of kaempferol include Brussels sprouts, broccoli, grapefruit and apples.

Furthermore, *resveratrol* from grapes and berries modulate nuclear factor-kappaB and transcription/Janus kinase pathways—which strengthens immunity. Good sources of resveratrol include peanuts, red grapes, cranberries and cocoa (wine is not advisable for cleansing as we'll discuss later).

Nearly every plant-food has some measure of phytonutrients discussed above and more. These phytonutrients alkalize the blood and increase the detoxification capabilities of the liver. They help clear the blood of toxins.

Foods that are particularly detoxifying and immunity-building include fresh pineapples, beets, cucumbers, apricots, apples, almonds, zucchini, artichokes, avocados, bananas, beans, collard greens, berries, casaba, celery, coconuts, cranberries, watercress, dandelion greens, grapes, raw honey, corn, kale, citrus fruits, watermelon, lettuce, mangos, mushrooms, oats, broccoli, okra, onions, papayas, parsley, peas, whole grains, radishes, raisins, spinach, tomatoes, walnuts, and many others.

These plant-based foods are also our primary source of soluble and insoluble fiber. Diets with significant fiber help clear the blood and tissues of toxins, and lipid peroxidation-friendly LDL cholesterol. Fiber is also critical to a healthy digestive tract and intestinal barrier. Fiber in the diet should range from about 35 to 45 grams per day according to the recommendations of many diet experts. Six to ten servings of raw fruits and vegetables per day should accomplish this—which is even part of the USDA's recommendations. This means raw, fibrous foods should be present at every meal.

Good fibrous plant sources also contain healthy *lignans* and *phytoestrogens* that help balance hormone levels, and help the body make its own natural corticoids. Foods that contain these include peas, garbanzo beans, soybeans, kidney beans and lentils.

Plant-based foods provide these immune-stimulating factors because these vary same factors make up the plants' own immune systems. For example, the red, blue and green flavonoid pigments in plants and fruits help protect the plant from oxidative damage from radiation. The proanthocyanidins in grains like oats, for example, help protect the oat plant from crown rust caused by the *Puccinia coronata* fungus. So the same biochemicals that stimulate immunity in humans are part of plants' immune systems.

These same whole food phytonutrients also neutralize oxidative radicals in our bodies—the reason they are called antioxidants. How do we know this? Scientists can measure the ability of a particular food to neutralize free radicals with specific laboratory testing. One such test is called the *Oxygen Radical Absorbance Capacity Test* (ORAC). This technical laboratory study is performed by a number of scientific organizations that include the USDA, as well as specialized labs such as Brunswick Laboratories in Massachusetts.

Research from the USDA's Jean Mayer Human Nutrition Research Center on Aging at Tufts University has suggested that a diet high in ORAC value may protect blood vessels and tissues from free radical damage that can result in inflammation (Sofic *et al.* 2001; Cao *et al.* 1998). These tissues, of course, include the airways. Research has confirmed that consuming 3,000 to 5,000 ORAC units per day can have protective benefits.

ORAC Values (100 grams) of Selected (raw) Fruits (USDA, 2007-2008)

Cranberry	9,382		Pomegranate	2,860
Plum	7,581		Orange	1,819
Blueberry	6,552		Tangerine	1,620
Blackberry	5,347		Grape (red)	1,260
Raspberry	4,882		Mango	1,002
Apple (Granny)	3,898		Kiwi	882
Strawberry	3,577		Banana	879
Cherry (sweet)	3,365		Tomato (plum)	389
Gooseberry	3,277		Pineapple	385
Pear	2,941		Watermelon	142

There is tremendous attention these days on two unique fruits from the Amazon rain forest and China called *açaí* and *goji berry* (or wolfberry) respectively. A recent ORAC test documented by Schauss *et al.* (2006) gives açaí a score of 102,700 and tests documented by Dr. Paul Gross gives goji berries a total ORAC of 30,300. However, subsequent tests done by Brunswick Laboratories, Inc. gave these two berries 53,600 (açaí) and 22,000 (goji) total-ORAC values.

In addition, we must remember that these are the dried berries being tested in the latter case, and a concentrate of açaí being tested in the former case. The numbers in the chart above are for fresh fruits. Dried fruits will naturally have higher ORAC values, because the water is evaporated—giving more density and more antioxidants per 100 grams.

For example, in the USDA database, dried apples have a 6,681 total-ORAC value, while fresh apples range from 2,210 to 3,898 in total-ORAC value. This equates to a two-to-three times increase from fresh to dried. In another example, fresh red grapes have a 1,260 total-ORAC value, while raisins have a 3,037 total-ORAC value. This comes close to an increase of three times the ORAC value following dehydration.

Part of the equation, naturally, is cost. Dried fruit and concentrates are often more expensive than fresh fruit. High-ORAC dried fruits or concentrates from açaí or goji will also be substantially more expensive than most fruits grown domestically (especially for Americans and Europeans). Our conclusion is that local or in-country grown fresh fruits with high total-ORAC values produce the best value. Local fresh fruit offers great free radical scavenging ability, support for local farmers, and pollen proteins we are most likely more tolerant to.

By comparison, spinach—an incredibly wholesome vegetable with a tremendous amount of nutrition—has a fraction of the ORAC content of some of these fruits, at 1,515 total ORAC. Spinach, of course, contains many other nutrients, including proteins lacking in many high-ORAC fruits.

Dehydrated spices can have incredibly high ORAC values. For example, USDA's database lists ground Turmeric's total ORAC value at 159,277 and oregano's at 200,129. However, while we might only consume a few hundred milligrams of a spice per day, we can eat many grams—if not pounds—of sweet colorful fruit every day.

Red tart cherries have even higher levels of ORAC than most other cherries. That's not all. Montmorency (red tart) cherries also have a number of other powerful phyto-nutrients, including melatonin, anthocyanins 1, 2 and 3, perillyl alcohol, quercetin, SOD (super oxide dismutase) and many others.

Melatonin has been connected to relaxation, sleep and healthy circadian rhythms. Anthocyanins have been linked to helping protect arteries from plaque build-up and other tissues from oxidative damage. Perillyl alcohol and ellagic acid have been studied for their cancer-protective qualities, while quercetin and SOD have been shown to support detoxification and healthy immune function.

Blueberries

Blueberries have a great reputation for being potent antioxidants and for improving metabolic syndrome, but their real benefit, according to new research, is protecting against DNA damage—which translates to damage to brain cells. The best part: Effects can be seen even after eating one two-cup portion.

Researchers from the University of Milano (Del Bo *et al.* 2013) gave 300 grams of ground blueberries to ten adult volunteers (human) or a control jelly in a crossover study design.

The researchers drew blood from the subjects before and after (one and two hours after and 24 hours after) their ingestion of the blueberries. They also conducted the same protocol using the control jam and compared the results.

The researchers found that in just one hour after consuming the ground blueberries, their cellular DNA damage—related to hydrogen peroxide—was reduced by 18% when compared to the control jelly.

The data—confirming other studies—showed that the protection to the cells were related to their antioxidant potential. The researchers stated in their conclusion that, "one portion of blueberries seems sufficient to improve cell antioxidant defense against DNA damage."

This ability of blueberries to protect cells from damage from free radicals has been seen in other studies, including those showing blueberries benefit memory and may help stave off Alzheimer's disease.

Other research has determined that blueberries can improve insulin resistance—linked closely to Alzheimer's disease as we've discussed.

A study from Louisiana State University (Stull *et al.* 2010) gave blueberry extract or a placebo twice daily to 32 obese patients with insulin resistance. After six weeks the researchers found that the blueberry group had significantly less insulin resistance.

In another study, from Appalachian State University (McAnulty *et al.* 2011) 12 human subjects were given 250 grams of blueberries a day while 13 others acted as controls. After six weeks the researchers found that the blueberry group had significantly higher natural killer cell counts—a sign of increased immunity.

In a study from Oklahoma State University (Basu *et al.* 2010) of 48 people with metabolic syndrome were given either 400 grams of blueberries a day or not. The blueberry group had significantly lower LDL-cholesterol levels and reduced symptoms of metabolic disease otherwise.

Blueberries contain judicious quantities of a special category of phytonutrients called anthocyanins. These include cyanidins, delphinidins, malvidins, pelargonidins and peonidins. Anthocyanins are significantly antioxidant and they help protect the cells from the damaging effects of free radicals.

Blueberries also contain other phytonutrients such as gallic acid, procathuic acid, caffeic acids, ferulic acids, kaempferol, quercetin, resveratrol, pterostilbene, myricetin and gallic acid. These phytonutrients provide a host of health effects, including anti-inflammatory and antioxidant effects as mentioned.

From a nutrient standpoint, blueberries also contain significant quantities of vitamin K (1 cup = 28 micrograms), manganese (1 cup = 500 micrograms), choline (1 cup—9 mg)and vitamin C (1 cup = 14 mg). They also contain a healthy amount of fiber (1 cup = 3.6 grams).

Açaí

The purple berries of the açaí (*Euterpe oleracea*) palm tree have received much acclaim over the recent years, specifically for their high antioxidant values. The ORAC (oxygen radical absorbance capacity) value of açaí berries has been measured at an astonishing 161,400 units. To give you a gauge of how high this is, the ORAC value of pomegranates is 2,860, and blueberries is 6,552. A food's ORAC value relates to its ability to neutralize and reduce free radicals in the body. Free radicals damage cells and tissues, and are the cause for many inflammatory diseases.

This tall palm grows throughout the tropics, and it is a staple for many in the Amazon region. This is because the fruit has significant protein content, at 8% by weight. It also contains significant calcium and vitamin A.

In addition, the fruit contains procyanidin oligomers, which have been shown to reduce the risk of heart disease and diabetes. Açaí also contains several other potent phytonutrients, such as ferulic acid, a potent antibacterial agent.

Olives and Olive Oil

Researchers from Greece's National Center for Scientific Research (Kostomoiri *et al.* 2012)—Oleuropein was found to inhibit the development of brain cell beta-amyloid protein precursor along with beta-amyloid metabolism. Remember, beta-amyloid oligomers has been linked to causing long-term memory loss and Alzheimer's disease.

The researchers treated human cells that had become subjected to the growth of beta-amyloid protein complex—duplicating what occurs within the brain of someone developing Alzheimer's. They treated the cells with Oleuropein and found that the olive extract interacted with the amyloid proteins in such a way that halted the Beta-amyloid metabolism process. In this case, Oleuropein stimulated MMP-9 activity amongst these beta-amyloid complexed cells. Increasing MMP-9 activity helps reduce the beta-amyloid oligomers amongst these cells.

The researchers concluded that:

> *"The experimental data reveal an anti-amyloidogenic effect of Oleuropein and suggest a possible protective role for Oleuropein against Alzheimer's disease, extending the spectrum of beneficial properties of this naturally occurring polyphenol."*

In a study related to one I discussed in the diet section, researchers (Martínez-Lapiscina *et al.* 2013) tested 285 people. Again, the subjects were divided into three equal and randomized groups.

Before and after the study, the patients were tested for cognition, which included memory testing and language fluency testing using a 14-point questionnaire. Their diets were also carefully validated using food extensive questionnaires.

The researchers found that the Mediterranean diet group that consumed the extra olive oil had a 66% reduced incidence of mild cognitive impairment at the end of the period compared to the control group—the conventional low-fat diet group.

And like the first study, this was after removing many other possible factors, such as smoking, alcohol intake, weight, diabetes and many others.

The olive oil result confirms another study done in 2009 (Berr *et al.*), where researchers from France's University of Montpellier followed 6,947 people, and found that consuming more olive oil resulted in a 17% reduction in cognitive decline and a 15% reduction of verbal fluency decline.

Olive oil is one of the healthiest oils because olives contain a number of medicinal phytonutrients. These include oleuropein, an antioxidant and anticancer agent shown to reduce blood pressure and inflammation. We reported on oleuropein's anti-cancer ability here. Other olive phytonutrients include hydroxytyrosol, tyrosol and verbascoside.

Extra-virgin is important for olive oil because this means the olives are freshly pressed without introducing heat into the process. The olives are being mechanically pressed, and there is no heating or addition of extraction chemicals into the process. This results in more polyphenol content within the olive oil.

While olives contain a number of polyphenols, Oleuropein is one of the best known. Other polyphenols within olives and olive oil can include hydroxytyrosol, tyrosol and verbascoside.

Along with these benefits, Oleuropein has been found to dilate the blood vessels, reducing blood pressure and increasing blood flow. Olive's high level of antioxidants also gives it a tremendous anti-inflammatory capacity, especially among the cardiovascular system. Olive leaf has been found to be antiviral. It appears to inhibit virus' ability to replicate, preventing viral shedding and budding within the cells and cell membrane.

Olives are also rich in a host of other beneficial nutrients, including copper, vitamin E and iron. The olive also contains a unique monounsaturated fatty acid called oleic acid. Olive oil also contains linoleic, palmitic, stearic and linolenic fatty acids. The combination of fats in olive helps balance pro-inflammatory fats such as saturated fats and arachidonic acids in other foods.

This blend of fatty acids, along with its antioxidants, gives olives and olive oil its proven ability to reduce the risk of cardiovascular disease and help prevent inflammatory diseases such as arthritis.

What about virgin or extra virgin olive oil?

Olive oil comes with a variety of labels, including virgin or extra virgin. Virgin oil must maintain a standard of less than 1.5-2% acidity (depending upon the country or origin), while extra virgin must maintain less than 0.8% acidity. A misnomer is that extra virgin is supposed to be from the first pressing. Rather, oil manufacturers find that certain seasonal pressings of certain olive varietals will produce the desired lower acid levels.

Many also assume that extra virgin oil utilizes only a mechanical press, but virgin olive oil also must be mechanically pressed. This contrasts to using chemical solvents to extract the oil. Most conventional vegetable oils are chemically extracted, while most olive oils are mechanically pressed. It should be noted that some mechanically pressed olive oils are blended with others to achieve the lower acidity—which is regulated by the Italian, Greece and government agencies.

In addition, high quality extra virgin olive oil is typically cold pressed, because it is mechanically pressed and utilizes less heat in the process. Most of the high quality extra virgin olive oils are cold pressed. Mechanical cold pressing helps preserve some of the heat-sensitive polyphenols and other nutrients contained within a fresh olive.

Pickling olives in a vinegar solution is one of the easiest and more delicious ways to preserve the polyphenol content of fresh olives.

Coconut Oil and MCT

The health community has been stirred by reports of coconut oil being a cure-all for Alzheimer's disease. Many report it is simply "anecdotal evidence." Is there really any scientific evidence for the notion that late-stage Alzheimer's disease can be reversed by coconut oil? Surprisingly, yes, but the evidence also points to an important caveat.

The Youtube videos and book by Dr. Mary T. Newport regarding Coconut oil and Alzheimer's have captured the attention of the health community. After her husband Steve was diagnosed with early onset Alzheimer's disease, Dr. Newport discovered the link between medium chain triglycerides and dementia.

In 2001, at the age of 51, Steve Newport began making memory mistakes. His memory and cognitive functions spiraled downward over the next eight years. By 2008, Steve's Alzheimer's had become severe.

So Dr. Newport developed a dosage of coconut oil to mimic the 60% middle chain triglyceride (MCT) product used in a study called AC-1202. She gave Steve seven teaspoons of coconut oil per day—or 3-4 servings per day of MCT oil. During the first month, Steve's tremors resolved and his cognition difficulties improved. His cognition test scores increased dramatically during the first few weeks of the coconut oil. And over the next few years, Dr. Newport reported that her husband "came back."

And his scores proved it. His cognition scores improved by 6 points of 75 point scale on cognitive, and 14 points of 78 on daily living activity tests.

Dr. Newport has since collected about 250 testimonies, about 90% of which were positive—though admittedly improved people would most likely write a testimony.

111

So is there any scientific evidence for taking coconut oil for Alzheimer's disease?

Dr. Newport's personal research established that Steve's early Alzheimer's disease was related to the inability of his brain cells to process glucose, or its alternative, ketones, for energy.

And shutting down that energy supply naturally shuts off those brain cells—spiraling a person into Alzheimer's disease.

But does this happen for everyone who is experiencing Alzheimer's disease? In a word, no.

Yet the ketonogenic diet—replacing glucose with ketone esters—has been shown to help epilepsy and other nervous disorders among those who have difficulty processing ketones from foods such as breast milk or dairy milk.

Breast milk, for example, contains 10-17% medium chain triglycerides (MCTs), which are converted to ketones in the form of Beta-hydroxybuterate. This is why MCTs are now added to any good baby formula.

Enter Dr. Samuel Henderson—who patented a product called AC-1202, made up of primarily medium chain triglyceride oil processed from either palm oil or coconut oil.

Like coconut oil, AC-1202 is taken up by the liver and released as ketones, which can be identified in the bloodstream as beta-hydroxybutyrate.

Research over the past 20 years has shown that beta-hydroxybutyrate reduces symptoms of Parkinson's, epilepsy and other nerve-related disorders, because these ketones are utilized for energy by glucose-starved brain and nerve cells.

One study (Neal *et al.* 2008) of children with epilepsy showed that a beta-hydroxybutyrate-rich ketogenic diet reduced seizures by as much as 75%.

The relationship between Alzheimer's and the need for ketones in brain and nerve cells has been related to a genetic variation, the epsilon-4 (E4) variant of the apolipoprotein E gene—also referred to as ApoE4. Because this variation seems to block the ability of the body to convert fats to ketones, the brain and nerve cells can become starved for energy.

Remember, having a genetic variant of the ApoE4 does not always result in Alzheimer's disease, but having one E4 allele can increase the risk of Alzheimer's disease. Furthermore, Alzheimer's is not always the result of the ApoE4 gene variant. It is often seen among those with vascular damage—which also leads to damaging the tiny blood vessels in the brain.

As we've discussed, diet is one of the greatest determinants for Alzheimer's. And vascular damage is also seen without the E4 gene variant.

But this E4 variation has provided the key to unlocking—at least for those who have this genetic variation and have some issue with processing ketones in the liver—the potential link between Alzheimer's disease and coconut oil.

The science is related to neurons being powered by ketones in the form of beta-hydroxybuterate, being taken up by brain cells that are starving for energy. For those who have difficulty producing ketones and/or have glucose resistance, mild ketosis has been shown to improve cognition, not only in animal and laboratory studies, but also in clinical research.

Over a decade ago Dr. Samuel Henderson patented a product called AC-1202—a medium chain triglyceride oil. The AC-1202 product contains glycerin with caprylic acid—a middle chain triglyceride, with a chemical name of 1,2,3-propanetriol trioctanoate.

The AC-1202 product underwent a clinical trial published in the medical journal *Nutrition and Metabolism* in August of 2009 (Henderson *et al.*). This study followed 152 Alzheimer's patients for 90 days using randomized, double-blind and placebo controls.

The Alzheimer's patients took the AC-1202 or the placebo for 90 days, and were given cognitive tests at 45 days and after the trial period. This included the gold standard ADAS-Cog test.

The research found that the AC-1202 significantly increased levels of beta-hydroxybutyrate, meaning they now had ketone-rich blood. As a whole, the AC-1202 group scored significantly higher in cognitive test scores compared to the placebo group. But this significant improvement took place primarily among those patients who had the ApoE4 variant. Those E4 variant patients saw a 5.73 point difference between the placebo group on the ADAS-cog testing, while there was little difference among those patients without the ApoE4 gene variant.

> *"While the cognitive effects were not significant in the overall sample, a pre-defined examination of cognitive effects stratified by genotype yielded significant effects in E4(-) [ApoE4 variant] participants,"* wrote the researchers in their discussion of the study.

The results of this clinical study clearly indicates that the potential for dramatic positive effects of coconut oil or any other source of MCT should take place primarily for those with the ApoE4 variant—or those having another form of glucose or insulin resistance that affects brain cells' receiving glucose or ketones from our diet.

This later condition—having glucose or insulin resistance—is also a looming issue that relates the ApoE genetic variant to our diet. There is a growing epidemic of type 2 diabetes in modern society, due to the ravages of the western diet.

Still, jumping to the conclusion that coconut oil is a cure-all for Alzheimer's Disease is short sighted. It is important to understand the science and the physiology of the process, and see the relationship between the ApoE4 variant and the need for inducing mild ketosis with MCT or coconut oil.

In their discussion of the MCT study, the researchers said:

> *"The positive effects of AC-1202 in E4(-) [ApoE4 variant] subjects is further supported by analysis of serum beta-hydroxybutyrate levels and cognitive performance. AC-1202 resulted in significant elevation of serum beta-hydroxybutyrate relative to Placebo at all study visits when investigational product was administered. In addition, a correlation between circulating beta-hydroxybutyrate levels at the two-hour time point and improvement in ADAS-Cog score was noted in E4(-) subjects at Day 90. No significant correlation was found in E4(+) [non-ApoE4 variant] participants. Hence, higher levels of ketosis appear to confer greater benefit in the E4(-) group."*

In other words, while coconut oil or MCT oil might help someone experiencing mild cognitive impairment due to glucose or insulin resistance, its more likely benefit to Alzheimer's disease will be for those with the ApoE4 gene variant and thus cannot process triglycerides in the liver normally—combined with a diet that produces glucose and/or insulin resistance among brain cells.

This last point is the likely key that ties the diet link between Alzheimer's disease and the ApoE4 variant. Those with the ApoE4 variant who also develop glucose or insulin resistance through poor dietary habits may experience cognitive issues and Alzheimer's due to their brain cells becoming energy-starved—having no energy source from either ketones or glucose. The research evidence illustrates that these folks (poor diet plus ApoE4) may have the greatest likelihood of benefiting from supplementing the diet with coconut oil and/or MCT oil.

Food sources of middle chain triglycerides (MCTs) include palm kernel oil, ghee, coconut oil, and the milk fat of goat milk, cow's milk and breast milk. Note that non-fat milk has had the MCTs removed. Supplemented MCT oil is a source for concentrated MCTs.

Quercetin Foods

A number of foods and herbs that reduce inflammation and toxicity contain quercetin. This is no coincidence. Multiple studies have shown that quercetin inhibits the release of inflammatory mediators histamine and leukotrienes. Foods rich in quercetin include onions, garlic, apples, capers, grapes, leafy greens, peppers, tomatoes and broccoli. In addition, many medicinal herbs also contain quercetin. This includes fennel, bilberry, green tea, lovage, dill weed and others.

Remember our earlier discussion of aluminum toxicity as a risk factor for Alzheimer's. Researchers from India's Postgraduate Institute of Medical Education and Research (Sharma *et al.* 2016) found that quercetin effectively helps to clear aluminum toxicity from the brain and help reverse its damage to neurons. The researchers stated:

> *"Further electron microscopic studies revealed that quercetin attenuates aluminum-induced mitochondrial swelling, loss of cristae and chromatin condensation. These results indicate that treatment with quercetin may represent a therapeutic strategy to attenuate the neuronal death against aluminum-induced neurodegeneration."*

Numerous studies have shown that quercetin stimulates the immune system, and neutralizes free radicals.

In one study, four weeks of quercetin reduced histamine levels and allergen-specific IgE levels. More importantly, quercetin inhibited anaphylaxis responses (Shishehbor *et al.* 2010).

Cairo researchers (Haggag *et al.* 2003) found that among mast cells exposed to allergens and chemicals in the laboratory, quercetin inhibited histamine release by 95% and 97%.

Over the past few years, an increasing amount of evidence is pointing to the conclusion that foods with quercetin slow inflammatory response and autoimmune derangement. Researchers from Italy's Catholic University (Crescente *et al.* 2009) found that quercetin inhibited arachidonic acid-induced platelet aggregation. Arachidonic acid-induced platelet aggregation is seen in inflammatory mechanisms, as we discussed earlier.

Organic foods contain higher levels of quercetin. A study from the University of California-Davis' Department of Food Science and Technology (Mitchell *et al.* 2007) tested flavonoid levels between organic and conventional tomatoes over a ten-year period. Their research concluded that quercetin levels were 79% higher for tomatoes grown organically under the same conditions as conventionally-grown tomatoes.

Root Foods

It is no coincidence that many antioxidants are roots, such as ginger, turmeric, onions garlic, beets, carrots, turnips, parsnips and others. These root foods are known for their ability to alkalize the bloodstream and stimulate detoxification. They are also known to help rejuvenate the liver and adrenal glands.

Beets, for example, contain, among other nutrients, betaine, betalains, betacyanin and betanin. They also contain generous portions of folate, iron and fiber. One of the primary fibers in beets is pectin, which is also found in apples. Pectin has a unique soluble and insoluble fiber content that maximizes the attachment of radical-producing LDL cholesterol in the intestines. Pectin also attaches to many other toxins, drawing them out of the body as well.

Meanwhile, betaine is known as stimulating liver health. Betaine has been shown to reduce liver injury (Okada *et al.* 2011). Betaine is also considered healthy for the bile ducts, because it helps draw out toxins. Beets are delicious foods that can be grated into salads, juiced, steamed, baked and simply eaten raw. Red beets are typically considered the healthiest, but pink and white beets also contain betaine.

We should note that while beets contain significant amounts of betaine, other betaine-rich foods include broccoli, spinach and some whole grains.

Each of the root foods listed above contain unique constituents that support liver health and detoxification.

Beetroot exemplifies this ability among roots.

Several recent studies have proven that beetroot increases not only athletic endurance and stamina, but also increases cardiovascular health by lowering blood pressure and reducing free radical damage.

One of the more recent studies comes from the UK's University of Exeter Sport and Health Sciences department (Kelly *et al.* 2013). The research tested team sport players in this double-blind study. Fourteen of the athletes were given 490 milliliters of beet juice and a matched group was given the same beet juice but without the nitrate content.

They found that the beet juice with nitrate group performed at significantly greater levels than the other group and had faster recovery rates. The researchers concluded:

> *"Dietary nitrate supplementation improves performance during intense intermittent exercise and may be a useful ergogenic aid for team sports players."*

Another study, this from the University of Exeter (Wylie *et al.* 2013) found in testing nine athletes during cycling training that 250 milliliters of beet juice twice a day significantly increased endurance during the most intense workouts. Several other studies from the same university have confirmed these findings.

As researchers have struggled to find the mechanism and active constituent, it appears beets supply some complex biomolecules that fuel the cell's energy producers—the mitochondria.

116

A study from Mexican researchers (Alcántar-Aguirre *et al.* 2013) found that beet juice stimulates the voltage-dependent anion channels within the mitochondria. This creates a more streamlined production of energy in a pathway called oxidative phosphorylation.

This mechanism proves out in practical endurance situations as well. Researchers at the Saint Louis University (Murphy *et al.* 2013) studied 11 athletes (men and women). The subjects were either given placebo or 200 grams of baked beets prior to their training workouts.

Those who ate the baked beets ran 0.4 kilometers faster than the athletes who ate the placebo on average for a five kilo run. And during the last mile, the beet eaters ran 5% faster than those who did not eat the beets.

The researchers concluded:

> *"Consumption of nitrate-rich, whole beetroot improves running performance in healthy adults."*

Mid Sweden University researchers (Engan *et al.* 2012) also found that the nitrate content in beets may help sleep apnea as well.

Research from the University of Reading (Hobbs *et al.* 2012) found that beetroot juice and even bread infused with beets significantly lowered both systolic and diastolic blood pressure among 32 adults.

Research from The Netherlands' Maastricht University Medical Centre (Engan *et al.* 2012) found that 140 milliliters of concentrated beet juice a day significantly improved the times and speeds during cycling workouts among competitive cyclists.

Meanwhile, Polish university researchers (Zielińska-Przyjemska *et al.* 2012) found that the betanin in beets stimulated developing immune cells—neutrophils—and reduced free radicals.

Other studies have found that the nitrate content in beetroot juice increases muscle efficiency and exercise intolerance (Cermak *et al.* 2012).

Beets also contain lutein, which has been shown to slow down age-related macular degeneration.

A study from Texas (Włodarek *et al.* 2011) showed that beets and other nitrate-containing foods can increase endothelial function.

Perhaps those cyclists and other athletes who want to somehow increase their performances might consider beets over steroids?

Other root foods have high nitrate levels, because roots typically fix nitrogen. Roots also contain numerous medicinal compounds. Other root foods to include in the Ancestors Diet are potatoes, carrots, onions, ginger, peanuts, turnips and others.

Cruciferae

The Cruciferae family, often termed cruciferous, includes broccoli, cabbage, bok choy, watercress, cauliflower, collards, kale, turnips, rutabaga, mustard, radish, daikon, wasabi, arugula, komatsuna, cress, horseradish and even rapeseed (canola is a rapeseed hybrid).

Cruciferous veggies contain numerous constituents that improve liver function and stimulate the immune system. These include sulforaphane and allyl isothiocyanate—which was shown in a study from the University of Pittsburgh to inhibit prostate cancer cells (Xiao *et al.* 2003).

Besides glucoraphanin, cruciferae contain indoles, glucosinolates, dithiolthiones, sulfoxides, isothiocyanates, sulforaphane and indole-carbinol.

Here we will discuss broccoli and cabbage, but the cruciferae family shares most of these benefits.

Broccoli

Researchers from Italy (Riso *et al.* 2013) have determined that eating broccoli for just ten days will cut inflammation in more than half. Other studies find it prevents and repairs DNA damage.

For ten days, the researchers—from Italy's University of Milan—gave 250 grams of broccoli to a group of young smokers.

Before and after the study the researchers collected blood from the subjects and conducted an extensive analysis of the blood. They measured the subjects' various immune cell status, including C-reactive protein (CRP) levels, tumor necrosis factor alpha (TNF-α) levels, interleukin 6 (IL-6) and adiponectin. They also analyzed levels of folate and lutein in the blood.

After the 10-day broccoli-enriched diet the subjects were re-tested and the researchers found that their CRP levels went down by 48%. This is a significant drop in CRP levels, indicating the smokers' inflammatory levels went down by nearly half.

The researchers found that circulating levels of lutein and folate went up as well. Note the drop in CRP levels was found independent of lutein and folate levels. The researchers did find that lycopene levels increased accompanied by a drop in IL6 levels—indicating a relationship between lycopene and inflammation factors—as other studies have confirmed.

This study confirms an earlier study done at the same university (Riso *et al.* 2010). In this study the researchers tested 27 young smokers who were otherwise healthy, and gave them either 250 grams of steamed broccoli per day or a control diet. In this study the researchers tested mRNA and DNA enzyme levels—which relate directly to the repair of DNA. They also measured DNA strand breaks within the blood.

The researchers found that those eating the broccoli had a 41% drop in strand breaks of DNA, and other changes in enzyme levels associated with DNA protection.

In a number of laboratory studies, broccoli has been shown to be anti-carcinogenic. Other studies have shown its antioxidant content is helpful in helping prevent heart and cardiovascular disease.

Broccoli is also a significant source of tocopherols, magnesium, selenium, thiamin, riboflavin and pantothenic acid.

Broccoli sprouts have been shown to have more of these anti-inflammatory and anti-cancer nutrients than conventional broccoli.

Cabbage

Cabbage contains a unique constituent, s-methylmethionine, also referred to as vitamin U. Through a pathway utilizing one of the body's natural enzymes, called Bhmt2, s-methylmethionine is converted to methionine and then to glutathione in several steps.

In this form, glutathione has been shown to stimulate the repair of the mucosal membranes within the stomach, intestines and airways. Glutathione has also been shown to increase the health and productivity of the liver. It also neutralizes lipid peroxide radicals.

Plants use s-methylmethionine to help heal cell membrane damage among their leaves and stems. This is reminiscent of antioxidants: Plants produce antioxidants to help to protect them from damage from the sun, insects and diseases. In other words, the very same biochemicals that protect plants also help heal our bodies.

Watercress

Watercress contains a host of antioxidant nutrients, including xanthophyll, beta-carotene, alpha-tocopherol and gamma-tocopherol (two forms of vitamin E), each of which have been shown to slow free radical formation in the body.

Strenuous exercise typically produces DNA damage, which a healthy body will hopefully repair. Watercress has been shown to reduce DNA damage and cancer growth.

Research from Britain's Edinburgh Napier University (Fogarty *et al.* 2012) found that watercress reduces DNA damage and oxidative stress induced by exercise, confirming other research showing watercress inhibits cancer.

The researchers studied ten healthy young men (average age 23) for four months. The men were tested before and after the study, and on a daily basis, before an after exhausting aerobic exercise. During one eight-week period, the subjects took watercress supplements daily, two hours before exercise. During the other eight-week period, they were given 85 grams of watercress two hours before their workouts.

When given the watercress supplement, the men showed a significant reduction in reactive oxygen species levels, and the damage to their DNA as a result of exercise.

Blood samples revealed that levels of lipid peroxidation—the major cause for artery disease—were also significantly lower when taking the watercress.

The researchers commented on this aspect of the study:

"The study demonstrates that exhaustive aerobic exercise may cause DNA damage and lipid peroxidation; however, these perturbations are attenuated by either short- or long-term watercress supplementation, possibly due to the higher concentration lipid-soluble antioxidants following watercress ingestion."

Previous research has established that watercress contains a nutrient called phenethyl isothiocyanate or PEITC. Georgetown University researchers (Wang *et al.* 2011) established that PEITC inhibited the growth of cervical cancer and breast cancer cells.

Adding cruciferae to our diet is often a matter of blending. The most obvious way is with a salad. But steaming and soup-making are good options as well. The issue with steamed or souped cruciferae is heat and nutrient loss. When steaming, separate the hot water from the food. When souping, add the vegetables last, just before serving.

Super Greens

Greenfoods are considered nutritionally superior to most fruits and vegetables. Greenfoods include the leafy greens, wheat grasses, sprouts, algae, sea vegetables, parsley and others. Here we will discuss only a few of these incredible foods.

Greenfoods provide practically every nutrient known, including enzymes, minerals, trace elements, essential and non-essential amino acids, vitamins, antioxidants and various phytonutrients. Many will provide over 1,000 nutrients.

A big benefit of greenfoods is their alkalinity. This gives them the ability to neutralize radicals and lipid peroxides.

Much of this alkalinity comes from greenfoods' bioavailable mineral content. Many of these minerals are also are colloidal. They tend to be hydrophobic, and maintain a positive electrical charge—rendering them alkaline.

Leafy Greens

Leafy greens include lettuce, kale, spinach, chard, beet leaves, cabbage, mustard greens and turnip greens. They are nutrition powerhouses, containing folates, antioxidants, minerals like iron, potassium and calcium, and a whole array of vitamins including vitamin K. They also contain beta-carotene, lutein, zeaxanthin and others.

The need for vitamin K is critical to immunity, as it helps regulate inflammation, healing and blood clotting.

But there's more.

Australian researchers (Rankin *et al.* 2013) determined that green leafy and cruciferous vegetables stimulate the immune system of the intestines by donating a gene that regulates the gut's defense mechanisms.

The research comes from the University of Melbourne and Melbourne's Walter and Eliza Hall Institute of Medical Research. The researchers studied the ingestion of leafy and cruciferous vegetables along with other foods. They measured and analyzed intestinal levels of interleukin 22—a critical element that regulates intestinal immunity through an immune cell called NKp46+. This is also called an innate lymphoid cell—or ILC.

IL-22 and the innate lymphoid cells play a critical part of the intestine's control of inflammatory conditions and food allergies. Low levels have been seen amongst various inflammatory diseases.

The genetic factor which stimulates these innate lymphoid cells from greens is called T-bet. T-bet is a genetic transcription factor that stimulates a type of signaling gene called a Notch gene. These Notch genes stimulate the conversion of from lymphoid tissue-inducers to innate lymphoid cells, according to the research.

The research was led by Dr. Gabrielle Belz from the Walter and Eliza Hall Institute. Dr. Belz commented on the research:

> *"we discovered that T-bet is the key gene that instructs precursor cells to develop into ILCs (innate lymphoid cells), which it does in response to signals in the food we eat and to bacteria in the gut. ILCs are essential for immune surveillance of the digestive system and this is the first time that we have identified a gene responsible for the production of ILCs."*

The research illustrated that leafy and cruciferous greens apparently donate key proteins. *"Proteins in these leafy greens could be part of the same signaling pathway that is used by T-bet to produce ILCs,"* added Dr. Belz in a later statement.

These powerful green vegetables apparently interact with cell surface receptors, which switch on the T-bet gene.

Celery

The Romans awarded wreaths of celery to winners of sporting events. Ancient Asian cultures harvested wild celery and brewed it to produce a tonic used for stomach difficulties and general vitality. Celery garlands were found inside tombs of ancient Egyptian pharaohs. While many other cultures used wild celery as a medicinal herb, cultivated celery is mentioned being grown in France in 1623, and celery began being grown commercially in the U.S. in the 1880s.

The famous Naturopath Dr. Paavo Airola recommended celery for blood purification, detoxification and for building immunity. Dr. Bernard Jensen has recommended it for neutralizing rheumatic acids within the body, detoxification, fevers, nervous conditions and cardiovascular conditions.

Celery is a member of the parsley family. It contains a host of nutrients, including potassium, vitamin K, vitamin A, folate and vitamin B6. It also contains a number of phytonutrients. Notably celery is also rich in sulfur, which has been shown to be useful for joint conditions.

Chinese medicine has used celery as a remedy to lower blood pressure. Dr. Quang Le and Dr. William Elliott from the University of Chicago found that one of celery's phytonutrients, 3-n-butyl phthalide, reduced blood pressure by 13-14% by eating the equivalent of four stalks per day. Dr. Le also tried this remedy himself and found that his blood pressure went from 158/96 to 118/82.

Celery also contains compounds called acetylenics. Acetylenics have been shown in several studies to inhibit tumor growth (Siddiq and Dembitsky 2008).

Celery also contains phenolic acids. Phenolic acids provide protection against free radical oxidative damage, and slow inflammation. Oxidative free radical damage causes arteriosclerosis, stroke, liver damage and heart disease in general.

In a study done by researchers from the Chinese Academy of Agricultural Sciences (Yao et al. 2010), 11 cultivars of celery from two different species were examined for their phenolic acid composition. The phenols found in the celeries included caffeic acid, p-coumaric acid, and ferulic acid. P-coumaric acid was the most abundant phenolic acid found amongst the samples. They also found several flavonoids, including apigenin, luteolin, and kaempferoland.

Furthermore, the researchers found the phenols and flavonoids in celery exhibited significant antioxidant potency. Of the 11 cultivars studied, Shengjie celery had the highest antioxidant activity, and the Tropica variety had the lowest levels of antioxidant potency.

Just as proposed by Dr. Airola decades earlier, the phenolic acids in celery stimulate phenolsulfotransferases (PSTs) within the body. PSTs are detoxifying metabolic enzymes that stimulate the removal of toxic compounds, including pharmaceutical chemicals and environmental chemicals.

In a study by researchers from Taiwan's National Chung Hsing University (Yeh and Yen 2005), phenolic acids were shown to directly increase the levels and activities of PST-P within the body. In a study using 20 different vegetables, celery was among the top five (along with asparagus, broccoli, cauliflower, celery and eggplant,) that stimulated PST-P the most among human HepG2 cells.

Celery is best eaten raw, but it can also be juiced and put into soups. Each of these methods will preserve most of the phytonutrient levels. A vegetable-barley soup with sliced celery is also delicious. Put the sliced fresh celery into the pot only after the barley has been cooked enough to be soft. After 10 more minutes on a low flame, the celery will be softened enough to eat, but not overcooked.

Celery also makes a fun and great snack for kids when combined with peanut butter and/or cream cheese. Just spread unsweetened natural peanut butter and/or fresh cream cheese into the chamber of the stalk to the brim and hand it over. It makes a delicious, satisfying and nutritious snack your child will never forget.

Parsley

Parsley is rich in numerous antioxidant nutrients, including vitamin A, vitamin C, vitamin E, beta carotene, lutein, cryptoxanthin, zeaxanthin, folate and is one of the greatest sources of vitamin K, with 1640 micrograms per gram—over 12 times the U.S. DRI (dietary reference intake) of 90-120 micrograms per day. One hundred grams of parsley also contains more than double the RDA for vitamin C and almost triple the RDA of vitamin A.

These antioxidant nutrients have been shown to reduce the effects of the oxidation of lipids, relating directly to reducing vision disorders, heart disease, dementia and other inflammation-related conditions.

Hungarian researchers (Pápay et al. 2012) confirmed that parsley (Petroselinum crispum) contains significant anti-inflammatory properties, boosts liver health, is antioxidant and even anti-carcinogenic. It also supplies numerous nutrients and relaxes smooth muscles.

The research found that parsley contained numerous nutrients and bioactive constituents, including several flavonoids and cumarins. One flavonoid called apigenin has been shown to provide significant anti-tumor properties, as well as the ability to slow inflammation and neutralize oxidative radicals (free radicals). Its ability to stop tumor growth lies in its ability to block tumors from creating blood vessels.

Research published from China's Jiangsu Polytechnic College of Agriculture and Forestry (Liu *et al.* 2011) found that apigenin also blocked the action of MEK kinase 1, which in turn prevented bladder cancer cells from migrating and thus inhibited tumor growth.

The ability of parsley to relax smooth muscles appears to come from its blocking of the polymerization of actin. This has significant importance to asthmatics, as a severe asthmatic attack will accompany the over-contraction of the smooth muscles around the lungs. Relaxing those smooth muscles is one key component of urgent care in asthmatic attacks.

Other bioactive constituents in parsley include eugenol, crisoeriol, luteolin and apiin. Eugenol has been used by traditional doctors as an antiseptic and pain-reliever in cases of gingivitis and periodontal disease, and has been shown to reduce blood sugar levels in diabetics.

Parsley's ability to encourage healing has also been shown in numerous studies.

For example, a study published from Turkey's Hacettepe University Faculty of Medicine (Tavil *et al.* 2012) found that increased parsley consumption was associated with fewer complications after hematopoietic (bone marrow) stem cell transplantation in children.

In this study, the diets of 41 children who underwent the stem cell transplantation were analyzed. Improved outcomes were seen among those eating more parsley, as well as those children who ate onions, bulgur, yogurt and bazlama (a Turkish yeast bread).

The Power of Sprouts

Sprouts and their powders are nutritional powerhouses. They have exponential nutritional value, well above the nutrient content of their seeds or the fully-grown plants. This was confirmed in 1970s experiments by former Hippocrates Health Institute Director of Research, Viktoras Kulvinskas, who found that ascorbic acid levels in soybean sprouts increased from zero to 103 milligrams per 100 grams by day six—about the ascorbic acid content found in lime juice. These levels fall off significantly within days.

Each sprouted seed has a different nutrient peak. Ascorbic acid content in broad bean sprouts—used to cure scurvy during World War I—peaks in three days, after which the levels fall off.

Many believe that sprouts produce this greater antioxidant content to defend themselves against threats from the soil.

During germination beans and seeds undergo a natural enzyme-intensive process, converting protein peptides and surrounding inorganic minerals to highly digestible chelated amino acid-mineral complexes. Various other nutrient levels increase during soy germination. Levels of vitamin C, riboflavin, niacin and biotin increase from 25% to 150% during germination (Kulvinskas *et al.* 1978). Highly antioxidative phenolic compounds also develop during sprouting according to other research (Lin *et al.* 2006).

Great nutritional sprouts include wheat grass sprouts, barley, oats, beans, broccoli and cabbage. The latter two provide a class of nutrients called glucosinolates. These glucosinolates yield sulfur compounds and indole-3 carbinols. Both have shown to have significant anticarcinogenic and anti-inflammatory effects in the body.

Researchers from Mexico's prestigious Monterrey Institute of Technology (Guajardo-Flores *et al.* 2013) determined that black bean sprouts are anticarcinogenic against breast cancer, liver cancer and colon cancer cells.

The researchers sprouted black beans (*Phaseolus vulgaris*) and tested them and their constituents against cancer cell lines of different types of cancers. The researchers found that after three and five days of germination, the sprouts were able to inhibit the growth of all the cancer cells tested.

They also tested the same sprouts against non-cancerous (healthy) cells as controls. After application, they found no negative impact upon these healthy cells.

The sprouts only inhibited the growth of the cancer cells.

The researchers then isolated some of the constituents of the sprouted beans, and found that the saponins and flavonoids had the greatest inhibition against liver and colon cancer cells. Meanwhile the genistein content of the sprouts was found to inhibit the growth of breast cancer cells.

The researchers also found the black bean sprouts to be particularly high in antioxidants.

In addition to Kulvinskas' work, other sprout research as documented by Hofsten (1979) and others has found that during the germination process many nutrients are increased, or made more available for assimilation. Other research (Chen and Pan 1977) found that phytic acid in soy beans decreased 22% while the enzyme phytase increased 227% after five days of soybean germination. Because phytic acid/phytate can bind minerals, nutrients like calcium and zinc are more assimilable. We will discuss phytic acid in more detail in Chapter Nine.

Also, the oligosaccharides that produce flatulence are hydrolyzed during germination, making bean sprouts easier to digest.

Seed or bean selection for sprouting is critical. A good quality seed or bean will germinate at least 50%. Heirloom seeds often germinate at much higher rates.

It is also important to wash sprouts often during the germination process, as microorganisms can grow along with the sprouts, especially in the warmer, wet environment that supports germination.

Sterol Foods

Plant sterols, also called phytosterols, are compounds found in most plant foods, including fruits, vegetables, seeds and nuts. There are a variety of different types of sterols, including avenasterol, campesterol and beta sitosterol.

These are the lipids that make up the cells membranes of plants. A healthy plant cell membrane made of these phytosterols helps protect the plant's cells from becoming vulnerable to free radicals.

Phytosterols also help reduce oxidized radicals in the human body as well. This means reducing lipid peroxidation, thus lowering the risk of Alzheimer's.

Foods high in sterols include fresh corn, with 952 milligrams per 100 grams, rice bran, with 1055 milligrams per 100 grams, wheat germ with 553 milligrams per 100 grams, and flax seed with 338 milligrams per 100 grams. Nuts also have good sterol content. Cashews have 146 milligrams per 100 grams and peanuts have 206 milligrams per 100 grams.

Researchers from Canada's University of Toronto and St Michael's Hospital (Jenkins *et al.* 2011) found that people who ate diets rich in plant-based foods known for lowering LDL-cholesterol, including plant sterols, soy foods, nuts and plant-based fibers showed reductions in LDL-cholesterol by 13% after six months. The average reduction in LDL-cholesterol went from 171 mg/dL on average down 25 mg/dL to 156 mg/dL of LCL-c.

The study was published in the *Journal of the American Medical Association.*

The study followed 345 volunteers who were either instructed to eat a low-saturated fat diet or were given specific dietary advice to eat certain foods known to lower cholesterol during clinic visits. Their LDL-cholesterol levels Those who ate the low-saturated fat diet showed a 3% reduction in LDL-cholesterol levels during the same period. Their levels reduced from the average of 171 mg/dL to 168 mg/dL.

The researchers also divided the specific-foods diet into two additional groups, one that was given two sessions of advice during the six months and the other, given seven clinical dietary sessions during the six months. These two groups showed little difference in their resulting LDL-cholesterol levels. The group given seven advice sessions had 13.8% average reduction in LDL-cholesterol, while the group given two advice sessions showed an average of 13.1% reduction in LDL-cholesterol.

This later result indicates that most people will adhere to diet advice when given occasionally as compared to frequently.

The overall result, however, is consistent with the multitude of research that has shown that plant sterols, cultured soy foods, nuts and high fiber foods specifically reduce LDL-cholesterol.

Higher LDL-cholesterol levels have been associated with higher incidence of heart disease, atherosclerosis (hardening of the arteries), strokes and other cardiovascular issues. This is because LDL-cholesterol is less stable, and readily oxidizes. This oxidation produces free radicals that damage the walls of the blood vessels. This causes scaring, which tends to harden the arteries, as well as releases scar tissue into the blood. This release is what causes thrombosis.

The Canadian researchers concluded that:

> *"Use of a dietary portfolio compared with the low-saturated fat dietary advice resulted in greater LDL-C lowering during 6 months of follow-up."*

The "dietary portfolio" was the specific foods mentioned, offered within nutrition counseling sessions that taught the volunteers how to incorporate these LDL-cholesterol-lowering foods into their diets.

Chapter Seven

Herbal Medicines for Alzheimer's

Now let's dig into a different class of curative strategy for Alzheimer's. Herbal medicines come from plants that have special curative properties. Some herbal medicines can be used as spices in foods. But herbal medicines are often concentrated to focus their healing compounds.

Herbal medicines have a long history of success in treating various conditions. It is for this reason that at least 60 percent of pharmaceutical medications were drawn from or are synthetic versions of herbal medicine-derived compounds.

In addition to their medicinal compounds, herbal medicines are particularly high in antioxidants. Antioxidant analysis methods such as ORAC (Oxygen Radical Absorbance Capacity) have found that herbs will often contain exponential levels of antioxidants compared with foods. This is because their medicinal constituents are antioxidant as well as medicinal.

Furthermore, a number of these herbal medicines have been shown to increase cognition and some even reverse Alzheimer's disease symptoms. Let's talk about some herbal medicines that science has proven out to help prevent, reduce or even treat Alzheimer's:

Ashwagandha

A flurry of new research from around the world on Ashwagandha is proving the medicinal effects of this ancient Ayurvedic herbal remedy are more than just anecdotal.

Numerous studies confirmed its healing properties in a variety of conditions, including stress, toxicity, heart disease, Alzheimer's disease, diabetes, Parkinson's and many others.

Researchers from the Defense Institute of Physiology and Allied Sciences (Ahmed *et al.* 2013) found that Ashwagandha supported memory and helped prevent nerve cell degeneration among rats.

Research from India's National Brain Research Center (Sehgal *et al.* 2012) found that Ashwagandha reduces beta-amyloid peptides within the brain—making it protective against Alzheimer's disease. The mechanism for this was quite novel: The herb increased receptors for low-density lipoproteins in the liver. This had the effect of reducing the oxidative lipoproteins—which we discussed above as linked to brain cell damage and Alzheimer's disease.

Research from India's Indian Institute of Technology (Grover *et al.* 2012) confirmed that the withanolide A compound—one of Ashwaghanda's many constituents—also reduced acetylcholinesterase. This, the researchers stated, makes Ashwagandha useful for Alzheimer's disease treatment and prevention:

> *"The study provides evidence for consideration of withanolide A as a valuable small ligand molecule in treatment and prevention of Alzheimer's disease associated pathology."*

Jamia Hamdard University researchers (Manjunath *et al.* 2012) found that Ashwagandha reduces oxidative damage related to brain cell damage—making it useful for reducing dementia and Alzheimer's risk.

Research from the Asha Hospital in Hyderbad (Chandrasekhar *et al.* 2012) found, in a study of 64 people with chronic stress, that Ashwagandha supplementation for two months decreased stress by 44% and decreased depression and/or anxiety by 72%.

Researchers from Jamia Hamdard University's Pharmacy Faculty (Anwer *et al.* 2012) found that Ashwagandha reduces oxidative stress related to type 2 diabetes, and thus insulin resistance.

Researchers from the Defence Institute of Physiology and Allied Sciences (Ahmed *et al.* 2013) found that Ashwagandha supported memory and helped prevent nerve cell degeneration among rats.

Another study (Manjunath *et al.* 2012) found in laboratory studies that Ashwagandha root powder significantly reduced signs of oxidative stress among brain regions. The researchers restored nitrate oxide levels and reduced inflammatory markers. The researchers found that Ashwagandha had significant "neuroprotective effects."

Researchers from Brooklyn's Woodhull Medical Center (Kalani *et al.* 2012) found that Ashwagandha increases circulating cortisol levels and improves insulin sensitivity.

Researchers from India's Cochin University of Science and Technology (Soman *et al.* 2012) found that Ashwagandha increased spatial memory and decreased oxidative brain stress among rats.

Human clinical studies from India's Banaras Hindu University (Upadhyay *et al.* 2011) found that Ashwagandha significantly reduced type II diabetes symptoms.

Scientists from the Indian Institute of Technology found further evidence of Ashwagandha's neuroprotective effects, in its ability to withanolide A to inhibit acetylcholinesterase.

Research from the Council of Scientific and Industrial Research Center found that Ashwagandha significantly stimulates the immune system.

Ashwagandha (Withania somnifera) contains a myriad of constituents, including withanolides named withanolide A, withanolide B, withaferin A, and withanone, along with 12-deoxy withastramonolide, withanoside V, withanoside IV. Other complex molecules include trihy-droxy-oxowitha-trienolide compounds.

Many of these compounds have independently been found to act synergistically to enable changes in gene expression within the cell—producing a variety of medicinal effects in addition to antioxidant effects.

Huperzine A

We have discussed numerous strategies that help prevent Alzheimer's disease in this text. But what about someone who is already suffering from the condition? Is there anything that can be done naturally to either slow or stop the continued cognitive impairment?

Huperzine A continues to show its clinical efficacy as a treatment for adults suffering of ongoing Alzheimer's disease—despite being virtually ignored by conventional medicine in the United States.

The effectiveness of huperzine A on current Alzheimer's and other dementia has been confirmed by a significant amount of clinical research.

Huperzine A is extracted from the Chinese moss plant (Huperzia ser-rata and other Huperzia species). These are collectively referred to as firmosses. There are numerous varieties of firmosses that grow on differ-ent continents.

Huperzine A, and its more newly-found molecular relatives huperzine B and huperzine U, is a sesquiterpene that has a mechanism of blocking the enzyme acetylcholinesterase. Acetylcholinesterase will break down acetylcholine, an important neurotransmitter that allows information to be carried from one nerve to another.

Excess acetylcholinesterase has been observed among a number of cognitive disorders, including Alzheimer's, Parkinson's and other dementia forms.

Yes, huperzine A is a natural acetylcholinesterase inhibitor. Four ace-tylcholinesterase inhibitors have been approved by the FDA—these are donepezil, rivastigmine, tacrine, rivastigmine and galantamine. Don't see a mention of huperzine in this list? So is huperzine A less effective? Nope.

Researchers from the Department of Neurology at the China-Jan Friendship Hospital in Beijing (Shao 2015) conducted a study of 110 patients with Alzheimer's disease. They were split into four groups and treated for six months with one of four possible treatments. These in-cluded three of the FDA-approved acetylcholinesterase inhibitors just mentioned, along with huperzine A.

One group was treated with the drug memantine with donepezil. An-other was given memantine and rivastigmine, and another group was given memantine and galantamine. And another group of 22 patients was given the memantine along with huperzine A. The last group was given the memantine together with a placebo.

The reason each group was given memantine is because other research has found that while memantine doesn't work so well for Alzheimer's disease by itself, for some reason it works great in combination with acetylcholinesterase inhibitors because they block acetylcholinesterase.

Anyway, the patients were tested at the beginning, after three months and after six months of their treatment protocols. The testing used the highly standardized Mini-Mental State Examination (MMSE), along with Activities of Daily Living (ADCS-ADL) scoring, which tests the ability of a person to do daily tasks without assistance—a test developed by the Alzheimer Disease Cooperative Study.

The researchers found that the group given the memantine with the huperzine A improved the most compared with the other groups.

The fact that huperzine A is not used in the U.S. is puzzling, given that even U.S. researchers have proven its efficacy in clinical studies. A study from the School of Medicine at the University of California, San Diego (Rafii *et al.* 2011) tested 177 Alzheimer's patients for up to four months. They treated half the patients with either 200 milligrams or 400 milligrams of huperzine A. The researchers gave 70 patients a placebo for the period.

The research found that while the 200 milligram dose of huperzine A had little effect, the 400 milligram dosage of huperzine resulted in a significant improvement in the Alzheimer's patients. Their scores in the Alzheimer's Disease Assessment Scale-cognitive test increased by 2.27 points at 11 weeks and 1.92 points at 16 weeks. This compares with little or no improvement among the placebo group.

We can add to these studies the reality that international research—most of it from China—has proven huperzine A's efficacy over two decades of research. A meta-study was conducted by researchers from the School of Public Health at China Medical University (Shu-huai Xing *et al.* 2014) has confirmed that the plant constituent called huperzine A can significantly improve cognitive function among Alzheimer's patients.

The researchers found and analyzed 42 clinical studies that have investigated Huperzine A. They eliminated all studies that did not fit inclusion criteria for quality research. The researchers were left with eight high-quality placebo-controlled and randomized studies—five being double-blind and three being single-blind—involving more than 10 human subjects each.

In all, the eight studies followed 733 patients with Alzheimer's disease. The fewest number of patients in a study was 28 and the most was 197. The studies ranged from 8 weeks to 24 weeks long.

All of the studies used the MMSE and the ADL tests to measure the results of the plant extract. These two tests together gauge the cognitive, consciousness and lifestyles of dementia patients. The MMSE test gauges orientation, repetition, attention, recall, language and complex commands.

The meta-analysis calculations of these studies found that huperzine A significantly increased cognition among those patients compared to those taking the placebo.

The average drop in MMSE scores among the Huperzine A groups compared with the placebo groups—indicating improved condition—was 4.84 points.

Among those subjects with vascular dementia, the rate of improvement in MMSE scores was similar—dropping 4.92 in comparison with the placebo group.

The point system on the MMSE goes up to 30, with the higher scores being indicative of cognitive decline. An improvement of nearly 5 out of 30 points is a significant change—though its percentage change does not necessarily indicate a straight-line relationship.

ADL scores also were significantly better among the huperzine A groups. The difference between the huperzine A and placebo groups among the vascular dementia cases was a significant 10.24 points lower.

The researchers added:

> "The results from our meta-analysis of eight randomized controlled trials showed that Huperzine A could significantly improve the MMSE and ADL score of Alzheimer's patients."

Cholinesterase inhibition

One of the mechanisms of this plant extract is that it naturally inhibits the enzyme acetylcholinesterase. This enzyme breaks down acetylcholine—which is necessary for the brain's ability to transmit electrical activity through the nervous system.

A study published by researchers from the Walter Reed Army Institute of Research (Alam *et al.* 2013) studied 84 healthy young adults to test the extent of blocking acetylcholinesterase and affecting neurological behavior.

The researchers tested the drugs galantamine (doses at 4 or 8 milligrams), donepezil (doses at 2.5 or 5 milligrams) along with huperzine A (at either 100 or 200 µg). They gave the last group a placebo.

The researchers found that the huperzine A blocked acetylcholinesterase as well as increased recall and memory tasks—illustrating its ability to treat dementia.

The first study I discussed above illustrates that huperzine A is a more effective acetylcholinesterase inhibitor compared with pharmaceutical acetylcholinesterase inhibitors. It is also smarter.

A study from India's Integral University (Alam *et al.* 2013) found that the acetylcholinesterase-inhibiting properties of huperzine B provides a more intelligent "docking" potential with acetylcholinesterase compared with pharmaceutical acetylcholinesterase-inhibitors, which can come with significant side effects including dizziness.

Studies on Huperzine A have indicated a history of safety, with the few side effects noted as minor stomach upsets.

Bacopa

A treatment known to ancient medical practitioners continues to provide both the most promising and the most scientifically valid approach to disorders related to dementia and cognitive impairment.

That's right. A simple herb that grows from the ground is outsmarting billions of dollars of research by pharmaceutical companies—focused upon finding a way to stimulate an increase in memory and cognition known to deteriorate in Alzheimer's disease.

Not only is their approach wrong—toxic chemicals which can harm brain tissues further—but their ammo is simply too light.

Nature's ammo swamps pharmaceutical drugs, because herbs contain sometimes hundreds of constituents that work synergistically to heal.

One of these is an Ayurvedic herb called Brahmi—botanical name *Bacopa monnieri*. This herb has been used for thousands of years to boost memory and cognition. Now we find it may also treat dementia and Alzheimer's disease.

Medical scientists from Thailand's Khon Kaen University Medical College (Peth-Nui *et al.* 2012) studied 60 elderly adults, with an average age of 63 years old. The researchers gave the adults the Ayurvedic herb bacopa or a placebo for three months.

Before and after the treatment period, the researchers tested the subjects' memory accuracy, attention span, cognitive processing speed and reaction time. They also measured their brain cell cholinergic and monoaminergic functions—which related to neuron firing speeds. The subjects were also tested every four weeks during the treatment as well as four weeks after the end of the treatment.

The herbal medicine-treated group were given either 300 milligrams or 500 milligrams of a whole-herb extract of the Bacopa monnieri herb.

The groups given the Bacopa had significant improvement in cognitive function, including increased memory, greater attention spans and better reaction times.

The researchers also found Bacopa altered their cholinergic and monoaminergic activity. The researchers concluded that these results:

> *"[The results] suggest that Bacopa monnieri can improve attention, cognitive processing, and working memory partly via the suppression of AChE activity."*

Another placebo-controlled clinical study of Brahmi was conducted by psychopharmacology researchers from Australia's Swinburne University of Technology (Downey *et al.* 2013). They gave 24 healthy adults either a placebo or standardized extracts of Bacopa. This study utilized two different dosages as well—320 milligrams or 640 milligrams—but also conducted a crossover design. This means that the adults given the placebo were tested and then given the herbal medicine and those given the Brahmi were then given the placebo.

In this study, the 320 milligram-treated groups showed significant increases in cognition and memory during three different intervals of testing.

A 2008 clinical study from Portland's National College of Natural Medicine (Calabrese *et al.*)—also a randomized, double-blind, placebo-controlled study—had similar results. Here 54 adults with an average age of 73 years old took either a placebo or 300 milligrams of a Bacopa standardized extract for three months. The Bacopa-treated group had increased word recall, less anxiety, decreased average heart rate and cognitive increases. The researchers concluded:

> *"This study provides further evidence that B. monnieri has potential for safely enhancing cognitive performance in the aging."*

Laboratory and animal research has concluded similar findings, using Brahmi and its constituents. These have also found that Brahmi prevented neurological damage related to oxidative damage. In a study conducted by India's National Institute of Mental Health and Neurosciences (George *et al.* 2012), researchers concluded:

> *"We infer that BM displays prophylactic effects against ACR induced oxidative damage and neurotoxicity with potential therapeutic application in human pathology associated with neuropathy."*

Swinburne University of Technology researchers (Downey *et al.*)conducted a study of Bacopa in 2013 with cognitive demand testing. The researchers tested 24 healthy elderly subjects. The researchers gave each subject 430 milligrams of Bacopa, 640 milligrams of Bacopa or a placebo. Each subject received each of the three treatments with a wash-out period in between. They gave the subjects a series of six cognitive demand tests—called a Cognitive Demand Battery.

The researchers found that the Bacopa treatments significantly improved cognitive performance—but not the placebo.

A 2008 study from Swinburne's Brain Science Institute (Stough *et al.*) studied the cognitive effects of Bacopa following three months of Bacopa treatment. Here 62 healthy elderly volunteers completed this double-blind, placebo-controlled study. They were given either a placebo or 150 milligrams of CDRI 08 twice a day—300 milligrams per day.

The subjects were given the Cognitive Drug Research cognitive assessment system before and after the 90 day treatment period. This battery of tests measures reaction times, number ordering, word recall and recognition, picture recognition, and spatial and numeric working memories.

The researchers found that the Bacopa significantly improved working memory and spatial working memory. This includes accuracy and context memory recognition. The researchers also found that rapid visual information processing tasking was improved.

Another double-blind, placebo-controlled study was conducted on Bacopa in 2001 (Stough *et al.*). Similar results were found using 300 milligrams of Bacopa, tested after five weeks and twelve weeks of treatment. The researchers concluded in this earlier study:

> *"These findings suggest that B. monniera may improve higher order cognitive processes that are critically dependent on the input of information from our environment such as learning and memory."*

These studies bear the obvious question of whether Bacopa can treat Alzheimer's disease. The answer is yes.

In a laboratory study using human brain cells at the pharmacy college of Thailand's Naresuan University (Limpeanchob *et al.* 2008), researchers duplicated the scenario of beta-amyloid-induced damage of Alzheimer's disease among brain cells.

When the researchers treated the brain cells with Bacopa monnieri, the beta-amyloid-induced Alzheimer's damage was halted. The researchers observed:

> *"Brahmi-treated neurons expressed lower level of reactive oxygen species suggesting that Brahmi restrained intracellular oxidative stress which in turn prolonged the lifespan of the culture neurons. Brahmi extract also exhibited both reducing and lipid peroxidation inhibitory activities."*

The results were convincing. In their paper, the researchers concluded:

> "From this study, the mode of action of neuroprotective effects of Brahmi appeared to be the results of its antioxidant to suppress neuronal oxidative stress and the acetylcholinesterase inhibitory activities. Therefore, treating patients with Brahmi extract may be an alternative direction for ameliorating neurodegenerative disorders associated with the overwhelming oxidative stress as well as Alzheimer's disease."

The overriding conclusion of all these studies—which are confirmed by others—is that Bacopa does significantly boost memory and cognition, and can be a valid Alzheimer's disease treatment. But this isn't all. Bacopa can also increase multi-tasking.

Increased multi-tasking is a hallmark for reducing dementia, as this stimulates brain activity and helps defer progression of the disease. Bacopa has been shown to boost multi-tasking. Research from Australia's Swinburne University of Technology (Benson *et al.* 2014) tested 17 healthy elderly adult volunteers.

In this cross-over design study, each patient was tested with the placebo and the Bacopa treatment with a clearance period in between.

The volunteers were tested for multi-tasking framework and then tested again one and two hours after taking two different doses of the Bacopa or a placebo.

The subjects were also tested for moods and salivary cortisol levels—which will indicate levels of stress and/or anxiety—before and after the dosing of the Bacopa or placebo.

Each of the subjects underwent the multitasking framework testing separated by a week—called the washout period. The first week the subjects were given the test, then given the placebo, and then tested again a week later before and after being given 320 milligrams of a commercial extract of Bacopa called CDRI 08—also labeled KeenMind®.

After another washout period of seven days, the subjects returned to receive 640 milligrams of the CDRI 08—followed and proceeded by a round of multitasking framework testing.

The results of the study determined the subjects' memory was significantly enhanced by the Bacopa, but not by the placebo.

This study also found the Bacopa elevated mood levels and reduced stress levels—indicated by the reduction of salivary cortisol levels. These also indicated adaptogenic effects of the Bacopa extract.

Another study from 2012 (Rastogi *et al.*) found that Bacopa helped to ameliorate brain injury—in effect helping to protect the brain from long-term brain damage.

Bacopa Monniera—also called Brahmi and Indian Pennywort—has been used for thousands of years in Ayurvedic medicine to boost moods, memory and related disorders. It has thus been used to relieve anxiety, stress, AD/HD-related issues, epilepsy and memory disorders such as Alzheimer's and other forms of dementia and mental diseases.

Outside of these uses, Brahmi has been used for irritable bowels, inflammation including joints, backache, headaches and some menstruation symptoms.

The plant is a small shrub that grows in wet and tropical regions, including South and Central America. Year-round ponds in warm climates will often support Bacopa.

All this research has noted few side effects among the study subjects. At most, slight stomach upset was noted in the Portland study.

While most pharmaceuticals—which typically have numerous harmful side effects—contain one or maybe two active constituents, Bacopa contains a host of medicinal compounds. These include multiple bacopasaponins, bacopasides, bacosides, jujubogenin, pseudojujubogenin, donepezil, deprenyl, brahmine, herpestine, D-mannitol, apigenin, hersaponin, cucurbitacins and plantainosides and other therapeutic phytochemicals.

How can pharmaceutical companies compete with this? Each of these—and other—components work synergistically to help different parts of our metabolism. Some affect our neurotransmitters. Some affect our liver. Some affect hormones. Why can't we admit that nature has designed the ultimate medicine for brain issues?

Garlic

Garlic (*Allium sativum*) is eaten in many cuisines as a spice. But it is also a potent medicinal herb.

Garlic's medicinal potential can be increased through aging or extraction. Aged garlic Aged garlic has either been dried in a dry storage or dried using ethanol. The natural drying process will convert its alliin and allicin content into derivatives, but it will also increase its sulfur compounds – for example, S-allylcysteine, which has been shown to reduce hypertension. Garlic contains hundreds of other medicinal compounds, many of which have been shown to protect the brain—such as thiacremonone and others.

Aged garlic extract and its medicinal components have been shown to help protect the brain from lipid peroxidation and the development of beta-amyloid oligomers. It has also been shown helpful for Parkinson's disease and Huntington's disease.

These benefits come from aged garlic's antioxidant and anti-inflammatory properties, along with the healing potential of garlic's sulfur compounds. Researchers from the University of Missouri School of Medicine (Qu *et al.* 2016) found that aged garlic extract stimulates changes among microglial cells by changing something called Nrf2-mediated signaling. This is a pathway for managing oxidative stress among brain cells.

Meanwhile, researchers from India's University of Delhi (Manral *et al.* 2016) found that the diallyl disulfide compound from garlic prevents APP processing within the brain. This interferes with the production of beta-amyloid oligomers. They also found that analogues of this compound protect against beta-amyloid-produced cell death. The compounds halted beta-amyloid-42 damage to brain cells, and even reversed damage caused by scopolamine to brain cells from the cerebral cortex and hippocampus.

Other research (Kumar 2015) has determined that allicin within garlic can significantly inhibit acetylcholinesterase and butyrylcholinesterase. This gives garlic the ability to slow beta-amyloid oligomer development and damage to brain cells, as we have discussed with other natural acetyl-cholinesterase-inhibitors. This research concluded:

> *"Allicin shows a potential to ameliorate the decline of cognitive function and memory loss associated with Alzheimer's disease by inhibiting cholinesterase enzymes and upregulate the levels of acetyl-choline in the brain. It can be used as a new lead to target acetyl-cholinesterase and butyrylcholinesterase to upregulate the level of acetylcholine which will be useful in alleviating the symptoms associated with Alzheimer's disease."*

Other research has found this ability of garlic. Researchers from Portugal's University of Lisboa (Keri *et al.* 2016) found that both S-allylcysteine and S-propargylcysteine from garlic successfully inhibited acetylcholinesterase.

In addition to these, other research (such as Zhu *et al.* 2015 and Yun *et al.* 2016; and Jeong *et al.* 2013) has determined that garlic and its constituents can protect the brain from beta-amyloid damage and help improve memory and cognitive function.

Turmeric

Turmeric is a powder ground from a root utilized for medicinal purposes and spicing food for thousands of years. Recent research has established it has anti-tumor, anti-inflammatory and antioxidant effects. Now researchers are discovering that it helps protect against the accumulation of amyloid plaque among brain cells, and other causes of nerve and brain cell damage.

A number of studies have revealed that turmeric and its central constituent, curcumin, may help prevent and even treat nerve cell and brain cell disorders such as Alzheimer's disease and Parkinson's disease.

A review of research from India's National Institute of Mental Health and Neurosciences (Mythri *et al.* 2012) reveals that curcumin crosses the blood-brain barrier to protect nerves from damage—this is called being "neuroprotective." The researchers stated:

> *"different experimental models of Parkinson's disease strongly support the clinical application of curcumin."*

Another study, this one from the University of Maryland School of Pharmacy (Mythri *et al.* 2012) found that curcumin protects the brain's cells from reactive oxygen species, and the A53T alpha-synuclein protein mutant, implicated in neuron damage found in both Alzheimer's and Parkinson's. The research also found that curcumin reduced mitochondrial damage among brain cells—another occurrence in Alzheimer's.

A study from India's Central Food Technological Research Institute (Gadad *et al.* 2012) found that curcumin-glucoside halts the formation of fibrils among nerve cells by binding to alpha-synuclein proteins. When this protein is expressed outside of the hippocampus and other inner brain regions, it can result in damage among brain cells.

University of Kentucky researchers (Mizwicki *et al.* 2011) found that curcumin reduced free radical oxidative stress damage among the brain and nerve cells, slowing down damage from and protecting against the progression of the build up of beta-amyloid and neurofibrillary tangles among the brain and nerve cells—evident among Alzheimer's patients.

Medical researchers from Thailand's Mahidol University (Mythri *et al.* 2011) found that curcumin prevents neurotoxicity by blocking 6-Hydroxydopamine damage to nerve and brain cells. This is the pathway said to occur among Parkinson's disease patients.

These researchers also found that curcumin protected nerve cells from free radical damage, and inhibited the p53 cell-death sequence following brain cell phosphorylation—another progression found in Parkinson's.

These and other studies all point to one general lesson: Turmeric helps protect the brain and nerves, and may well help prevent Alzheimer's and Parkinson's disease. Care for a little curry rice with tonight's dinner?

Seaweeds and Algae

There are numerous herbal medicines that grow in marine environments. Some grow wild in lakes and oceans, and others have been cultivated in ponds. Many of these have unique medicinal compounds that can stimulate the growth of brain cells as well as help protect the brain from oxidative stress.

There are about 70,000 known algae of three general types: Chlorophyta or green algae, Phaeophyta or brown algae and Rhodophyta, or red marine algae. These range from single-celled microalgae to giant broad-leafed kelps.

AFA

Aphanizomenon flos-aquae—or simply AFA—is an alga that grows on the pristine volcanic waters of the Klamath Lake of Oregon. AFA's nutrients are readily available because of its soft cell wall. The rich volcanic lakebed of Klamath Lake renders it an available source of vitamins, minerals, phytonutrients, and all the essential and non-essential amino acids. Like spirulina and chlorella, AFA is a complete protein with 60% protein by weight. AFA also contains up to 58 trace minerals.

Astaxanthin

Another exciting pond-grown microalga is Haematococcus pluvialis, noted for containing astaxanthin. Astaxanthin is an oxygenated carotenoid with significant antioxidant properties, some hundreds of times the antioxidant value of vitamin E. Recent studies have shown astaxanthin to be effective in reducing inflammation and stimulating the immune system. Studies have shown astaxanthin's ability to prevent and treat retinal oxidative damage and macular degeneration, with activity greater than beta-carotene. Reports from marathoners and tri-athletes also reveal that astaxanthin increases recovery rates from rigorous exercise.

Several studies have suggested that a nutrient derived from this commercially farmed green algae species may treat and even reverse cognitive impairment and conditions relating to neuron damage. This of course includes Alzheimer's disease.

Researchers from China's Fujian Medical University (Ye *et al.* 2012) tested a nutrient called Astaxanthin with nerve cells and found that the nutrient blocked the type of oxidative stress that has been identified as the primary cause of neuron damage that result in brain and nerve damage.

The researchers found that Astaxanthin blocked the MPP+ related Heme oxygenase process implicated in nerve and brain cell damage. This type of oxidative damage has been linked to Parkinson's disease, Huntington's disease and Alzheimer's disease.

Other research has found that Astaxanthin comes with antioxidant properties from an estimated one hundred to one thousand times the antioxidant level of vitamin E. One of the richest natural sources of Astaxanthin is the algae *Haematococcus pluvialis*—which we'll discuss later.

The Fujian Medical University researchers' conclusion:

> *"ATX suppresses MPP+-induced oxidative stress in PC12 cells via the HO-1/NOX2 axis. ATX should be strongly considered as a potential neuroprotectant and adjuvant therapy for patients with Parkinson's disease."*

Clinical research has supported this finding and more. Last year, researchers from the Graduate School of Medicine at Japan's Juntendo University (Katagiri *et al.* 2012) tested Astaxanthin using 96 elderly adult volunteers. In this randomized, double-blind and placebo-controlled study, the researchers gave the subjects either a capsule with Astaxanthin extract or a placebo for three months.

Before, after and every four weeks during the study, the researchers tested the subjects' cognition, and found that those who took both dosages of Astaxanthin extract—12 milligrams or 6 milligrams—scored significantly higher on learning and cognition testing than the placebo group.

The researchers concluded:

> *"The results suggested that astaxanthin-rich Haematococcus pluvialis extract improves cognitive function in the healthy aged individuals."*

Another study from Japan (Ikeda *et al.* 2008)—this from the Life Science Institute—found among ten healthy adults that 12 milligrams a day of Astaxanthin significantly improves cognitive function and psychomotor functions.

Another clinical study (Miyazawa *et al.* 2011) found that Astaxanthin treatment significantly raises blood levels of carotene, and improves the health of circulating red blood cells—reducing free radical related damage that can eventually produce nerve and brain cell damage. Even low dosages of one and three milligrams a day have shown a strengthening effect among red blood cells.

Research headed up by Dr. Mark Tso from the University of Illinois determined that the antioxidant Astaxanthin concentrations in the blood stream effectively cross the blood-brain barrier, allowing its protective factors to become available directly to brain cells and central nervous system cells.

Research from the Tokyo Metropolitan Institute of Gerontology (Ye *et al.* 2012) found that Astaxanthin inhibited this oxidative process, concluding that Astaxanthin, *"markedly abolished 6-OHDA-induced reactive oxygen species generation."*

A 2009 study from Taiwan's Hungkuang University (Satoh *et al.*) using brain cells, found that Astaxanthin suppressed about 75% of the reactive oxygen species production along with other parts of the oxidative process involved in the beta-amyloid production process found in Alzheimer's disease.

Kelps and Sea Grasses

Kelps might be called seaweeds, but these phytonutrient powerhouses are anything but weeds. About 1,500 species of sea kelps flourish, many in the North Pacific and North Atlantic oceans.

Most kelps are stationary, and sustainably harvested in the wild. This means they must be allowed to regrow to guarantee future harvests. *Ascophyllum nodosum* kelp contains an impressive array of vitamins—more than many vegetables. They include over 60 essential minerals, amino acids and vitamins. They also contain growth promoters, according to kelp researchers.

Most kelps also contain fucoidan, a sulfated polysaccharide. Laboratory studies have indicated fucoidan has anti-tumor, anticoagulant and anti-angiogenic effects. Fucoidan inhibits beta-amyloid oligomer formation, implicated in Alzheimer's. It also down-regulates Th2, which inhibits allergic response, inhibits proteinuria in Heymann nephritis and decreases artery platelet deposits.

There are about 1,500 species of kelp-like brown algae, many of which flourish in the cold waters of the North Pacific and Atlantic oceans. Well known kelp-like sea veggies include nori, wakame, dulse, kombu, Irish moss, sea palm, and several species of laminaria. Kelps are harvested periodically and managed carefully—easy to do since kelp beds are stationary. Out of necessity, kelp farmers maintain a sustainable supply.

Kelps have an impressive array of vitamins—more than most land-based vegetables, with A, B1, B2, B5, B12, C, B6, B3, folic acid, E, K, and a steroid vitamin D precursor. Nori and dulse have beta-carotene levels as high as 50,000 IU per 100 grams. Certified organic kelps show 60 minerals at ppm levels. They are also good sources of calcium and magnesium. Most brown algae also contain all the essential amino acids. Nori is 30% protein by weight and other kelps average about 9%. Laminaria also produces the sugar substitute mannitol.

Kelps also contain a number of beneficial polysaccharides and polyphenols. One such sulfated polysaccharide, fucoidan, has been shown to have anti-tumor, anticoagulant and anti-angiogenic properties. Research shows it also inhibits allergic response, inhibits beta-amyloid formation (linked to Alzheimer's), and decreases artery platelet deposits.

While vegetables from the sea are often overlooked as viable food and supplement sources, they are some of the most nutritious foods on the planet. They can be used to increase well-being and stamina, rendering a stronger, healthier body and mind.

As to the effect of seaweed (the primary algae eaten in the Japanese diet), a recent study from Russia (Besednova *et al.* 2013) has concluded that seaweed contains compounds that prevent and possibly reverse oxidative damage to brain and nerve cells. The primary group of nutrients in seaweeds having these effects are called sulfated polysaccharides. These have been shown in laboratory and animal studies to reverse degeneration of nerve cells among the brain and central nervous system. According to the researchers:

"Sulfated polysaccharides can arrest a number of secondary pathological effects observed in neurodegenerative diseases (oxidative stress, inflammation, the phenomenon of increased neuronal apoptosis, toxic effects etc.)."

They also suggested that:

"sulfated polysaccharides may be the basis for the creation of next-generation drugs for the treatment of neurodegenerative diseases."

Red marine algae

Red marine algae research has confirmed some potentially amazing health benefits. Dumontiae, a larger-leaf Rhodaphyte typically harvested in colder oceans by either wildcrafting or rope farming, has been shown to inhibit growth of several viruses, notably herpes simplex I and II, and HIV. Most studies have pointed to their heparin-like sulfated polysaccharide content for antiviral effects, which blocks DNA and retroviral replication.

Michael Neushul, Ph.D. from University of California Santa Barbara's biology department has reported antiviral properties among all of the 39 California red marine algae varieties tested. Sulfated polysaccharides such as carrageenan are considered the central antiviral constituents, along with dextran sulfate and other heparinoids. Retrovirus inhibition has also been illustrated by the research.

Spirulina

Commercial spirulina is harvested from huge dedicated ponds in sunny areas and typically freeze-dried. Spirulina is a good source of carotenoids, vitamins, minerals, and important fatty acids like gamma linolenic acid—known to help reduce inflammation. Spirulina also contains all the essential and most non-essential amino acids, with 55-65% protein by weight. It also has a variety of phytonutrients such as zeaxanthin, myxoxanthophyll and lutein. Clinical studies have indicated spirulina can increase brain cell health, reduce inflammation, and help prevent cancer. It also contains antioxidant phytonutrients such as zeaxanthin, myxoxanthophyll and lutein.

Spirulina also contains phycobiliprotein, a unique blue pigment anti-inflammatory and antioxidant. Research has showed that phycobiliproteins can protect the liver and kidney from toxins. They are also anti-viral, and stimulate the immune system.

In one study from the University of California-Davis, 12 weeks of 3,000 milligrams of Hawaiian spirulina per day significantly increased hemoglobin concentration and mean corpuscular hemoglobin among 30 adults over the age of 50. IDO (indoleamine 2,3-dioxygenase) enzyme activity—a sign of increased immune function—was also higher among the subjects.

Chlorella

Chlorella pyrensoidosa, or simply chlorella, is also cultured in outdoor ponds. Over 800 published studies have confirmed its safety and efficacy for various health issues. Chlorella's ability to detoxify heavy metals and other toxins make it a favorite of natural health practitioners. Chlorella's phytonutrients include beta-carotene, various vitamins, and a substance called Chlorella Growth Factor—which seems to increase cell growth. Chlorella is also a complete protein at 40%-60% by weight with every essential and non-essential amino acid. Clinical studies have shown that chlorella stimulates T-cell and B-cell activity and increases macrophage activity. Chlorella has been shown to help fibromyalgia, hypertension, and ulcerative colitis. Its cell wall is tough, but most producers crush it. This releases polysaccharides and fiber, giving chlorella its unique ability to bind to toxins in the body.

Chlorella contains a special compound called chlorella growth factor (CGF), known to stimulate nerve cell growth. Another study showed that chlorella increases IgA levels and lowers dioxin levels in breast milk.

Chlorella's tough cell wall must be broken down mechanically to allow these nutrients' bioavailability. Our digestive enzymes cannot digest these outer cell walls. For this reason, quality chlorella growers will pulverize this tough outer cell wall.

DHA Algae

Some algae also produce a potent and pure form of docosahexaenoic acid, or DHA—a fatty acid recommended by medical doctors and naturopaths alike for reducing inflammation and increasing cardiovascular health. Commercial DHA-producing microalgae are cultured in tanks, so their DHA is harvested without the risk of mercury or DDT toxicity. Algal DHA doesn't put pressure on fish populations. The two algal DHA microorganisms commercially produced are Crypthecodinium cohnii and Schizochytrium spp. They are now used in many supplements and infant formulas. Eicosapentaenoic acid or EPA is produced in the human body from DHA, so no need to add EPA.

Aloe Vera

Scientists from the University of Miami's School of Medicine (Lewis *et al.* 2013) determined that an a constituent of Aloe vera was able to reduce Alzheimer's disease symptoms and increase cognition scores. The researchers gave a supplement with aloe polymannose—also called acemannan—to Alzheimer's patients over a one year period. They tested them every three months.

The researchers found that the cognitive improvements occurred in 46% of the patients taking the supplement. They also found that several cytokines and other inflammatory factors significantly decreased as well—indicating a reduction in neuro-inflammation among the patients.

The researchers concluded:

> *"Participants tolerated the aloe polymannose supplement with few, temporary adverse reactions. Our results showed improvements in both clinical and physiological outcomes for a disease that otherwise has no standard ameliorative remedy."*

Chili pepper

Chili peppers contain a special ingredient called capsaicin. This significantly increases circulation in other studies. For this reason, chili pepper and capsaicin decreases the risk of heart disease, hardening of the blood vessels (atherosclerosis), obesity, hypertension gastrointestinal conditions, inflammatory conditions and circulatory disorders.

In a study published in the Journal of Alzheimer's Disease, (Liu *et al.* 2016) researchers tested 338 people who were 40 years old or older. The researchers used a Food Frequency Questionnaire to determine their dietary habits. The researchers also tested the subjects' cognitive functions using the Mini-Mental State Examination (MMSE). They also tested each subjects' blood beta-amyloid-40 and beta-amyloid-42 levels.

The researchers found that those with more chili pepper in their diet had higher MMSE scores, lower levels of beta-amyloid-40. This of course was after other potential associations were removed—such as age, gender, educational level, smoking history, alcohol consumption, body mass index (BMI) and other common associations.

The researchers concluded:

> *"These findings suggest that a capsaicin-rich diet may exert favorable effects on Alzheimer's disease blood biomarkers and cognitive function in middle-aged and elderly adults."*

Sacred Lotus

The hypnotically beautiful Sacred Lotus flower is certainly pleasing to the eyes. Depending upon the location and genetics, lotus flowers can be white, pink, yellow or even rainbow-colored.

Turns out the Sacred Lotus (Nelumbo nucifera) is not only pleasing to the eyes. The plant contains natural compounds that give it numerous healing powers—to both the body and the mind.

The leaves, stem, seeds, roots and flowers of the lotus have been used medicinally for thousands of years. The Mandarin name for the Sacred Lotus (seed) is Lian Zi and its Japanese name is Renshi, and in Korean, Yoncha.

Ancient Chinese and Ayurvedic texts indicate the stems and leaves of the plant are helpful for stomach aches, ulcers and intestinal cramping, increasing circulation, and improving the condition of the heart (cardiotonic). It is also known for strengthening the spleen.

The seeds and flowers of the lotus flower—and to a lesser degree the leaves—also have a range of other effects. These include being hypnotic and calming. The seeds contain alkaloid constituents that relax the nerves and the muscles. They also promote sleep. Restlessness and nervousness—even depression—have been treated traditionally using the seeds, flowers and leaves of the Sacred Lotus.

Then you have the roots of the lotus. These have been used to treat numerous infections, including intestinal infections and diarrhea. The dried roots have also been used for various issues of bleeding as well.

These are not theoretical uses either. These are recorded uses of the plant in clinical settings. Science has been recently confirming these uses.

Researchers from Korea's Kyung Hee University (Ahn *et al.* 2014) studied one of the Lotus' constituents, called Allantoin. They analyzed the compound in the laboratory and found that it stimulated the proliferation of brain cells in the hippocampus.

This of course is a major finding for Alzheimer's disease. For this reason, the researchers stated:

"In conclusion, allantoin has memory-enhancing effects, and these effects may be partly mediated by the PI3K-Akt-GSK-3β signal pathway. These findings suggest that allantoin has therapeutic potential for the cognitive dysfunctions observed in Alzheimer's disease."

A study from the Republic of Korea's Kangwon National University (Kim *et al.* 2014) found that Sacred Lotus seeds exhibited several anti-Alzheimer's effects. One extract of Lotus inhibited acetylcholinesterase and butyrylcholinesterase enzymes. Acetylcholinesterase inhibitors are used to treat a myriad of conditions, from tachycardia, to Alzheimer's and other dementias, to Parkinson's and schizophrenia.

The researchers explained the connection:

"The cholinergic system is important for memory function, and scopolamine induces memory impairment through blockade of the cholinergic system. Previous studies have shown that Nelumbo nucifera semen and Nelumbo nucifera seedpod inhibit acetylcholinesterase activity. Choline acetyltransferase (CHAT) is an enzyme that is synthesized by acetylcholine, and Nelumbo nucifera semen improves memory by inducing CHAT expression. Moreover, neferine, one of the major compounds in ENS, has an antiamnesic effect due to AChE inhibition. Further, we found that ENS inhibited AChE activity in the hippocampus."

The researchers also found 19 medicinal constituents in the seeds, including saponins, flavonoids, steroids, alkaloids, terpenoids and cardiac glycosides. Some of these were found to reduce oxidative stress, and thus help protect brain cells.

Alzheimer's disease is often associated with anxiety and stress. Researchers have confirmed the hypnotic and sedative effects of the lotus plant. In a study published in the *Journal of Agricultural and Food Chemistry* (Yan *et al.* 2015) found that alkaloids of the plant increased the production of gamma-amino butyric acid (GABA), along with serotonin, 5-hydroxyindoleacetic acid and dopamine.

The researchers stated:

"These data demonstrated that the alkaloids from lotus leaf exert sedative-hypnotic and anxiolytic effects via binding to GABA receptor and activates the monoaminergic system."

Another study found that an extract of the flower of the Sacred Lotus had elements that bound to several key receptors in the brain and nervous system known for encouraging relaxation: two cannabinoid receptors, and four opiod receptors.

A study from the Yokohama College of Pharmacy (Sugimoto *et al.* 2015) extracted two special alkaloids from the Sacred Lotus: liensinine and isoliensinine. Each of these were found to have anti-depressant effects.

The researchers concluded:

> *"These data suggest that liensinine and isoliensinine from Nelumbo nucifera Gaertner have antidepressant-like effects and that antidepressant-like effects of liensinine and its analogues are closely related to serotonergic mechanisms."*

Sacred Lotus also produces a number of medicinal effects in the body. These include general anticancer and antioxidant effects, as well as improving the health of the liver, kidney and skin. Some of these effects are simply because Sacred Lotus is an extreme free radical scavenger. But other effects follow its complex blend of medicinal constituents.

Rosemary

The Rosemary plant not only smells nice and looks nice when growing in our garden. It also appears that it increases our brain power.

Studies over the past few years have shown that *Rosmarinus officinalis*—the common herb Rosemary and its essential oil—can boost memory and help prevent Alzheimer's disease.

Researchers (Ramachandran *et al.* 2014) from Miami Children's Hospital's Research Institute, studied extracts of Rosemary and Bacopa separately and together using human brain and nerve cells.

They found that each extract inhibited the phosphorylation of tau tangles. Tau tangles have been linked with Alzheimer's progression. But the combination of the two produced an even greater inhibitory effect.

This took place by halting the production of beta-amyloid proteins. Amyloid protein production precedes the tau tangle formations as we have discussed.

The researchers stated:

> *"These results suggest that the extract of Bacopa monnieri plus rosemary antioxidant is more neuroprotective than Bacopa monnieri or rosemary antioxidant extract."*

In a study from Maryland's Tai Sophia Institute (Pengelly *et al.* 2012), researchers gave 28 elderly adults with an average age of 75 years old either a placebo powder or a rosemary leaf powder of different doses spread with weekly wash-out periods in between.

The subjects were tested using the Cognitive Drug Research computerized assessment system. The doses ranged from 750 milligrams to 6,000 milligrams.

The researchers found that the lowest doses produced a significant improvement in cognitive scores, while the higher doses actually had an impairing effect upon the subjects.

In a study from Japan's Tottori University medical school (Jimbo *et al.* 2009), researchers tested 28 elderly people including 17 Alzheimer's patients using aromatherapy.

During a 28-day period preceded and followed by two wash-out periods of 28 days, the researchers gave the subjects aromatherapy using rosemary and lemon essential oils in the morning and lavender and orange essential oils in the evening.

The study found a significant increase in cognition scores in the Touch Panel-type Dementia Assessment Scale (TDAS) test. The researchers stated:

> *"In conclusion, we found aromatherapy an efficacious non-pharmacological therapy for dementia. Aromatherapy may have some potential for improving cognitive function, especially in Alzheimer's patients."*

Psychology researchers from the UK's Lancaster University (Ball *et al.* 2010) studied rosemary aromatherapy in a series of experiments that tested environmental context-dependent memory (ECDM). The research found that rosemary provided a *"striking ECDM effect."*

Furthermore, researchers from the Human Cognitive Neuroscience Unit at the UK's University of Northumbria (Moss *et al.* 2003) studied 144 healthy volunteers. They divided the volunteers into three groups. One was given aromatherapy with lavender essential oil. The other was given aromatherapy with rosemary essential oil. The last group was given no aromatherapy.

The researchers conducted Cognitive Drug Research (CDR) testing found that the lavender oil depressed working memory and reaction times. This included memory and attention tasking.

The research found rosemary aromatherapy significantly boosted memory and cognition. The researchers stated that the rosemary aromatherapy:

> *"...produced a significant enhancement of performance for overall quality of memory and secondary memory factors, but also produced an impairment of speed of memory compared to controls."*

These studies illustrate that consuming fresh or powdered rosemary in culinary doses can help boost memory. The Tai Sophia Institute study found that 750 milligram doses had the most therapeutic effect, but not higher. Higher doses had the opposite effect.

Even more promising is the use of rosemary essential oil as aromatherapy. This can boost memory function almost immediately. Sprinkling a drop or two onto a crumpled tissue is a quick and easy way to diffuse an essential oil. Essential oil diffusers are also available if you want a more permanent instrument.

Rosemary is very easy to grow in the garden. It is also a great drought-tolerant plant. It needs very little water and in fact hates being over-watered.

Cannabinoids and Hemp Oil

Growing evidence indicates that deranged amyloid-beta oligomers within the brain and central nervous system may be to some degree mitigated or reduced by plant compounds called cannabinoids.

In particular, microglia cells of the brain and nervous system—which help the brain fight inflammation and brain cell damage—contain what are called cannabinoid receptors. More specifically, these are called CB2 receptors.

When these receptors become attached to cannabinoid molecules, they apparently balance the production of inflammatory cytokines with the needs of the brain cells to fight off inflammation and the eventual production of amyloid-beta oligomers.

Some of the mice studies have shown that cannabinoid agonists promote the clearance of amyloid-beta oligomers from the brain. This may provide a mechanism for blocking the process, though it may not precisely correct the cause.

In addition, some of the research has shown that cannabinoid infusion increase cognitive function and even memory capacity. The mechanisms for this effect appear to come from agonizing (attaching to) CB1 and CB2 receptors (Martín-Moreno *et al.* 2012 and others).

This research is preliminary. There is no hard clinical evidence that hemp oil or any other cannabinoid provider helps prevent or treat Alzheimer's. Rather, what we have are a collection of cell and mice studies that show some promise for cannabinoid therapy in the prevention and treatment of Alzheimer's disease (Aso *et al.* 2016).

One of the best sources of cannabinoids is hemp oil. Supercritical hemp oil extract provides a wealth of cannabinoids without any of the THC molecules that produce intoxication.

Other foods can also attach to cannabinoid receptors. One study (Rousseaux *et al.* 2007) found that Lactobacillus acidophilus from yogurt produced cannabinoid agonists.

Medicinal Mushrooms

A mushroom is a fungus that feeds off of the soil, the bark of a tree or any number of other natural elements. Mushrooms are one of the richest sources of nutrition. They are also medicinal.

Edible mushrooms offer a significant tool to cleanse out toxins and boost our immunity. These include Shiitake, Buttons or Chanterelles. Medicinal mushrooms are available in supplement form. These include Reishi (*Ganderma lucidum*), Hoelen (*Wolfiporia extensas*), Maitake (*Grifola frondosa*), Shiitake (*Lentinula elodes*), Turkey Tails (*Coriolus versicolor or Trametes versicolor*), Agaricus (*Agaricus blazeil*), Cordyceps (*Cordyceps sinensis*) and Lion's Mane (*Hericium erinaceus*). All of these significantly stimulate the immune system, and their constituents bind to toxins within our bodies.

Mushrooms that have been found to improve memory and cognitive function include *Poria cocos, Hericium erinaceus, Ganoderma lucidum, Sarcodon spp., Antrodia camphorata, Pleurotus giganteus, Lignosus rhinocerotis, Grifola frondosa, Agaricus bisporus* (Phan *et al.* 2015; Bennet *et al.* 2014; May *et al.* 2016; many others).

The Agaricus species is the most popular eating mushroom, and this species contains the Button mushroom. But there are many, many others. Scientists have cataloged some 50,000 mushrooms, and identified less than 20,000 different mushroom species. Some estimate there may be over 150,000 mushroom species within the Fungi kingdom, which likely encompasses more than 1.5 million total species. Biologists have described less than 5% of Fungi species.

Over 600 mushroom species have been documented to stimulate the immune system. However, the ones mentioned above have received the most attention. Research on these mushrooms have revealed their effects as being antimicrobial, cholesterol-lowering, anti-inflammatory, antioxidant, anti-mutagenic, anti-tumor, adaptogenic and immunostimulating.

A few medicinal mushrooms have been noted in research as being potentially able to prevent or reduce the progression of Alzheimer's disease. Here is a summary:

Research from the College of Pharmacy at Korea's Kyungpook National University (Chon *et al.* 2016) found that the *Polyozellus multiplex* mushroom contains compounds called p-terphenyls. These were found to inhibit beta-secretase activity. Remember that beta-secretase is an enzyme involved in deranging beta-amyloid proteins, turning them into beta-amyloid oligomers. The researchers also found the mushroom significantly reduced lipid peroxidation. By doing this, and blocking the activity of these enzymes, the researchers agreed that the mushroom could be used to fight Alzheimer's disease.

A study from Korea's Incheon National University (Im *et al.* 2016) tested the mushroom *Trametes pubescens* and found it to have anti-diabetic effects and anti-dementia effects. Some of it's anti-dementia effects seemed to have come from its ability to inhibit acetylcholinesterase and butyrylcholinesterase. It also inhibited some of the enzymes known to be involved in beta-amyloid oligomer production.

Australian researchers (Bennett *et al.* 2013) found that *Auricularia polytricha* was able to block the beta-amyloid oligomer producing beta-secretase enzymes known to be involved in Alzheimer's disease.

A study from Malaysia's University of Malaya (Samberkar *et al.* 2015) studied Lion's Mane (*Hericium erinaceus*) and Tiger Milk (*Lignosus rhinocerotis*) mushrooms, and found they stimulated new nerve cell and brain cell production. This gave them, according to the researchers, regenerative capacity.

Another mushroom found to have this capacity to increase the regeneration of new brain cells was *Ganoderma lucidum* (Ling-Sing Seow *et al.* 2013).

Research from Italy's University of Catania (Trovato *et al.* 2016) studied the Coriolus versicolor mushroom and found that it released an anti-inflammation substance called lipoxin A4, which produced a "braking signal" for inflammation within the brain's of rats.

Research from China (Wang *et al.* 2012) found that the fruiting body of the *Antrodia camphorata* mushroom blocked brain cell damage from beta-amyloid oligomers and enhanced memory.

Research from Germany's Leibniz Institute of Plant Biochemistry (Geissler *et al.* 2010) found that the *Cortinarius infractus* mushroom also inhibited acetylcholinesterase. But they found this inhibition was selective, meaning a lack of side effects, such as those produced pharmaceutical acetylcholinesterase-inhibitors often used to treat Alzheimer's disease.

Certainly, medicinal mushrooms often have similar medicinal benefits. Therefore, combinations can often be synergistic. For example, researchers from Ewha Womans University in Korea (Seo *et al.* 2010) studied the 12-mushroom extract called Jangwonhwan. The researchers found a modified version of the extract significantly reversed levels of beta-amyloid within the brains of mice.

Mushroom radical scavengers

Remember that peroxidative free radicals are the primary cause for damaging cellular DNA and giving rise to deranged secretases that turn beta-amyloid proteins into brain cell wreckers.

Medicinal mushrooms are incredible radical scavengers. For example, Lion's Mane mushroom has been shown to reduce the risk of Alzheimer's and senility by virtue of radical neutralization. The mushroom also stimulates nerve growth factor, a substance that can reduce dementia and benefit Alzheimer's patients.

An immune-boosting compound called AHCC—Active Hexose Correlated Compound—has been is derived from Shiitake mushroom and its sub-species. This has been shown to stimulate the activity of white blood cells. Further research has showed AHCC stimulates interferon (IFN-y) and tumor necrosis factor (TNF-a) as well.

Much of the dramatic scavenging and immunity effects of mushrooms are due to their polysaccharides and polysaccharide-protein complexes. Laboratory research has isolated multiple polysaccharide types within each species. Twenty-nine unique polysaccharides have been isolated in Maitake, for example.

Mushroom polysaccharides are primarily glucans with different glycosidic linkages, including 1->3 and 1->6 beta glucans, and 1->3 alpha glucans. The complex branching and even helical nature of mushroom glucans appears to be significant. Schizophyllan polysaccharides with (1,3)-b-glucans with 1,3-b-d-linked glucose with 1,6-b-d-glucosyl side groups have been described as "stiff triple-stranded" helices in laboratory research, for example. Schizophyllan (SPG) is an active macrophage stimulator, increasing T cell and NK cell activity and inhibiting various infective agents.

Various immunostimulatory effects have been also attributed to mushrooms' polysaccharide-protein complexes such as PSK (krestin), PSP, lentinan and others. While many varieties contain different levels of the various beta glucans, researchers believe it is their unique protein sequencing that differentiates effects among species.

Medicinal mushrooms also contain a variety of nutrients. Many mushrooms contain significant amounts of protein. Shiitake can be as much as 17% protein while oyster mushrooms can be 30% protein by weight. Several also contain vitamin B complexes. Most edible mushrooms also contain a variety of macro-minerals and trace elements. Shiitake also can contain as much as 126 mg of calcium, and 247 mg of magnesium per serving, for example. Reishi also contains magnesium, calcium, zinc, iron, copper and trace minerals. Many are good sources of selenium.

Maitake and a number of other mushrooms also contain ergosterols (provitamin D2), along with phosphatidylcholine and phosphatidylserine. Shiitake, Reishi and Maitake have been known to increase from less than 500 IU of D2 in indoor growing conditions to 46,000 IU, 2760 IU, and 31,900 IU respectively, following six to eight hours of sunlight exposure (Stamets 2005).

Various antioxidants have been isolated among popular mushroom varieties. Constituents such as ganoderic acid (*G. lucidum*), cordycepic acid (*C. sinensis*), linzhi (*G. frondosa*), agaric acid (several), sizofilan and sizofiran (*S. commune*), galactomannan (*C. sinesis*), and various triterpenoids (several) can actively reduce oxidative radicals and stimulate the immune system.

The density of these in mushrooms is quite incredible. Reishi has over 100 ethanol-soluble triterpenoids. Most of these are antioxidant, and many are anti-inflammatory agents.

Some of the mechanisms of mushrooms to safely stimulate the immune system and produce long-term cleansing benefits are quite complicated. For example, differently branched beta glucans have been observed stimulating immune cells in different ways. For example, certain beta glucans from Maitake will stimulate T-cell production, while differently bonded-chain beta glucans from *Agaricus blazei* stimulate natural killer (NK) cells. Others stimulate B-cells, T-helper cells, lymphokine activated killer cells [LAK], macrophages; and the cytokines interferon gamma, interleukin-2, -12 and tumor necrosis factor [TNF].

Mushrooms significantly detoxify heavy metals inside our bodies, and in their natural environments. Their proteins will bind to certain heavy metals within the soil. These same metabolites become active within the body when eaten, and thus help chelate minerals in our bodies.

For this reason, Cordyceps, Reishi, *Agaricus blazei* and Maitake have been used in China to reduce effects of heavy metal and radiation poisoning.

Mushrooms can be eaten fresh, frozen, drank as teas, cooked with sauces or eaten as supplements. Parts used include the fruiting body (cap and stem) and the mycelia (colonizing rooting network).

While each form will stimulate our immune system, fresh or freeze-dried are preferable. Some supplements are hot-water extracted, and some are alcohol extracted. Hot water extracts likely retain more constituents, although alcohol can extract specific medicinal constituents as well.

Even the common culinary mushrooms have medicinal properties. Oyster mushrooms, Button mushrooms, Agaricus mushrooms, and Shiitake mushrooms all provide incredible nutrition and healing effects.

Panex Ginseng

Ginseng has been used in Traditional Chinese Medicine for centuries for a myriad of cognitive issues. Often it is combined with other herbs or potents, but it has also been used effectively alone.

Panex ginseng is an immune stimulant. *Panax ginseng* will come in white forms and red forms. The color depends upon the aging or drying technique used.

When Ginseng is cultivated and steamed, it is called 'red root' or Hong Shen. Ginseng root will turn red when it is oxidized or processed with steaming. Some feel that red root is better than white, but this really depends upon its intended use, the age of the root, and how it was processed. Soaking Ginseng in rock candy produces a white Ginseng that is called Bai shen. This soaking seems odd, but this has been known to increase some of its constituent levels such as superoxide and nitric oxide. When the root is simply dried, it is called 'dry root' or Sheng shaii shen. Korean Red Ginseng is soaked in a special herbal broth and then dried.

There are a number of species within the *Panax* genus, most of which also contain most of the same adaptogens, referred to as gensenosides. Most notable in the *Panex* genus is American Ginseng, *Panax quinquefolius.*

Ginseng contains camphor, mucilage, panaxosides, resins, saponins, gensenosides, arabinose and polysaccharides, among others.

One study (Heo *et al.* 2012) followed 40 patients with Alzheimer's disease for 24 months—about six months. The patients were split into four groups. One was given 1.5 grams per day of a heat-processed form of ginseng, with a higher concentration of ginsenosides. Another 10 patients were given 3 grams per day of the ginseng and a third group of ten were given 4.5 grams per day. The fourth group was the control group.

The researchers found that all the groups given the ginseng showed significant improvements in memory and Alzheimer's disease symptoms according to ADAS (Alzheimer's Disease Assessment Scale) testing and MMSE (Mini-Mental State Examination) cognitive scores.

Of the three groups, the group given the 4.5 grams per day had the move improvement, and showed improved scores as early as three months after treatment began.

Another study done by some of the same researchers (Heo *et al.* 2008) tested 61 Alzheimer's patients. They were divided into three groups. One group was given 4.5 grams per day of whole red panex ginseng (dried and steamed). Another group was given 9 grams per day. The third group was the control group.

After three months of treatment, the researchers found the groups given either Ginseng dose had higher MMSE scores compared to the control group—1.42 versus -.48. But those given the higher dose had significantly better MMSE scores, as well as ADAS scores.

A study from the Seoul National University Hospital (Lee *et al.* 2008) tested 97 Alzheimer's patients for 12 weeks. They gave 58 patients 4.5 grams per day of Panax ginseng powder. The other patients were the control group.

The researchers found that cognitive scores (MMSE) and Alzheimer's disease symptom scores (ADAS) both improved significantly, to levels higher than the control group.

This and the other studies confirm the usefulness of Panax Ginseng in the treatment of Alzheimer's disease. The researchers in the first (2008) studied stated:

> *"These results suggest that Panax ginseng is clinically effective in the cognitive performance of Alzheimer's patients."*

Davaie loban

Research from Iran's Shahid Beheshti University of Medical Sciences (Tajadini *et al.* 2015) studied 44 Alzheimer's patients for 12 weeks. In a double-blind placebo study, they gave 24 patients 1,500 milligrams per day of the *Davaie loban* and 20 patients took the placebo.

The researchers found that the group treated with the *Davaie loban* had significantly improved ADAS cognitive scores. The treated group also had higher average CDR-SOB (Clinical Dementia Rating Sum of Boxes) problem-solving scores.

FoTi

One of the particularly beneficial herbs of the GETO formulation discussed below is FoTi (*Polygonum multiflorum*). This promising Chinese herb shows clear evidence for the potential to treat Alzheimer's disease.

Researchers from China's Central South University (Chen *et al.* 2010) treated 180 patients with Polygonum multiflorum extract, and 29 patients with the drug piracetam. The FoTi herb significantly increased memory scores and daily living scores using the Mini-Mental State Examination (MMSE) and Ability of Daily Living Scale (ADL) indices. The researchers found a 93% effective rate among the FoTi herbal treatment group, compared to 69% among the piracetam group.

Celery Seed Extract

Researchers from Harvard University and China's Zhengzhou University (Peng *et al.* 2012, 2011, 2010; Tian *et al.* 2016, Zhao *et al.* 2016; Yang *et al.* 2015) have been researching a celery seed extract that prevents Alzheimer's disease pathology and significantly improves memory and cognition.

The early series of studies were led by Ying Peng, PhD, a Postdoctoral Fellow at Harvard Medical School and China's research Institute of Materia Medica. In these, Dr. Peng and associates determined that L-3-n-butylphthalide (L-NBP) extracted from celery seed (*Apium graveolens* Linn) inhibits brain injury and oxidation, while increasing cognition and memory. The research is revealing that the celery seed extract may be a treatment to prevent and possibly reverse Alzheimer's disease.

The laboratory studies have found that the celery seed extract reduces oxidative injury via its ability to decrease tau phosphorylation within brain cells. Tau proteins provide the foundation for microtubule transmissions, which provide the conduits for the instant transfer of information between brain cells. The phosphorylation of the tau proteins slows microtubule transmissions, thereby destabilizing microtubule-MAPT genes.

One study found the celery seed extract reduces beta-amyloid plaque, and illustrated its mechanism was related to blocking the tau protein phosphorylation, which may then prevent future beta-amyloid oligomer and plaque build-up.

Besides this effect, celery seeds have also been shown to increase vascular circulation. This is particularly important when it comes to brain cells. Celery seed is also a significant antioxidant.

Multiple studies have found that mice given the celery seed extract showed significant improvements in spatial learning and decreases in memory deficits.

As of this writing, the research hasn't graduated to human clinical studies. However, celery seed has been used in Ayurveda and Chinese Medicine for thousands of years for a variety of circulatory and nerve issues.

Herbal Combinations

Research has been suggesting that combinations of herbs used in traditional medicines can improve memory and possibly treat Alzheimer's disease. Here are a couple of these that have been clinically examined:

GETO Formula

A study from doctors at the Hubei University of Chinese Medicine (Liu *et al.* 2013) tested 60 Alzheimer's patients with a Chinese medicine formula. The formula is called Bushenhuatanyizhi, with the research acronym GETO. The formula was given to the patients in the form of six grams of granules twice per day for twelve weeks. The researchers gave a control group piracetam.

The researchers found that the Bushenhuatanyizhi treatment significantly improved cognitive function and improved daily life of the Alzheimer's patients.

The formula contains the following herbs:

- Radix Polygoni Multiflori (Heshouwu)—*Polygonum multiflorum*—also called FoTi
- Rhizoma Panacis Japonici (Zhujieshen)—*Panax japonicum*—Panax Ginseng
- Rhizoma Acori Tatarinowii (Shichangpu)—*Acorus tatarinowii*—Grassleaf sweetflag
- Caulis Bambusae In Taeniam (Zhuru)—*Bambusa tuldoides*—Bamboo stem shavings
- Rhizoma Pinelliae (Banxia)—*Pinellia ternate*—Crow dipper / Pinellia
- Poria (Fuling)—Poria mushroom
- Radix palygalae (Yuanzhi)—Thinleaf Milkwort Root

Several of these herbs have been shown to improve memory and cognitive skills in other studies

The GETO formula also contains some of these herbs. In a clinical study presented at the First Alzheimer's Association International Conference on Prevention of Dementia in Washington, D.C., 70 Alzheimer's patients 65 years old and older were given GETO, a placebo or piracetam. The researchers found that GETO resulted in higher memory scores than the placebo groups or the piracetam group.

In addition to these studies, other research on GETO on brain cells and animals have shown similar results—a reversal of plaque and increase cognition symptoms.

According to other research the FoTi, the Poria mushroom and the Thinleaf milkwort root appear to offer the most scientifically verifiable benefits for improving memory and cognition in Alzheimer's disease. But the synergy presented by the various herbs within the GATO and Bushenhuatanyizhi formulas offers another dimension. These incorporate issues related to mood and nervous system improvements that are often overlooked by focusing strictly upon memory loss and the beta-amyloid oligomers, and the resulting plaque.

This said, Chinese herbal medicine is typically applied differently for different people according to the diagnostic study by the Chinese physician. The Chinese physician will typically review the flow of Qi and the relative flows or stagnations among the various organs and meridians of the body before concluding on a treatment that fits the individual patient.

Illustrating the effectiveness of this individual approach in Chinese medicine, researchers from China's Shanghai Geriatric Institute of Chinese Medicine (Yu *et al.* 2012) followed 131 Alzheimer's patients who were given individual Chinese medicine treatments, comparing them to those patients given the Western medicine standard treatment of 5 milligrams of donepezil per day.

Those Alzheimer's patients given the individual Chinese medicine treatments improved in 71% of the cases, while only 20% of the cases worsened. Among those Alzheimer's patients given the donepezil, 56% improved and 35% worsened.

The researchers also tested the patients using functional magnetic resonance imaging (fMRI) testing to determine the relative neuron connectivity between brain centers. Both treatments resulted in improved connectivity. The researchers concluded:

> *"TCM treatment based on syndrome differentiation is effective in improving cognitive function of patients with mild to moderate Alzheimer's disease and increasing the brain function by increasing connectivity between posterior cingulated gyrus and specific areas in the brain."*

PGRJ Formula

A study from Egypt's Green Clinic and Research Center (Yakoot *et al.* 2013) tested a combination of Ginkgo biloba (120 milligrams), Panax ginseng (150 milligrams) and 75- grams of Royal jelly per day. The researchers tested 66 people with mild cognitive impairment for four weeks, plus a control group who were given a placebo.

After the four weeks, the researchers found the group treated with the herbal formula had significantly higher MMSE scores compared with the control group (+2.07 versus +0.13)

The researchers concluded:

> *"This combined triple formula may be beneficial in treating the cognitive decline that occurs during the aging process as well as in the early phases of pathologic cognitive impairment typical of insidious-onset vascular dementia and in the early stages of Alzheimer's disease. Larger-sized studies with longer treatment durations are needed to confirm this."*

Do Cholinesterase Inhibitors Work?

In the past two chapters we've mentioned a few natural remedies that inhibit cholinesterase. Do cholinesterase (also acetylcholinesterase) inhibitors really help Alzheimer's patients?

A 2006 Cochrane review from Oxford University (Birks *et al.*) conducted a meta-analysis of 13 clinical studies of pharmaceutical (synthetic) cholinesterase inhibitors on Alzheimer's patients. The study found that the drugs - donepezil, galantamine or rivastigmine – did result in improvements in cognitive function among Alzheimer's patients. Cognitive function using the Alzheimer's disease ADAS-cog scale, improved an average of 2.7 points in treatments that lasted between six months to a year.

The problem is there was a huge drop-out rate among these studies, due to significant side effects. The study found that a full 29 percent— nearly a third—of the patients suffered from side effects. These included nausea, vomiting and diarrhea.

So we find that natural cholinesterase inhibitors offer an advantage over these pharmaceutical cholinesterase inhibitors: Most come with little or no side effects.

Natural cholinesterase inhibitors also do not act within a vacuum. Pharmaceutical cholinesterase inhibitors have one metabolic effect because they are typically made of one isolated active compound. Herbs and superfoods contain dozens—even hundreds of active compounds. A few of these might inhibit cholinesterase, but others will have other medicinal effects, often buffering or balancing what might typically cause side effects in a pharmaceutical drug.

This is why herbal medicines have been each been used for centuries for a myriad of conditions. Because they have so many constituents— each of which exert medicinal metabolic effects, along with few if any adverse side effects.

Other natural acetylcholinesterase inhibitors

Besides the natural acetylcholinesterase inhibitors mentioned elsewhere in this text, there are a number of other medicinal plants that contain natural acetylcholinesterase inhibiting compounds. Numerous plants contain alkaloids such as quinolizidine, isoquinoline and indoles. For example, willow bark (*Salix alba*) was found to with a 50% inhibition for acetylcholinesterase (Konrath *et al.* 2013, Jukic *et al.* 2012)

Researchers from Turkey's Gazi University (Şenol *et al.* 2010) found that *Heptaptera triquetra*—also named *Colladonia triquetra*, a Mediterranean flowering plant in the parsley family—inhibited acetylcholinesterase at more than 80% in their laboratory studies.

Chapter Eight

Lifestyle Strategies for Alzheimer's

Sleep

Research has found that lack of sleep increases the risk of Alzheimer's disease, increases the risk of dying from the disease, and increases the risk of dementia.

Researchers from Johns Hopkins School of Public Health (Spira *et al.* 2014) studied 70 elderly adults with an average age of 76 years old. They conducted examinations on each, which included positron emission tomography on their brains to determine their "beta-amyloid burden."

Other research from Johns Hopkins (Spira *et al.* 2013) has linked a greater build up of beta-amyloid plaque to the incidence of Alzheimer's disease. This and tau protein fibers tangles within the brain are both recognized as key characteristics of Alzheimer's disease.

The positron emission tomography allowed the researchers to observe these symptoms in the patients. Before this technique, the beta-amyloid protein load and neuron tangles could only be seen during autopsy.

In addition to this analysis, the researchers also conducted questionnaires to determine the sleep habits of the elderly subjects.

They found that greater beta-amyloid deposits were linked with lower sleep quality and greater sleep disturbances. They concluded:

> *"Among community-dwelling older adults, reports of shorter sleep duration and poorer sleep quality are associated with greater beta-amyloid burden."*

Another study also found this same connection. Here University of Toronto medical researchers(Lim *et al.* 2013) followed 698 elderly adults without dementia were followed for six years. Their average age was 82 years old, and 77% were women. The subjects were examined yearly and their sleep habits were recorded.

In this study, beta-amyloid burden and neurofibrillary tangles were identified only among the 201 patients who died during the six years.

The researchers found that among those 201 people who died, 98 of them had developed Alzheimer's disease.

The researchers compared the dead subjects' records of sleep quality with the incidence of Alzheimer's disease. They found that better sleep reduced the incidence of Alzheimer's disease by 33%.

They also specifically linked better sleep with the ε4 gene allele neurofibrillary tangle interaction. Here better sleep reduced the interaction—connected with beta-amyloid buildup—by 42%.

A study on dementia with Lewy bodies confirms the importance of sleep and its effect on dementia. In this study, Mayo Clinic researchers (Murray *et al.* 2013) studied 75 patients with dementia with Lewy bodies together with their sleep histories. They found that 35 of the patients had probable REM sleep behavior disorder.

The existence of Lewy bodies among the brain is also prevalent in Alzheimer's disease. While the mechanisms of the Lewy bodies are still not well understood, they almost always occur with beta-amyloid plaque build up and neurofibril tangles.

The researchers graded the patients using MRIs to estimate their beta-amyloid deposit and neuron tangles burden. Among those with "high-likelihood" dementia—more beta-amyloid and tangles—60% had REM sleep problems. Among those with "low-likelihood" dementia—only 6% had REM sleep behavior disorder.

They concluded that REM sleep difficulties were related to greater risk of dementia.

Other research has found that sleeping helps brain cells clear toxins and consolidate memories. Much of this takes place in REM (rapid eye movement) sleep.

Research from the Sleep and Neuroimaging Laboratory at the University of California at Berkeley (Mander *et al.* 2013) confirmed that memory is linked to poor sleep quality and atrophy of the brain's prefrontal lobe.

While previous studies have confirmed the relationship between cognition and sleep quality, the Berkeley researchers, led by UC Berkeley associate professor of psychology and neuroscience Matthew Walker, Ph.D., compared memory, sleep quality and frontal lobe size among 18 healthy young adults and 15 healthy older adults.

The young adults were primarily in their 20s while the older adults were primarily in their 70s. Before they went to bed they were given 120 word sets to remember. They were tested for memorization of the word sets.

As they were sleeping, brainwave tests using electroencephalopathy (EEG) equipment were measured. This measures the brain's waveforms, illustrating the extent and potential lack of slow wave activity associated with good quality sleep.

In the morning the subjects were then tested once again on the same word pairs, while being given MRI scans (magnetic resonance imaging).

In comparing the MRI scans with the EEG tests, the researchers found an association between the lack of slow wave activity during sleep and the deterioration of the middle frontal lobe of the prefrontal cortex.

On average the older adults had 75% less slow wave sleep. In other words, their sleep quality was 75% worse than the younger subjects. Their word recall was also 55% worse than the word recall of the younger subjects.

According to the researchers, this illustrated that the increased slow wave sleep allowed the younger subjects to likely more efficiently transfer memories from the hippocampus to the prefrontal cortex.

> *"What we have discovered is a dysfunctional pathway that helps explain the relationship between brain deterioration, sleep disruption and memory loss as we get older," commented Dr. Walker. "When we are young, we have deep sleep that helps the brain store and retain new facts and information. But as we get older, the quality of our sleep deteriorates and prevents those memories from being saved by the brain at night."*

This is not the first study that has connected frontal lobe function with sleep quality. In 2001, researchers from Liverpool's John Moores University (Jones *et al.*) also found a link between the frontal lobe tasking and sleep.

The fact that the frontal lobe decreases in size as a person ages has also been established in previous research. In 2009, University of Oslo researchers (Fjell *et al.*) found that the prefrontal cortices deteriorated an average of 0.5% among healthy adults, and significantly more among adults with Alzheimer's disease.

A large review of research at Finland's University of Turku (Alhola *et al.* 2007) clearly established that poor sleep quality is linked to cognitive impairment.

A 2012 study from Germany's Max Planck Institute of Psychiatry (Ahrberg *et al.*) confirmed that academic performance is linked with sleep quality. In this study, 144 medical students underwent sleep studies before taking board exams. The research found that poor exam performance was connected to poor sleep quality among the students. This study also confirmed the association between sleep quality, frontal lobe size and memory.

My book on sleep, *"Natural Sleep Insomnia Solutions"* contains more than 200 natural remedies to help fall asleep and improve sleep quality.

Exercise

A German study (Geidl *et al.* 2011) found that 90 minutes a week of vigorous aerobic exercise or 150 minutes per week of moderate-intensity aerobic exercise dramatically decreased diabetes risk.

A systematic review from researchers from France's University of Toulouse (Barreto Pde *et al.* 2015) found that among 18 studies, exercise training significantly reduced depression levels among dementia patients. They also found that exercise improved most other symptoms of dementia.

Remember the research presented earlier showing the connection between type-2 diabetes and Alzheimer's disease. Since type-2 diabetes is linked with Alzheimer's, it makes sense that strategies that reduce type-2 diabetes will also reduce our risk of Alzheimer's disease. A number of studies have linked type 2 diabetes with exercise.

In a study from the Britain's University of Bristol (Andrews *et al.* 2011) studied 593 type 2 diabetes patients, and found that while the control group (no diet or exercise regimen) worsened over a six month period, those who underwent diet therapy had 28% increased glycemic control, and those who underwent diet and exercise therapy had 31% increased glycemic control after six months.

A study from Canada's University of Western Ontario (Heath *et al.* 2016) tested 23 mature people with a six-month exercise program. One group underwent a moderate-to-high intensity daily workout program on a treadmill. The researchers found this group had improved executive function and improved motor control as gauged by goal-directed eye movement.

A study from the University of Helsinki (Iso-Markku *et al.* 2016) followed 3,050 Finnish twins over a 25 year period and found that those who participated in vigorous physical activity during their midlife years had a 31 percent reduced risk of cognitive decline compared to those with less exercise.

Many other studies have showed the benefits of exercise as a prevention and curative strategy for Alzheimer's.

A meta-analysis of research from Spain's European University Miguel de Cervantes (Santos-Lozano *et al.* 2016) calculated the benefits of exercise for Alzheimer's among 10 high-quality studies on 23,345 people between 70 and 80 years old. The researchers pooled results calculated that physical activity reduces the risk of Alzheimer's disease by 40 percent.

A review of the research from Canada's prestigious Sunnybrook Research Institute (Maliszewska-Cyna *et al.* 2016) concluded:

"Physical activity has the potential to improve overall brain health, which could delay or lessen Alzheimer's disease-related cognitive

deficits and pathology. Ultimately, physical activity influences cognitive function, vascular health and brain metabolism, which taken together offers benefits in both the healthy aging population as well as in Alzheimer's disease patients."

Music and Dance Therapy

This element of exercise brings up two other related strategies: Music Therapy and Dance Therapy. Both have been shown to have significant effects upon Alzheimer's patients.

For example, in a study of five patients with early Alzheimer's disease from France's CHU de Montpellier (Guetin *et al.* 2009), patients underwent 44 sessions of music therapy over a period of 10 weeks. Tests before and after the therapy sessions found that the patients were more relaxed, less anxious and had a greater sense of well-being. Depression levels dropped significantly using the Cornell scale. The researchers concluded:

> *"This preliminary study demonstrates the feasibility as well as the initial efficacy of music therapy in terms of its impact on the overall care for patients suffering from Alzheimer's disease. This easily applicable technique can be useful in treating anxiety and depression in a patient with Alzheimer's disease and also in relieving the emotional and physical burden experienced by the main caregiver."*

Researchers from Sweden's Karolinska Institutet (Palo-Bengtsson *et al.* 1998) studied the effects of social dancing among those with dementia among six patients. They found that the dancing improved moods, communication and behavior. Their retention levels also improved.

One of the more convincing displays for the use of music therapy and dancing is found in the 2014 documentary, *"Alive Inside: A Story of Music and Memory."* This documentary observes Alzheimer's patients' memories being revitalized through the use of listening to music. It shows how practically mute and depressed patients became animated and suddenly able to recall numerous memories as a result of listening to music.

It is a stunning documentary—one that anyone interested in this topic should watch.

Pollution and Chemical Exposure

Remember Dr. Zeiliger's research, as we discussed in the risk factors section. Dr. Zeiliger's research determined that lipophilic chemicals will invade cells by breaking down their fat-containing cells membranes. This will provide further entry for the many other chemicals that may not be fat-soluble, but are water-soluble (hydrophilic).

165

These include so many cancer-causing chemicals and neurotoxins win our waters, air, households and foods including many pesticides and herbicides. Some of the most damaging were fat-soluble toxins present in many products found around the home and business. These include polychlorinated bisphenols (PCBs), organochlorine pesticides, dioxins, polybrominated bisphenyl ethers (PBDEs) and perfluorooctanoic acid esters (PAEs).

Dr. Zeiliger's research found that these hydrophilic toxins gain access into our nerve cells through the increase in lipophilic chemical exposure. As lipophilic exposure damages cell membranes, there is little defense left for the cells to protect themselves from other toxins.

The increase of such lipophilic chemical exposures over the last half-century also correlates precisely with the increase in many neurological diseases among first-world countries, including multiple sclerosis, Alzheimer's, ALS, AD/HD, autism and others.

This is consistent with findings of many other human and animal research (such as Winneke 2011) illustrating the neurotoxicity of these chemicals.

The research also found that many of these lipophilic chemicals will remain in our fat cells for decades, accumulating to produce neuropathic diseases later in life:

> "Persistent organic pollutants (POPs) are long-lived and accumulate in white adipose tissue from which they can pass to the blood and be transported around the body. Due to the slow rates of metabolism and elimination, once absorbed, POPs can persist in the body for 30 years or longer and can build up with time to toxic concentrations. This bioaccumulation of POPs with time over many years accounts for the delayed onset of disease following initial exposure."

Much of the research exposing the link between lipophilic chemicals and neuropathies comes from pharmaceutical studies. Pharmaceutical companies have been blending lipophilic chemicals with hydrophilic chemicals in their medicines in order to increase the absorption and entry of their chemical medicines—many of which are hydrophilic—into cells.

The research has also determined that hydrophilic toxic compounds do not require lipophilic compound exposure concurrently: We don't have to be exposed to both simultaneously.

Rather, lipophilic compounds will build up in the system and increase assimilation of hydrophilic toxins long after the initial lipophilic toxin exposures.

This, according to Dr. Zeiliger's research, will allow many toxins that produce neural damage to penetrate the blood-brain barrier due to the lipophilic toxin accumulation:

> "Lipophilic chemicals were found to facilitate the absorption of hydrophilic chemicals across the body's lipophilic membranes. It is proposed here that the lipophilia of these exogenous chemicals induces neurological disorders by permeating lipophilic membranes, including the blood brain barrier, thus enabling the entry for toxic hydrophilic species that would otherwise not be absorbed."

It is ironic that the very substances—toxic chemicals—that humanity thought it was so smart in inventing and producing are in turn damaging our intelligence in the end in form of dementia and other neurological disorders.

Air Pollution

Remember also the correlation discussed between Alzheimer's disease and air pollution. Researchers from Mexico City, Boise State University and the University of Montana (Calderón-Garcidueñas *et al.* 2016) found that people exposed to fine particular matter (PM2.5) within air pollution, along with ozone, at levels abot the Environmental Protection Agency standards is associated with greater incidence of Alzheimer's disease.

This study also found that even younger people from Mexico City showed signs of deranged beta-amyloid plaque along with tau tangles and other signs of Alzheimer's disease.

In a review of research from George Washington University (Power *et al.* 2016), 18 different studies found an association between at least one air pollutant and one form of dementia—with some linking Alzheimer's to air pollution.

Air pollution includes smoking. Many studies (Hausinkveld *et al.* 2016) have linked Alzheimer's with smoking. The fine particles associated with cigarette smoke are the most damaging. This combined with the risk of lung cancer should help motivate any smoker to quit.

By the way, healthy indoor air can be aided with the use of indoor plants (Wolverton 1997).

Pesticides

Today over five billion pounds of pesticides are applied to our crops, households and other areas we share with insects. Many of these pesticides have been shown to be neurotoxic—they damage nerves and nerve transmission. Three-quarters of the twelve most dangerous chemicals (aka the "dirty dozen") used by man are pesticides according to the Stockholm Convention on Persistent Organic Pollutants.

Many of these pesticides have been proven to be neurotoxins. Organochlorine hydrocarbons are one of the most widely used types of pesticides in commercial farming enterprises. These include DDT (dichlorodiphenyltrichloroethane), which is banned in the U.S. but not in many other countries where lots of our food is grown. DDT's analogs such as dicofol and methoxychlor are also in use. Other neurotoxic organochlorine hydrocarbons include hexachlorocyclohexane, lindane, gamma-hexachlorocyclohexane, endosulfan, chlordane, heptachlor, aldrin, dieldrin, endrin, kelevan, mirex, chlordecone, toxaphene and isobenzan. Most of these will cause changes to the central nervous system by altering potassium, sodium or calcium ion channels.

Today many of the organochlorines have been replaced by organophosphates, but these will alter neurons by blocking acetylcholinesterase enzymes. Cholinesterase enzymes are acetylcholine inhibitors. Increased acetylcholine availability leads to excessive to neuron firing, resulting in nerve excitability, long term nervousness, nerve weakness and even paralysis.

We have heard about the toxicity of pesticides. Let's look at an example of just how real this toxicity is.

A review of research from Belgium's Catholic University of Louvain (Van Maele-Fabry et al. 2012) found that Parkinson's disease is linked to occupational exposure to pesticides.

The researchers, working with the Louvain Center for Toxicology and Applied Pharmacology, analyzed studies between 1985 and 2011 that looked at pesticide exposure by workers who handled pesticides. These included farm workers who sprayed pesticides.

The research found that those who handled pesticides were significantly more likely to contract Parkinson's disease. In four studies, where the Parkinson's diagnoses were confirmed by neurologists, those handling pesticides had an average of over two-and-a-half times the risk of contracting Parkinson's disease. The increased risk ranged from 46% higher to almost four-and-a-half times higher among the workers.

Three cohort studies, which followed larger populations and compared them to the general population, concluded that workers handling pesticides had close to twice the risk of contracting Parkinson's disease than the rest of the population. It should also be noted that the general population typically also has constant contact with pesticide residue in the form of foods and household pesticides.

One of these cohort studies showed workers handling pesticides had almost three times the rate of contracting Parkinson's disease.

The researchers found significant rates of increased Parkinson's disease risk among workers in banana plantations, sugarcane fields and pineapple farms.

Another study, this from the University of California (Gonzalez *et al.* 2012), tested Mexican-American mothers and their children living in agricultural regions with higher pesticide exposure. The researchers monitored 202 mother-and-daughter pairs for relative levels of paraoxonase, acetylcholinesterase, and butyrylcholinesterase enzymes and their respective activity among neurons.

The researchers confirmed that pesticide exposures not only affect adult acetylcholinesterase levels, but also affect children under the age of nine years old more than adults. They also concluded that children born of pesticide-exposed parents have even lower levels of acetylcholinesterase—relating to the higher risks of nerve disorders.

Other pesticides, such as imidacloprid and related neonicotinoids are neurotoxins in turn bind to nicotinic acetylcholine receptors—important to healthy nerve firing. These pesticides are also suspected in bee colony collapse disorder.

Manufacturers of neonicotinoid pesticides have claimed that the chemicals will not affect human acetylcholine receptors. However, a study by researchers from the Tokyo Metropolitan Institute of Medical Science (Kimura-Kuroda *et al.* 2012) found that the neonicotinoids imidacloprid and acetamiprid *"had greater effects on mammalian neurons than those previously reported in binding assay studies."*

As for those of us not handling pesticides on the job or at home, pesticide residues are found on a majority of commercially grown foods. In a review of the research by Cornell University's Dr. David Pimentel (2005), 73% to 90% of conventional fruits and vegetables contain pesticide residues, with at least 5% of those pesticide levels above FDA tolerance amounts.

While the cost of organic foods might be a tad higher in the store, the price paid in the long run for pesticides in terms of liver disorders and nervous disorders such as Alzheimer's and Parkinson's—as well as environmental damage to our bees, waterways and soils—makes the real price for organic foods cheap in comparison.

Oral Health Care

As pointed out in the risk section, Alzheimer's disease had been linked to periodontal disease and gingivitis. The mechanism is that when disease-causing bacteria overload our teeth, they will leak their endotoxins into the blood stream. Some of these toxins cause lipid peroxidation. This of course is linked to the pathway of cells producing the enzymes that derange the beta-amyloid proteins, producing brain-damaging oligomers.

Certainly, brushing and flossing after meals are important strategies. Adding periodic water pik cleansing and regular cleanings at the dental hygienist will help prevent the build up of bacteria and the plaque they cause in our teeth and gums.

However, another productive strategy is to help defend ourselves against these bacteria using oral probiotics.

I have discussed these strategies extensively in my book on the subject, *"Oral Probiotics."*

Leaky Gut and Dysbiosis

We discussed this topic in the Anti-Alzheimer's Diet chapter earlier, but it makes sense to elaborate on the element of gut permeability. When the intestines host an abundance of pathogenic bacteria combined with increased intestinal permeability—also called leaky gut syndrome—the risk of Alzheimer's disease increases. This has been established among several studies, of which were reviewed by scientists (Hu *et al.* 2016), who stated:

> *"The increased permeability of intestine and blood-brain barrier induced by gut microbiota disturbance will increase the incidence of neurodegeneration disorders. Gut microbial metabolites and their effects on host neurochemical changes may increase or decrease the risk of Alzheimer's disease."*

In another study, researchers from German scientists (Leblhuber *et al.* 2015) studied 22 Alzheimer's patients. They found that 73 percent of them (16 patients) had above-normal levels of calprotectin in their bloodstreams. Other studies have confirmed that high levels of calprotectin in the blood indicate a condition of abnormally increased intestinal permeability—leaky gut syndrome.

Besides the supplementation of probiotics and probiotic foods, there are a number of strategies that can be employed to reduce gut permeability or leaky gut syndrome. This is a big topic. A detailed explanation of strategies to reduce increased intestinal permeability can be found in my book, *"The Science of Leaky Gut Syndrome."*

Hydration

Dehydration (lack of sufficient fluid intake) can contribute to systemic inflammation and toxicity. Fluids are critical for the body's ability to neutralize and remove peroxidative radicals. This has been confirmed by research.

In a dehydrated state, our mucosal membranes and tissues weaken. Every cell is stressed. It is for this reason that some research has found that many ulcerated conditions can be cured simply by drinking adequate water.

Water is directly involved in inflammatory metabolism. Research has revealed that increased levels of inflammatory mediators such as histamine are released during periods of dehydration in order to help balance fluid levels within the bloodstream, tissues, kidneys and other organs.

Research by Fereydoon Batmanghelidj, M.D. (1987; 1990) led to the realization that the blood becomes more concentrated during dehydration. As this concentrated blood enters the capillaries of the respiratory system, histamine is released in an attempt to balance the blood dilution.

The immune system is also irrevocably aligned with the body's water availability. The immune system utilizes water to produce lymph fluid. Lymph fluid circulates immune cells throughout the body, enabling them to target specific intruders. The lymph is also used to escort toxins out of the body.

Intracellular and intercellular fluids are necessary for the removal of nearly all toxins—and pretty much every metabolic function of every cell, every organ and every tissue system.

Water also increases the availability of oxygen to cells. Water balances the level of free radicals. Water flushes and replenishes the digestive tract. Thus, water is necessary for the proper digestion of food, as well as nutrition utilization. The gastric cells of the stomach and the intestinal wall cells require water for proper digestive function. The health of every cell depends upon water.

There is certainly reason to believe that dehydration is a key factor for toxicity and inflammation.

As Dr. Jethro Kloss pointed out decades ago (1939), the average person loses about 550 cubic centimeters of water through the skin, 440 cc through the lungs, 1550 cc through the urine, and another 150 cc through the stool. This adds up to 2650 cc per day, equivalent to a little over 2-½ quarts (about 85 fluid ounces).

Meanwhile many have suggested drinking eight 8-oz glasses per day. This 64 ounces would result in a state of dehydration.

In 2004, the National Academy of Sciences released a study indicating that women typically meet their hydration needs with approximately 91 ounces of water per day, while men meet their needs with about 125 ounces per day. This study also indicated that approximately 80% of water intake comes from water/beverages and 20% comes from food. Therefore, we can assume a minimum of 73 ounces of fresh water for the average adult woman and 100 ounces of fresh water for the average adult man should cover our hydration needs. That is significantly more water than the standard eight glasses per day—especially for men.

The data suggests that 50-75% of Americans have chronic dehydration. Dr. Batmanghelidj, probably the world's foremost researcher on water, suggests a ½ ounce of water per pound of body weight. Drinking an additional 16-32 ounces for each 45 minutes to an hour of strenuous activity is also a good idea, with some before and some after exercising. More water should accompany temperature and elevation extremes, and extra sweating or fevers. Note also that alcohol is dehydrating.

A glass of room-temperature water first thing in the morning on an empty stomach can significantly hydrate our mucosal membranes. Then we should be drinking water throughout the day. Our evening should accompany reduced water consumption, so our sleep is not disrupted by urination.

There are easy ways to tell whether we are dehydrated. A sensation of being thirsty indicates that we are already dehydrated. A person with toxicity and/or inflammation should thus be drinking enough water to never feel thirsty. Dark yellow urine also indicates dehydration. Our urine color should be either clear, or bright yellow after taking multivitamins.

Drinking just any water is not advised. Municipal water and even bottled water can contain many contaminants that can burden the immune system and trigger inflammation. Care must be taken to drink water that has been filtered of most toxins yet is naturally mineralized. Research has confirmed that distilled water and soft water are not advisable. Natural mineral water is best. Please refer to the author's book, *"Pure Water"* for more information on water content, filters and water therapy.

Sunshine and Vitamin D

The medical need for adequate sunshine has been revealed in numerous studies, where deficiencies in vitamin D have been linked with at least 70 medical conditions. Alzheimer's is no exception. A number of studies have found that those with Alzheimer's tend to also have low levels of vitamin D in their bloodstreams (Landel *et al.* 2016 and others).

A study from the University of Edinburgh (Russ *et al.* 2016) analyzed mortality rates from deaths related to Alzheimer's disease and other forms of dementia from around the world. They found that dementia mortality is higher among regions furthest from the equator—notably those regions that receive the least amount of sunshine. Other studies (such as Grant 2016) have had similar findings.

A study from Korea's Gyeongsang National University (Raha *et al.* 2016) found that vitamin D directly blocked the pathway for production of deranged beta-amyloid oligomers, through the suppression of lipid peroxidation. Other studies have also shown that vitamin D helps neutralize lipid radicals.

Supplemented vitamin D may be useful for those who are deficient. A study published in the *Journal of Alzheimer's Disease* (Miller *et al.* 2016) found that supplementing 50,000 IU of vitamin D per week significantly increased levels of beta-amyloid proteins in the bloodstream. As discussed earlier, higher levels in the bloodstream correlate with lower levels in the brain, and a reduced incidence of Alzheimer's disease.

As I discussed in depth in my book, *"The Healing Power of Sunshine,"* not all vitamin D is alike. The best form of vitamin D is produced by the skin and liver as a result of ultraviolet-B exposure. This can be accomplished by outdoor sun exposure during certain times of the day and year. For those in environments with less UV-B exposure, there is an easy option: UV-B bulbs and lamps. Learn more in my book mentioned above.

Synthetic Living

The assumption of modern chemistry is there is no inherent difference between a chemical synthesized in a lab or manufacturing facility from one made in nature by living processes. This assumption has led humankind to haphazardly invent new synthetic chemical combinations with reckless abandon. Blinded by patents and profits, the industrial chemical complex has assumed there is no environmental cost.

When we interfere with any one part of nature's cycling of molecules, we can interrupt the balance of the rest of the cycle, often causing reverberations on an exponential basis. This is precisely what humans have unfortunately arrived at after two hundred years of industrial technological development.

Spectroscopy tests show that when two different ions with different atomic character are brought together, the resulting compound will display different spectra than either did independently. The combination's waveforms are not necessarily a composite of the two. It is a new waveform combination resulting from the resonating interference of the combining elements together with its natural catalysts and environment.

Most biological combinations require a catalyst (a facilitator) to complete. These catalysts may supply or borrow electrons in an oxidizing or reducing mechanism to assist in the combination. They will also supply the needed electromagnetic energy to speed up the reaction. Nature's catalysts provide specific changes in molecular structure—creating a unique *fingerprint* of sorts.

Synthetic catalysts will produce a different molecular combination, even if the original ions or compounds are the same as found in nature.

Even if the combination may be similar to nature's version, often the molecular orientation—as with trans fats—will be subtly different.

Because it is not cohesive—or stable—with the body's components, a synthetically combined compound throws off the balance between oxidizers and reducers in the body. This produces increased levels of oxidized or oxidative radicals, which will rob electrons or ions from the molecules that make up our tissues—notably our cell membranes, and the membranes that make up our mitochondria.

This later point—damage to the membranes of our mitochondria—is now implicated as the functional event that causes dementia, chronic fatigue and fibromyalgia. When the mitochondria within our brain cells are damaged by free radicals, these brain cells begin to shut down.

In chronic fatigue and fibromyalgia—often considered the same condition—damage to the membranes of mitochondria shuts down the energy production of cells.

This is because mitochondria is where are energy is produced. The mitochondria house the Krebs cycle, which converts glucose and oxygen to heat and energy. As they become damaged and dysfunctional, we experience fatigue.

While our bodies are built to handle moderate levels of free radicals, our chemical industrial complex is overloading our body with synthetics, which produce these oxidized or oxidative radicals within the body. This oxidizing potency of toxins leads to an overload of acids (H+), causing excessive acidosis, and the subsequent degeneration of our brain tissues.

Consider fats. When palm and coconut oils are cooled, they become hardened. This makes them good thickening agents for cooking and good for frying. In an attempt to match nature, in 1902 German Wilhelm Normann patented the first hydrogenation process, which was eventually purchased by Proctor and Gamble, leading to Crisco® oil and eventually margarine. When nutritionists convinced us that *"all saturated fats are bad"* in the sixties and seventies, margarine sales took off. Processors also found that frying oil had a better shelf life and was cheaper if cottonseed oil and soybean oil were *partially hydrogenated*. Because these oils do not normally harden at room temperature as does palm, coconut and lard, hydrogenation allowed processors to use the less expensive oils for frying, spreading and cooking.

Hydrogenation means to *saturate* hydrogen onto all of the available bonds of the central molecule. Whereas a natural substance might have a double bond between carbon and other atoms, hydrogen gas can be bubbled through the substance—using a catalyst to spark the reaction—to attach more hydrogen to the molecule. To saturate carbon bonds with hydrogen, catalyst is added, and the oil undergoes the bubbling of hydrogen within a heated catalytic environment. This saturation synthetically changes the oil's melting point, giving it more versatility at a lower cost.

Let's review. Food scientists took real foods—oil extracted from soybeans or cottonseed—and synthetically converted them into what appeared to be the same molecular structure, but with a different melting point. Harmless, yes? Think again. After decades of use and millions of heart attacks and strokes later, health researchers began realizing that partially hydrogenated oils have damaging effects upon the cardiovascular system.

While the saturated or partially saturated molecule was the same formula, the synthetic process of hydrogenation created an unusual (transversed) molecular structure called a *trans- at*. Trans fat is now implicated in a various degenerative disorders, including atherosclerosis, dementia, liver disease, irritable bowel syndrome, and Alzheimer's disease among others. While the epidemic increase in cardiovascular disease has focused billions of dollars into research, the consumption of trans fats was altogether overlooked. Why? Because researchers assumed that hydrogenated soybean oil was harmless because its molecularly-identical cousin—raw soybean oil—was harmless, and even healthy because it was a polyunsaturated oil.

The mechanism whereby trans fats produce damage in the body is lipid peroxidation. Because trans fats are less stable than cis-fats, and because fats make up our cell membranes, trans fats become more readily damaged, producing what is called lipid peroxides. Lipid peroxides damage blood vessel walls and other tissue systems, producing cardiovascular disease and other degenerative disorders.

So now researchers realize that the orientation—polarity and spin—of a molecule can have altogether different effects from the same molecule rotated in the orientation nature designed.

Nature normally orients healthy oil molecules—and many other nutrients—in *cis* formation: They are oriented so that the hydrogens are on the same side with the other molecular bonds. A *trans* configuration has hydrogens on the opposite side of the bonds.

This *cis* and *trans* orientation issue is also evident from the opposite perspective in the case of resveratrol. Resveratrol is a phytochemical constituent of more than seventy different plant species, including many fruits such as berries and grapes. Studies have shown natural resveratrol has many biological properties important to health. These include antioxidant, anti-bacterial, anti-viral, anti-fungal, liver-cleansing, mood-elevation, and amyloid-plaque-removal properties. Resveratrol also activates an enzyme-protein called sirtuin 1, which appears to promote DNA repair.

However, these effects are exclusive to the natural form: *trans*-resveratrol. Not surprisingly, pasteurization and other processing will convert the *trans*-resveratrol molecule to its less effective cousin, *cis*-resveratrol.

Another example of human meddling is vitamin E. While natural vitamin E is d-alpha-tocopherol, the synthetic version is dl-alpha-tocopherol. While d-alpha-tocopherol has one isomer, dl-alpha-tocopherol has eight. One of those eight is similar to the one natural isomer. The difference is that the natural version is more readily bioavailable than the dl-alpha version.

Illustrating this, in one study (Burton *et al*. 1998), subjects took either natural vitamin E or the synthetic vitamin E. Natural vitamin E levels in the bloodstream for all subjects were at least twice as high as levels of the synthetic versions. After twenty-three days, tissue levels were also significantly higher for the natural vitamin E group, compared to the synthetic vitamin E group. These tests illustrated that nature's form of vitamin E is more readily absorbed and utilized than the synthetic version.

Furthermore, Oregon State University researchers (Traber *et al*. 1998) found that humans excrete synthetic vitamin E three times faster than natural vitamin E. So not only does the human body not readily absorb the synthetic version, but it wants to rid the body of this version three times faster.

This ratio was confirmed in another test (Kiyose *et al*. 1997) showing that it took three times the quantity of synthetic vitamin E to reach the same levels achieved by natural vitamin E among seven women.

Vitamin C provides another example. Gas chromatography has revealed several structural differences between synthetic vitamin C (isolated ascorbic acid) and natural forms of vitamin C. While many people supplement with isolated ascorbic acid, nature provides a completely different structure. Not only is the molecule itself different, but natural vitamin C is naturally bonded—or *chelated*—to other natural compounds called biofactors. These include bioflavonoids, minerals, rutin, and other biochemicals produced by living organisms or nature's ecology. These are often referred to as *ascorbates*.

Synthetic vitamin D—referred to as vitamin D_2 or ergocalciferol—is also molecularly different from naturally produced cholecalciferol. In a study published in 2004 by Armas *et al*., twenty healthy male subjects were given single doses of 50,000 IU of either vitamin D_2 or nature's form, vitamin D_3.

After supplementation, their 25-hydroxyvitamin D (25-ODH) levels in the blood were measured over a twenty-nine day period. The measured 25-ODH levels were the same between the D_2 and D_3 in subjects for the first three days. However, blood levels of 25-OHD fell dramatically after that for the D_2 subjects. The D_3 group's 25-OHD levels continued to rise, and peaked fourteen days after the initial dose was given.

After 29 days, the subjects taking D_2 had concentrations of less than a third of the levels of the D_3 subjects. Using a calculation called the *area under the plasma curve* (AUC), this translated to the synthetic D_2's potency being about one-tenth of the potency of the more natural form of vitamin D_3. In reality, our bodies produce a sulfated form of vitamin D_3 from the sun's UVB rays.

In a recent study from Washington University's School of Medicine (Nicola *et al.* 2007), 168 healthy postmenopausal women were tested for supplemented calcium versus dietary (natural) sources of calcium. Women whose calcium intake was primarily from supplementation—even though their dosages were higher—had lower bone mineral density levels than the women whose calcium intake was primarily from dietary sources. Those taking supplements plus good dietary sources had the highest totals.

Naturally occurring nutrients are electromagnetically different than synthesized chemicals. The resulting quanta of spin, angular momentum and so on will vary between nature's version and a version synthesized in a lab or processed beyond nature's intended course.

The same goes for anything we are exposing our bodies to. Whether it is clothing, furniture, sheets, water, air or food, synthetic chemistry produces toxic radicals that burdens our body's immune and detoxification systems. This in turn adds to our inflammatory stress, and our body's ability to remove free radicals.

The equation relates specifically to Alzheimer's disease because as we've proven here, Alzheimer's disease is a conditional result of an imbalance between free radicals and our body's ability to neutralize them.

Brain Training

There are a bunch of different computer brain training courses out there that pitch they can reduce dementia risk. Can brain training really stave off dementia and Alzheimer's disease? This question has been posed variously over the past couple of decades. With Alzheimer's disease running rampant among aging generations, researchers, doctors and anyone over 50 are asking this question.

The answers have varied, depending upon the source and the date of the source. A decade ago the answer from everyone was most certainly.

And initial testing—depending upon the program—showed immediate cognitive benefits: Emphasis on immediate.

But the question soon became: Are there lasting benefits to cognitive training?

177

Cognitive Activity

In 2007, a study from Chicago's Rush University Medical Center, led by Robert Wilson, PhD and associates, studied 700 older people for up to five years. The researchers rated their cognitive activity during annual examinations.

After they died, the researchers tested their brains for Alzheimer's beta-amyloid brain plaque, Lewy bodies or cerebral blockages. They also assessed the patients for other forms of dementia as well as mild cognitive impairment through the years.

The researchers found that more frequent cognitive activity resulted in a 42 percent reduced incidence of Alzheimer's disease. They also found that those with low cognitive activity had 2.6 times the incidence of Alzheimer's disease. Increased cognitive activity also reduced mild cognitive impairment incidence.

This and similar studies seemed to assure others that brain training exercises would certainly stave off Alzheimer's disease.

The researchers concluded:

"Level of cognitively stimulating activity in old age is related to risk of developing dementia."

Does brain training work?

Then in 2010, researchers started seeing cracks in the ice. Another study led by Dr. Wilson of Rush University followed 1,157 mature folks for about 11 years. Of the total population studied, 148 had Alzheimer's disease and 395 had mild cognitive impairment.

The research found that cognitive activity reduces cognitive decline by a robust 52% for every one percent increase in cognitive activity. But this was only among those with no cognitive impairment.

But for those who had mild cognitive impairment, there was no improvement as a result of greater cognitive activity.

And for those who had Alzheimer's disease, the study found for each one percent increase in cognitive activity, cognitive decline advanced by 42 percent.

Yes. Somehow, the increased cognitive training also advanced the Alzheimer's patients' rate of decline.

In these studies, cognitive activity was considered as activity related to lifestyle, but also included games and puzzles. For example, in this last study, cognitive activities included reading newspapers, magazines and books; playing games like cards, checkers, crosswords or other puzzles; or educational trips such as museum visits.

The early assumption was that if cognitive activity decreases risk of dementia, then brain training will surely help.

Not so fast. Other research has found little or no improvement among brain training exercises. The issue is long-term results. In the near term there might be some improvement just after completing the training. But few long-term effects have been found.

Illustrating the progression of the science, in January of 2016, the Federal Trade Commission settled with Luma Labs – maker of Luminosity. The company elected to refund $2 million back to its subscribers, in response to a charge of deceptive advertising.

The point is that Luma made claims that brain training staves off Alzheimer's and dementia, while little proof exists for such a claim.

"There's little evidence that playing brain-training games improves overall cognitive ability."

So said Peter V. Rabins, M.D., a professor at the University of Maryland and a director of geriatric psychiatry at Johns Hopkins University School of Medicine.

"When you use these games, you may see improvements in how well you play those games. Unfortunately, the benefit has not been shown to improve memory or thinking in general. This means that, at least as of now, the benefits will not generalize to other activities in your life." "Spending even 100 hours playing brain games isn't enough to build cognitive capacity," Rabins adds.

In a study of 60 Alzheimer's patients between 2004 and 2012, Spanish researchers (Martínez-Moreno *et al.* 2016) found that only 52 percent of the responder group (a portion of the whole group) saw any improved cognitive performance. Many of the Alzheimer's patients were non-responders, meaning they didn't respond to the training at all. The researchers concluded that some Alzheimer's patients will benefit from cognitive training while others won't:

"The response to a cognitive stimulation treatment of some subjects over others is linked to cognitive and functional capacity. This research contributes to characterize the neuropsychological profile that differentiates subjects who respond better than others before and after the treatment. This should contribute to customize and optimize neuropsychological interventions in patients with Alzheimer's disease."

Speed of Processing Training

The mistake of many studies could be that not all brain training is alike. According to Jerri Edwards, PhD of the University of South Florida:

"The mistake some people make is thinking that all brain training is the same."

While many forms of brain training have uncertain continuing bene-fits, the exception appears to be a particular type of training, called Speed of Processing Training — also called Useful Field of View training or UFOV.

The researchers (Edwards *et al.* 2016) conducted a meta-analysis re-view of more than 50 studies examining speed of processing training over extended periods. The study followed 2,832 people between 65 and 94 for an average of 10 years.

The researchers found that when 11 or more sessions of this training was completed, the risk of dementia was decreased by 48 percent over a 10 year period.

The risk of dementia was decreased by eight percent for every session of speed training completed.

"This highly specific exercise is designed to improve the speed and accuracy of visual attention or someone's mental quickness," says Dr. Edwards.

The training tests both reaction speed and accuracy. In one task, the person must identify an object at the center of a screen while locating a target. This may be a related object in peripheral vision. The task of locat-ing the peripheral object improves as the training continues. Or the pe-ripheral target might be surrounded by distracting objects. This forces the person to work harder to stay focused, according to Dr. Edwards.

In their study, those completing speed of processing training had im-proved performance across cognitive, behavioral, functional and real world measurements. These included improvements in attention, moods, quality of life and function.

Some of the research showed that speed of processing training im-proved reaction time. While driving, the brain training yielded an extra 22 feet of stopping distance at 55 mph - and a 36 percent decrease in dan-gerous maneuvers.

"Some brain training does work, but not all of it," Edwards con-cluded. "People should seek out training backed by multiple peer-reviewed studies. The meta-analysis of this particular speed of processing training shows it can improve how people function in their everyday lives."

The speed of processing training (UFOV) program was developed by Karlene Ball, PhD, and Daniel Roenker, PhD at the University of Alabama Birmingham and Western Kentucky University. It is exclusively licensed to Posit Science Inc.

Learning Another Language

Research has found that learning or knowing a second language delays the onset of Alzheimer's disease symptoms.

A study from Toronto's York University (Bailystok *et al.* 2007) followed 184 Alzheimer's patients, of whom 51 percent were bilingual. The researchers found that the bilinguals showed dementia symptoms four years later than those who spoke only one language.

In addition, the rate of decline using the MMSE examination illustrated that their rate of progression of the disease was also slower than those who spoke only one language.

This research was confirmed by other studies.

Cognitive Reserve: Raising our Consciousness

In general, cognitive training has not shown much benefit, but cognitive stimulation has. For example, a review of research from London's King College (Huntley *et al.* 2015) conducted a meta-analysis of multiple studies on cognitive training versus cognitive stimulation. Cognitive training means standardized brain games and tasks that target specific functions. Cognitive stimulation means a range of different social and cognitive activities that stimulate intellectual thinking and engagement.

Anyway, the researchers found—consistent with the previously mentioned research—that cognitive training had little evidence of significant benefit to reducing Alzheimer's disease or dementia.

However, cognitive stimulation did produce significant benefits, in terms of accomplishing better MMSE scores and ADAS-cog scores. This means reducing the incidence and symptoms of Alzheimer's and other forms of dementias.

Like others, University of Iowa researchers (Guzmán-Vélez and Tranel 2015) found multiple studies confirming that learning or knowing a second language can stave off symptoms of Alzheimer's. But analyzing the realm of cognitive research reveals an important issue for Alzheimer's: The notion of cognitive reserve.

Cognitive reserve is the connection between several intellectual variables and Alzheimer's risk. The more education one has; better reading skills; and intellectual skills one has, the lower the risk of developing Alzheimer's symptoms.

These variables include, as we've discussed earlier, greater education, intelligence and socioeconomic status. Multiple studies have confirmed this:

A 2004 study from Sweden followed 931 people 75 years old or older. They found that the incidence of dementia among less-educated people was 3.4 times those who were better educated. Those with a lower socio-economic status (lower income) had a 60 percent higher incidence of dementia.

A 2012 study from Germany's University of Heidelberg (Sattler *et al.* 2012) followed 500 people and found that those who were "cognitively active" had a significantly reduced risk of developing Alzheimer's disease. They also found that higher education and higher socioeconomic status reduced the risk of Alzheimer's, as well as mild cognitive impairment.

Researchers from the School of Medicine at Boston University (Jefferson *et al.* 2011) studied 951 older people (average age 79) and found those who had a higher education had significantly lower risk of Alzheimer's. Those with higher reading scores—tested with the National Adult Reading Test—also had a significantly lower risk of Alzheimer's.

The question now becomes how to make the appropriate changes to take advantage of these findings. Higher socioeconomic status has been investigated from various angles in innumerable studies over the past three decades. The ongoing conclusion of why higher socioeconomic status affects disease is education: Those with a higher socioeconomic status are in that condition primarily because they are better educated. Or they are better educated as a result of being born into a family of higher socioeconomic status.

This is a practical matter. People who get higher degrees typically get better paying jobs. And kids in families with higher paying jobs typically become better educated.

Certainly learning a new language, reading more and some continuing our education would improve our status. Why? Because these have the ability to raise our consciousness.

But we must be careful about this. Gathering a bunch of details about things that don't really interest us doesn't exercise our frontal lobes very much. We must learn things that we are interested in learning—things that raise our consciousness.

Raising our intellectual function to a higher state of awareness is the key. This means utilizing our mental resources to search the meaning of life. Understanding who we are and our purpose for existing. Such a mission would effectively raise our consciousness. It would require learning new languages—languages relating to philosophy and spiritual life. This engagement of our intellectual abilities goes straight to the frontal lobe. This endeavor is, in other words, to exercise both our frontal lobe and our hippocampus.

Yes, the frontal lobe and hippocampus—these critical brain regions—are like muscles. They have to be exercised.

The research showing that 'cognitive reserve' reduces Alzheimer's incidence and symptoms illustrates that raising our consciousness to a higher state of awareness is a practical step for anyone concerned about delaying or preventing the onset of Alzheimers.

The researchers mentioned above stated in their conclusion about cognitive reserve:

> *"In sum, because cognitive reserve cannot be measured directly, and in vivo measures of neuropathology are often unavailable, operationalizing and studying how cognitive reserve moderates the relationship between neuropathology and clinical outcome has proven to be quite challenging. Moreover, it is extremely challenging to establish cause-and-effect relationships between measures of cognitive reserve and outcome variables (usually onset of diagnosis), given the nature of these variables, and thus far, only correlations have been established."*

The reason it is hard to measure directly is because raising ones consciousness is a difficult thing to quantify.

Part III: Consciousness and Alzheimer's

Chapter Nine

The Brain and the Self

Alzheimer's disease is a mystery condition to researchers, doctors, family members and patients alike. The question relates to consciousness. What is going on with the consciousness of the Alzheimer's patient? Is this simply a mechanical problem of the brain? Or is there a deeper component involved?

This, together with the lack of clear prevention and treatment strategies, creates hopelessness. This condition devastates not just the sufferers, but the family and friends of the sufferers. This leads to a loss of hope. It leads to broken hearts and broken families.

The purpose of this last section and chapter is to comb the current science to better understand this condition in relation to consciousness.

This chapter will show reason for renewed hope and understanding: Hope from the reality that this condition does not destroy the person within. Understanding from learning the condition is not a permanent reality.

To fully comprehend Alzheimer's Disease, we need to be clear from a scientific perspective, just what the brain and mind is—and just what memory is. After all, Alzheimer's disease is memory dysfunction. And memory dysfunction relates to not just a dysfunction of the brain: It is also a dysfunction of the mind.

But what about the beta-amyloid plaque and oligomers found in the brains of most Alzheimer's patients?

We discussed these in detail in this book. There is no doubt that the physiological processes involved in Alzheimer's disease are complex. The information discussed earlier certainly confirms this. But there are still missing pieces to the mechanisms. This relates to the larger picture of how the brain and the mind functions with respect to consciousness.

With these points in mind, let's start by discussing the key elements of the brain's anatomy and some of their basic functions. Then we can piece together these elements as we discuss some of the practical issues related to consciousness and Alzheimer's disease.

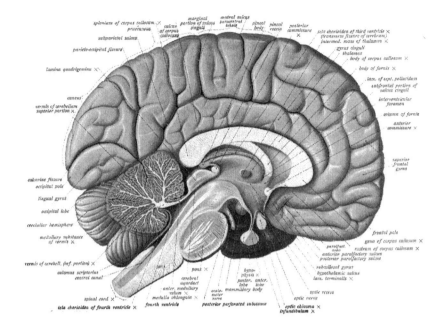

Neural Matter

The brain is made up of billions of neurons. These are networked into bundles of groupings, which include nerve tracts, gyri, fissures, sulci, cortices and cerebrum lobes. These groupings of specialized neurons work conjunctively to accomplish specialized tasks, while transmitting information back and forth through neural superhighways.

The brain is divided into four general regions, called lobes, each consisting of several ridged convolutions (also called gyri or gyrus in the singular) of brain tissue and various cortices. The front part of the brain, behind the forehead, is the frontal lobe. There are four convolutions within the frontal lobe, and key cortices including the frontal cortex and prefrontal cortex. The frontal lobe contains neurons associated with focus, short term tasking, planning and execution. The prefrontal cortex is associated with intelligence and decision-making.

Behind the frontal lobe, over the top side of the brain and about halfway back and to the middle, is the parietal lobe. The parietal lobe contains three convolutions and several sensory cortices. These sensory cortices include part of the visual cortex called the posterior parietal cortex, the somatosensory cortex and vestibular cortex. In addition, the parietal lobe contains sensory regions that accommodate orientation among the hands, fingers, toes and so on. The front of this lobe and along each side contains the motor cortex. At the back of this lies the premotor cortex and the posterior parietal cortex. These coordinate the movements of the body and receive feedback from those movements.

Behind the parietal lobe at the back of the brain, is the occipital lobe. This lobe is at the very back of the head and contains three convolutions. The occipital lobe contains most of the visual cortex. This region typically processes visual signals, and translates those into images using a complex mapping system. We'll discuss the mapping system later on.

Below the parietal lobe and between the frontal and the occipital lobe is the temporal lobe. The temporal lobe sits behind the temples. This lobe also comprises much of what is considered the cerebral cortex, containing the hippocampus and associated parts of the limbic system. The occipital lobe also contains the auditory cortex, which processes sounds, words, language, and semantics. In addition to processing auditory information, this cortex also processes visually-gathered language and semantics information.

The brain grows and develops in the fetus from a tubular canal called the neural tube. The cortices expand outward from this tube. We can also review the brain's hierarchical activity with a discussion of the cortices. The brain's commanding region lies in the frontal cortex. Here the various inputs provided by the senses and the body's feedback are taken in to the command center, the prefrontal cortex. This cortex is behind and on top of the forehead.

The motor cortex lies just behind the frontal cortex as we comb back over the head. It normally resides within a band of neural grey matter (neuron cells) that wrap around the top of the head onto the two sides. Within the motor cortex reside specialized networks of neurons, each network coordinated with specific types of motor activity.

The premotor region contains billions of specialized mirroring neurons, which mirror and sort the executive decisions transmitted from the frontal cortex. Behind the premotor cortex is the primary motor cortex. This region contains specialized neurons that are able to broadcast specific neural impulses out through the neural network for specific parts of the body. One section will govern the toes, while another will govern the feet, and so on. This organized vertical arrangement of specialized motor neurons is also referred to as the homunculus motor region, because each location is connected to specific body locations.

Behind the region of the motor cortex neurons is another set of regions grouped into what is called the sensory cortex. This region has several individual cortices, and spreads from the top of the head (parietal lobe) through the back of the head (occipital lobe) and along the sides (temporal lobe). Among these lobes lie the visual cortex, the auditory cortex, the olfactory cortex, the postcentral gyrus, and the gustatory cortex.

In these respective regions, the various incoming sensory impulses are translated and processed. The first three cortices—the visual, auditory and olfactory—are self-explanatory, being the centers that process impulses of seeing, hearing and smelling, respectively. The postcentral gyrus processes the sensory impulses of touch and balance, while the gustatory cortex processes taste impulses from the tongue. Into each sensory cortex, specialized neural tracts conduct in and blend impulses from the sense organs. The interference patterns of these impulses blend together to provide an image screen of sorts for the personality to observe.

The limbic system is positioned inside these cortex regions, towards the center of the brain. The limbic system is made up of the thalamus, the hypothalamus, the hippocampus, the cingulates, the fomix and the amygdala. Each of these has a slightly different function, but together they translate nerve impulse data from the body into memories and instructions. The limbic system's role is to prioritize and sort information. The hypothalamus and thalamus are the central translation stations. They also stimulate endocrine release of hormones and neurotransmitters, and translate incoming communications from around the body.

The cingulates are programmed to govern the autonomic systems such as the heartbeat, breathing, hunger, and so on. The amygdala on the other hand, provides a gateway to the lower nerve centers, channeling the personality's focus upon survival into fear and anger into the information processing. The hippocampus sorts and prioritizes all this information for memory storage. The fomix channels the waveform information from the hippocampus through a circuitry of memory processing called the Papex circuit.

Together the limbic system provides a translation and staging service for information. We might compare the limbic system to a computer's operating system.

We might also compare the anatomical elements of the brain to the hardware and physical circuitry of the computer.

The Brain's Software and the Personality Within

But what about the brain's software? The software in a computer is differentiated from the hardware of the computer. The circuit boards and the memory chips are the hardware, and the software lies on another plane. The software of a computer is contained in a machine language that gives instructions to the hardware.

In the same way, the software of the brain lies on another plane. The neural cells and the brain tissues do not provide the software. Rather, the software is located within the mind—which essentially gives instructions for the operations of brain and its cells.

The existence of software that is loaded onto a computer using an interface (such as a disk drive or download from the internet) illustrates that the computer is a tool. It is a human tool. Humans created the software that runs our computers. The software provided the means for the computer to be under the control and instruction of the human.

We can make the same case for the brain. When a person dies, the brain stops working. All the brain cells and brain 'hardware' are still there, but they are no longer operating. What changed?

The personality has left the body. The personality who utilized the brain has gone. This personality set up instructions through the mind, which sent those instructions to the brain. This is why we instinctively say that someone "passed away." Because we see the entire physical body is still there at the time of death, but something is missing: The personality.

The reality of a personality or self separate from the body and the brain has been established scientifically by a number of studies regarding clinical death (Ring 1982; Sabom 1982, 1998; Moody 1975, 1972; Blackmore 1996; Kubler-Ross 1991; and others). These studies found consistently that at the time of death, most people experience a separation from the body and brain—after the body and brain are clinically dead. This means not only that the heart and breathing stopped: It also means brain activity stopped as well.

Understanding this clearly provides the means for another view of memory and the brain, one that provides scientific consistency.

The hypothesis that we are each simply cellular machines driven by the brain is not consistent with scientific observation. If we are simply machines, then Alzheimer's disease would merely be a mechanical process. Losing ones memory would not be very problematic if we were simply machines. There would be no heart-wrenching emotions to contend with.

But we're not machines. Each of us seeks love and relationships with others. These are not symptoms of a machine. These are symptoms of a deeper person who is operating the machine.

A machine that is coded with software can certainly perform the tasks it was programmed to do. But love is another matter. Love is not consistent with mechanical activity. Due to love, we do things that are often illogical, and contrary to survival. If we were simply machines programmed for survival, none of us would be willing to put our bodies in danger in the name of love.

We are not brains. Rather, what we find within the brain is a process, indicating the involvement of another variable. That variable is a living personality—one might refer to this as the soul or the spirit of the person—who is operating the body much as a computer operator would operate a computer.

But just as the computer operator cannot effectively run the computer if the hardware starts breaking down, the personality within cannot operate and access the brain and its memory storage systems if there is a disease process damaging the brain's cells.

But because the personality is alive, and because the interface between the personality and the brain is changeable—that is, the mind—the personality can often find workarounds to access the brain's operations.

This might be compared to the computer operator who finds the hardware of the computer becoming inadequate, and programs some software to instruct the computer hardware to circumvent the damaged regions and essentially redirect operations to healthy cells.

This understanding of the brain and personality also explains many of the mysterious things doctors and researchers have observed over the past century.

Neural Plasticity

For example, many people have strokes as they age, and sometimes these strokes can damage entire regions of the brain. Yet in many cases, the brain will redevelop the ability to perform the functions that used to be performed by the damaged region of the brain.

This is called neural plasticity—the ability of the brain's processing to be moved around from one region to another to accommodate the brain's required activities.

Another example of neural plasticity occurs with hemidecortication—the loss or surgical removal of one side of the brain. A cancer or other form of damage to one side of the brain may necessitate the removal of one of the brain's hemispheres. A few decades ago, hemidecortication surgery was conducted on many epileptic children.

Yet doctors have found that in most cases, after hemidecortication surgery, the patient will recover most of those functions that used to require both hemispheres to perform.

For example, saccade eye movements are typically run by coordinating each hemisphere of the brain—opposite to each eye. But patients who have one hemisphere of the brain removed will quickly recover saccade eye movements.

How? Because the personality within still wants to see. The personality will then send instructions through the mind to reconfigure the brain to process these functions with different brain regions. This is quintessential neural plasticity.

This also explains those rare cases where a person is born without a brain—yet still can learn, remember things and function normally in many ways.

Yes, hydranencephaly is a reality. A few people are born without functioning brains every year. Some will die during childhood, but some have survived. Without a brain.

Take Alex Simpson, for example. She is over ten years old now. Born with hydranencephaly ten years ago, she is still functioning. He communicates with his parents.

Aaron Murray is two years old now. He was also born without a brain. Last fall he spoke his first word—about the time a normal baby would. He looked at his mom and said, "mummy."

Many people born with this will die in childhood. But one person lived to the age of 33 without a functioning brain.

Like many other babies born with hydranencephaly, the functions that are normally performed by the brain are performed by neural cells in the brainstem. This is yet another example of brain function being the result of instructions coming through the mind from a personality within. A personality of another composition.

The operator of the body, so to speak.

The question now changes slightly. Yes, we can understand that the brains of most Alzheimer's patients have been damaged by beta-amyloid plaque. But what else is going on, since many healthy people also have this damage?

Okay, some of these points are simplified. But there is some solid evidence to substantiate them. As a reader, you can choose to accept this more simplified explanation of the "other variable" of Alzheimer's disease and skip the rest of this chapter if you like. Or you can read through the rest of this chapter to gain further insight into the mechanics of the brain, the mind and the personality within.

Chapter Ten

Brainwave Transmissions

Over the past 150 years, researchers have tried to understand the electrical nature of the brain's physiology. The electric quality of the body was hard to deny even in the early days of electricity exploration. Gradually the apparatus for this probing were refined. Though crudely applied, Dr. Hans Berger is credited to be the first researcher to use the electroencephalogram (or EEG) to record brainwaves in the early 1920s. These efforts gradually gave brainwave testing credibility in psychological research. Today the EEG is utilized for medical diagnostics, psychological testing, biofeedback testing and polygraph detection.

Several types of brainwaves, each with unique frequencies, were discovered using EEG testing. Further testing using the later-discovered magnetoencephalograph indicated that a variety of subtle magnetic pulses also pulse through the body. First used by Dr. David Cohen in 1968, the MEG picked up another dimension of magnetic polarity among waveform transmission. MEG technology was further developed using superconductors. This equipment has been referred to as superconducting quantum interference devices (or SQUID).

The multitude of EEG and MEG studies over the years has confirmed the existence of several major brainwave pulses, ranging from one to sixty cycles per second. Our neurons pulse with waveforms with frequency bandwidths that correspond to particular moods, stress levels, and physiological status. As we focus on the complexities of daily life, our brains reflect and emit shorter-frequency alpha or beta brainwaves. A relaxing mood tends to accompany the deeper delta or even the more meditative theta waves.

The greater the stress, the higher frequencies tend to get. Just as higher-pitched sounds tend to indicate intensity or urgency, higher frequency brainwaves reflect a mind hustling to keep up with life's details. Because initial EEG and MEG research predominantly focused upon the brain, these waves were tagged as brainwaves. Actually, we find these waves resonating throughout the body. They tend to be more predominant among the central nervous system and the brain because the brain and spinal cord tend to be the main collection foci for these waves. As will be detailed further, the central nervous system provides freeways for high-speed wave transit.

Researchers have divided the millions of possible brainwave combinations into five general ranges. Alpha waves are the typical dominant cycle during dream states and light meditation. The alpha waves are oscillations with between eight and thirteen cycles per second (same as hertz). Beta brainwaves are dominant during normal waking consciousness, and range from fourteen to thirty cycles per second.

Theta waves range from four to seven cycles per second and dominate during normal sleep and meditation. On the lower frequency side are the delta waves, which range from less than one cycle per second to about three cycles per second. These slow waves tend to be dominating during the deepest sleep and meditation states.

On the other side of the spectrum, some of the fastest rhythms recorded in the brain are the gamma waves. The high-energy gamma waveforms typically dominate during periods of advanced problem solving or critical thinking. They oscillate at between thirty and sixty cycles per second. Over the past decade, researchers have discovered the existence of even shorter-wavelength and faster brainwaves. Ranging from sixty to two hundred cycles per second or more, these high-speed waves are referred to as high gamma waves. The high gamma waves are thought to accompany critical thought processes and brain functions.

Multiple brainwave types occur simultaneously in our body. One type will often predominate, however. Just as multiple tuning forks will align to one dominate tone, the body will typically tune—harmonically—to the predominant waveform driven from the pervading consciousness.

A 2006 study from the University of California at Berkeley and San Francisco (Sanders *et al.*) concluded that it is likely these brainwaves are conduits for signaling between the various regions of the brain. Dr. Robert Knight, professor of neuroscience at the University of California at Berkeley, and a director of the research observed that some regions of the brain emitted waves, others reflected waves, and still others modulated waves. Meanwhile, a confluence of these waves corresponded with particular activities, indicating different brain centers were using brainwaves as a sort of information exchange system.

As these respected researchers correlated the type of wave with the part of the brain involved in some functions and thought processes, they began to see longer-wavelength theta waves synchronizing or coupling with shorter-wavelength gamma waves. They considered this coupling as part of a hierarchical signaling process. Regions of coordinated neurons produce resonant coherent wave patterns, which provide the means for one group of neurons to communicate with another group. Synchronizing impulses between neurons appear to coordinate firing patterns. The brainwave synchronization provides a process for ranking between brain regions in operational order. Theta waves appear to provide an executive control mechanism, which bridge the operations of various neuron groups.

Using epileptic subjects, the researchers found consistent relationships between cognition and the occurrence of coherent theta and gamma waves. These two types of waves provide a locked resonation process. As cognitive processes change, one wave from one region first couples with, then transitions into the next type of waveform. A congruent harmonic becomes apparent between these brainwave transitions.

Biofeedback therapy has focused on the relationship between stress and brainwave types for a number of decades. Biofeedback research has confirmed that stress directly influences brainwave activity and vice versa. Researchers have tested brainwave activity with patients in a number of different circumstances. Stressful conditions are linked to higher beta wave levels and lower alpha and theta wave levels. Consequently, a person who feels more relaxed and less stressed will produce more alpha and theta impulses.

Many of us are aware that certain sounds influence relaxation. Most of us have experienced greater relaxation as we listen to soothing music or the songs of birds for example. Melinda Maxfield, PhD (2006) determined that slowly beating a drum at 4.5 beats per second readily brings about a state of theta brainwave activity.

In 2006, Stanford University's Center for Computer Research in Music and Acoustics held a symposium with a purpose of "interdisciplinary dialogue on the hypothesis that brainwaves entrain to rhythmic auditory stimuli, a phenomenon known as auditory driving."

This symposium brought together some of the nation's leading sound researchers. Many discussed the implications of auditory driving as it relates to our mental and physical wellbeing. The implications of the research, reflected by the consensus at the symposium, were that we are merely at the tip of the iceberg of this research.

The applications of brainwave entrainment through auditory driving are numerous. Successful auditory driving and brainwave entrainment treatments have contributed to resolving psychological trauma, chronic pain, stress, and weakened immune systems. Research comparing normal subjects with schizophrenic subjects (Vierling-Claasen *et al.* 2008) has illustrated how gamma and beta waves interface and guide cognitive processes.

Normal subjects will tune to a 40 Hz wave in response to either 20 or 40 Hz driving frequencies. Schizophrenic subjects will typically respond with 20 Hz impulses. The study's authors comment that these results illustrate "how biophysical mechanisms can impact cognitive function." This research confirms that brainwaves provide a mechanism for signaling specific information throughout the physical anatomy.

Biofeedback testing has further demonstrated that with practice and proper feedback access, human subjects can consciously change their brainwave levels. As a stress-reduction technique for example, a person can decrease their beta wave activity and increase their alpha and theta activity.

The procedure entails the subject sitting down in front of a computer screen visually displaying rates from an electroencephalograph, photoplethysmograph (PPG—heart rate and blood flow), and/or possibly an electromyograph (EMG—muscle tension) to read waveform activity feeding back from different body parts connected to a variety of electrodes. Electrodes may be placed around the head, typically either on the scalp or in some cases around the cerebral cortex.

Skin electrodes may also be applied to the arm, and PPG electrodes may be connected to the chest. The computer will monitor the waveform output of these different locations—displaying the results on a graphic display screen for the subject and therapist to monitor.

Most of us will generate brainwave signals reflecting our mental or emotional state—be it anxious, focused, relaxed, tired, angry or asleep. A good biofeedback machine will register several of these waves and their relative strengths around the body. Using a good biofeedback machine, most people can gradually learn to significantly lower or increase their alpha and theta wave strengths. For a few people, there will be an almost immediate ability to influence their waves as soon as the monitoring begins.

For most of us, it will take a bit of practice—a number of sessions usually—to be able to effectively modulate our brainwaves. Researchers have found that most everyone is able to modulate their brainwaves at one point or other. Researchers have yet to understand why there is such a variance among people's ability to control their brainwaves.

Nonetheless, once people do learn to change their brainwaves using the biofeedback, they can usually transition successfully into being able to adjust their brainwaves without the biofeedback equipment. Bringing about a relaxed mental state through visualizing relaxing situations or hearing relaxing sounds are probably the most effective techniques used for this result. Auditory driving with rhythmic sounds has been increasingly used in biofeedback therapy.

Biofeedback therapy illustrates that our brainwaves are expressions of the role of consciousness within the body. An alteration of brainwaves from primarily beta to theta waves will almost invariably result in a lower heart rate, a slower, deeper rate of breathing, and a lowering of blood pressure.

Conversely, a lower heart rate, and slower breathing—as long as there is no mental disruption—will also tend to induce a theta brainwave state. We thus have an intersection between consciousness and the cascade of brainwaves with physiological states.

The reality that our brainwaves reflect our consciousness was confirmed in a 2015 study from Canada's Baycrest Center for Geriatric Care (Rondina *et al.*). This study tested the brain waves of a younger group of people and an older group. The younger people averaged 25 years old and the older group averaged 66 years old.

The researchers found in general, that the younger people had a greater volume of theta waves, while the older folks had a greater volume of alpha waves. The theta waves are slower, and are linked with greater levels of memory. Alpha waves are linked with more immediate reaction recall. Dr. Renante Rondina from the University of Toronto, who led the study, commented on the results:

> *"We know that our brains change over time, but fully understanding how we make and recall memories as we age has been a mystery."*

An example of a cascading messaging system is the response stimulated by sensory sensation occurring somewhere in the body and transmitted through the neurons to the brain. The pre-programmed sympathetic response (the reflex arc) is typically accompanied by conscious reception of the sensation via the limbic system.

The focal point of this stimulation is the thalamus, which acts as a waveform message translator and decoder. Waveform-transmitting neurons deep within the thalamus are engaged, stimulating waves that combine with others to form an interference pattern—also referred to as a neural mapping.

As these waveform interference patterns are decoded, some are reflected back to the cerebral cortex. Here an exchange of waveform patterns takes place. A relay of information is conducted between the cerebral cortex and the thalamus, reflecting the information back onto the prefrontal cortex.

Here the information is responded to, followed by a return of pulses that stimulate the hypothalamus gland to secrete biochemicals. These biochemical messengers either stimulate endocrine or cellular function directly, or stimulate the pituitary gland to in turn secrete biochemical messengers that precisely activate endocrine glands and physical response.

The hypothalamus, located at the base of the brain under the thalamus, encapsulates part of the third ventricle. The body's autonomic responses are processed here, some of which in turn stimulate the pituitary gland to release key master hormones. These master hormones signal responses that control the critical phase cycles of metabolism, body core temperature, appetite, thirst and so on.

The hypothalamus responds to waveform inputs from the brain centers and limbic system. These brain centers provide the platforms for conscious interaction with waveform messaging. Waveform interference patterns are created from the various sensory nerve transmissions and response neurotransmitter biochemicals. These interactive interference patterns form the basis for information.

This facilitates perspective, and allows a sorting process to prioritize the information within the limbic system. Stresses on the body such as infection and immune response also feed into the limbic system for response. For these waveforms, the hypothalamus activates immediate response cascades using the limbic system's programming.

The hypothalamus and limbic system thus respond to a wide range of stimuli, and construct biochemical responses by activating an orchestrated flow of biochemical messengers to stimulate particular physical responses around the body. Dispatched messengers include dopamine, melatonin, somatostatin and others. The hypothalamus also secretes hypothalamic hormones that stimulate the pituitary to produce a number of master endocrine hormones.

Neurotransmitter Waves

Information transmissions travel from neuron to neuron as they travel through the nervous system. Neurons stretched end to end make up the nerves—and the nerves are the pipelines for neural transmission.

These transmissions are in effect, waveforms.

Waveform transmissions pass between neighboring neural cell bodies through arms called dendrites. The dendrites of neighboring neurons do not touch, however. Rather, between them exists a space called the synaptic cleft within a region called the synapse. This region contains a special fluid called the neurotransmitter fluid. The chemistry of this fluid provides the medium for the specific waveform signals that travel between neurons.

Scientists have authenticated hundreds of different proteins that inhabit the synapses between the neurons. Neurons are typically divided into inhibitory and excitatory. Traditionally, the inhibitory neuron synapses have been considered to be rather simple. But recently, 140 previously unknown proteins have been discovered within inhibitory synapses (Uezu et al. 2016). This indicates that both types of neurons are extremely complex. This variety of different proteins provide the means for different sorts of waveforms.

One might compare it to a stained glass window. Each section of the stain glass window provides a different color as the sunlight passes through each one.

This variety of different proteins within synapses relates directly to different types of mood and cognitive processes. Because these proteins are expressed and produced as a result of the neuron's genes, the types of proteins in the synapses relates directly to the health of the neuron.

Central nervous system (CNS) neurons can also have a multitude of dendrites and synapses. Large neurons might have several thousand while others have significantly less. Through these synapses, each neuron may be firing up to 100,000 electromagnetic pulse inputs into this fluid concurrently.

This tiny sea of neurotransmitter fluid also contains various other biochemical components, many of which are ionic in nature. These ions combine with the protein neurotransmitters to create a medium that can buffer, accelerate or malign transmissions. The overall conducting ability of the neurotransmitter fluid is considered its electromagnetic synaptic potential.

The neurotransmitter fluid chemistry facilitates particular waves of different frequencies, wavelengths and amplitudes. At the same time, the fluid chemistry provides filtering mechanisms to buffer and screen out some transmission elements. Depending upon its particular makeup at the time, the fluid will provide a combination of excitatory potential and inhibitory potential. This balance serves to escort or conduct waveform information from one nerve to another, while at the same time dampening or filtering these impulses to prevent overload and over-stimulation.

This process might well be compared to the process of transistors and resistors we see in integrated circuits. Neurotransmitters are tremendous semiconductors. Their precise molecular structures allow them to buffer and/or amplify waveform transmissions within a particular spectrum.

Two examples of active neurotransmitters are acetylcholine and adrenaline (or epinephrine). These two biomolecules conduct and/or magnify impulses that relate to autonomic function and physical response. Acetylcholine will accelerate instructions to muscle fibers to contract, while adrenaline will amplify internal conditions that perpetuate the 'fight or flight' response: Causing a quickening of heart rate and blood flow, immediate motor muscle response, visual acuity, and so on.

These two biochemicals are interactive throughout the body. They impact the functioning of digestion, the secretion of mucus, defecation, the immune system, and many other processes around the body. They occupy the neurotransmitter fluid chemistry, but they also interact with processes outside the confines of the synaptic fluid. For example, acetylcholine also stimulates skeletal muscle cells directly. This means the body's autonomic response programming is facilitated through these chemicals, much as a key might facilitate the unlocking of the front door and our passage into the house.

Neurotransmitters and hormones have similar actions in the body, and some hormones are also neurotransmitters. By definition, a neurotransmitter is released by a nerve cell into the synapse, while a hormone is produced by an endocrine gland. For example, when epinephrine is secreted by the adrenal gland, it is a hormone. When it is secreted by the synapse it is a neurotransmitter.

Most hormone secretions of the body follow a chain of command. Their secretions are stimulated by other secreted conductors, produced in turn by the pituitary gland. The pituitary gland is the master gland stimulating most of the various hormones. Neurotransmitters, on the other hand, are produced through waveform-nerve reception. While hormones will stimulate a variety of responses in cells throughout the body, neurotransmitters are typically associated with the effects of the nerves.

At the same time, both hormones and neurotransmitters are waveform conductors. They both facilitate the transmission of electromagnetically-generated information from location to location around the body. The pituitary gland is considered the master gland for hormone productivity. The pituitary is about the size of a cherry. It is located behind the eyes in a depression of the sphenoid bone, just behind where the optic nerves cross.

The pituitary produces master hormones that directly stimulate the body, such as growth hormone (GH), vasopressin, oxytocin and others. The pituitary gland connects to the hypothalamus by the infudibulum, a stalk of portal veins and nerves tracts. It is through this stalk that the pituitary gland's activities are regulated by the hypothalamus. The hypothalamus sends releasing hormones to the pituitary. These stimulate the releases of the pituitary.

The hormone's chemistry provides a conductor for the body's instructional signals. Hormones are in essence tiny crystals that resonate particular types of impulses. These resonations are passed on to cells and organs by stimulating the gateways of tiny receptors that sit on the surface of cell membranes. We'll discuss this interaction between ligands and receptors in more detail shortly.

We must be careful not to confuse chemicals with waves, however. Waves are informational, and conduct through chemicals. Their interference patterns can be stored within biochemicals in the form of standing waves between atoms. This is why biomolecules have unique properties.

Biochemicals serve primarily as echo chambers, reflecting the informational impulses being transmitted around the body.

We might compare this to hearing a radio playing a song broadcast from a distant station. The radio does not contain the song, nor is it the source of the radiowaves that are being broadcast to millions of radios from the same radio station. The radio does not contain the singer either. Rather, the radio is simply a conducting vehicle, which temporary crystallizes and transforms the radiowaves into the speaker sounds that we can hear. In the same way, biochemicals reacting throughout the body during metabolism are merely vehicles of wave conduction. Waves and their informational interference patterns are being broadcast in multiple bandwidths as they are released and move through the body.

Neurotransmitter and hormone conduction also might be compared to opening our eyes under water. Were we to dive into a river during a rain storm and attempt to open our eyes and look through its murky, muddy waters, we would not see much. We would be lucky to see our hand in front of our face underneath the muddy brown waters. That same river during a warm summer day might be so clear that we could see the bottom ten feet down. The difference between seeing within the two rivers is due to the muddy river mud being stirred up by the rain and stormy weather. It is not that our vision has gotten worse.

In the same way, an imbalanced chemistry among the neurotransmitter fluid and/or hormones within the bloodstream will alter the transmissions passing from neuron to neuron. Some chemicals will interfere in the waveform transmissions. Others will facilitate them, while still others may subdue or distort the transmissions.

Case in point: When we drink alcohol, the alcohol will affect the chemistry of the synaptic junction—the neurotransmitter fluid—in such a way that distorts the electromagnetic signals that travel from one neuron to another. This produces an altered synaptic state that affects how nerve cells control motor functions. The motor cells may receive slow or even inaccurate signals. The same ethanol neurochemistry will distort sense and feedback signals as they are sent to the brain. The distortion can cause disorientation, coordination impairment, irrational behavior and mood swings: A potentially disastrous combination we often refer to as being drunk.

The key role of the neurotransmitter is to create a potential for the electromagnetic transmission. This creates a bridge of sorts for the waveforms to transverse. The type of neurotransmitter also dictates which type of channel gateway will be opened on the post-synaptic nerve—the receiving nerve. The type of ion channel will typically dictate what kind of information will be transduced through the linkage of neurons.

One of the more interesting players in neurotransmitter biochemistry is GABA, which stands for gamma-aminobutyric acid. GABA is considered an inhibitory neurotransmitter in that it slightly slows down wave conduction. This actually has a positive effect upon the synaptic transmissions, allowing nerve signals to pass through without as much distortion. As a result, GABA is known for producing feelings of relaxation and alertness.

Research has indicated that various mood disorders such as depression, anxiety and even insomnia are related to the body having lower GABA levels within neurotransmitter fluids. Epileptics typically have insufficient amounts of this neurotransmitter as well. Many of the popular anti-depressant pharmaceuticals increase GABA levels. It should be noted, however, that these drugs also produce various side effects as well.

Healthy amounts of GABA in the neurotransmitter fluid are also associated with an increase in alpha brainwaves. L-theanine (a GABA precursor) directly was given to thirteen subjects in one study (Abdou 2006). Electroencephalography examinations were conducted, and each subject given L-theanine had heightened levels of alpha waves and reduced beta waves. Remember that beta waves are associated with nervousness and anxiety while alpha waves accompany increased concentration.

Dr. Abdou's research also demonstrated the effect chemical neurotransmitters have upon the biocommunication of fear around the body. Two groups of eight volunteers were divided into a non-GABA (placebo) group and a GABA group. Both groups were monitored for IgA immunoglobulin levels following the crossing of a suspension bridge. Because IgA levels tend to shut down during anxious or fearful moments as the adrenal gland prepares for 'fight or flight,' this test illustrated GABA's effects upon fear-based immune response.

The GABA group had normal IgA levels while the non-GABA group experienced significantly lower IgA levels. It was thus concluded that GABA levels are associated with reducing inappropriate fear responses as well as facilitating alpha waves.

As we assess this last trial, we can conclude that GABA's effect upon the neurotransmitter fluid allowed the subjects to realistically assess the dangers involved. Using the senses to realistically assess the strength of the bridge and the likelihood of the bridge actually collapsing would be considered a clear-headed response. On the other hand, a heightened fear of falling simply by looking down (acrophobia) would not be considered a realistic assessment of the situation, simply because the bridge could be easily crossed and obviously was strong enough to handle all of the walkers.

A normalized neurotransmitter environment at the synapse (including GABA) allows for a clearer broadcasting of waveform information through the neural pathways. Just as clear water allows us to see the bottom of a stream, normalized neurotransmitter fluid produces less resistance and distortion along the conducting synapses placed along the transmission pipelines of the neural network.

What's this have to do with memory, you ask?

Research from Canada's McGill University (Boyce *et al.* 2016) studied spatial and emotional memory consolidation and REM-stage sleep. They confirmed, as many studies have, that these memories are consolidated during REM-stage sleep. But they also found this consolidation occurred during theta brainwaves.

Furthermore, they found that a neurotransmitter is utilized during this memory consolidation process. The neurotransmitter is a form of GABA called medial septum γ-aminobutyric acid-releasing, or MS-GABA.

The researchers found that if the MS-GABA activity was blocked, this would affect object-place recognition. At the same time, however, other neuron activity—and other types of memories—were unaffected.

The lesson here is that neurotransmitter chemicals and brainwaves provide facilities for transmission, just as do most neurons. We can see such a scenario with a computer. A circuit board on a computer is set up to provide electrical transmissions from one circuit to another. The circuitry is not set up to retain the information. It is simply communicating on- and off-states from one circuit to another—just as electrical and brainwave states are being transmitted from one neuron to another.

Let's look more closely at how brain transmission is affected in Alzheimer's disease.

Alzheimer's disease and Neural Transmission

The significance of this discussion of the brain's neural signaling becomes apparent as we understand that Alzheimer's disease interferes in these processes of waveform transmission. Sensory impulses will still occur in a person with Alzheimer's disease. An Alzheimer's disease patient will still be seeing. They will still be hearing. But their brain will not process those sensory inputs the same. Due to brain cell damage, the transmissions are not being passed along. They may or may not reach the cortex intact. But the transmission and assembly of sensory inputs between the sensory cortices, the cerebrum and the limbic system, will become damaged.

In Alzheimer's, some of the more important neuron damage will occur in the frontal lobe, the hippocampus and the amygdala regions. The frontal lobe is the region that helps process language and working memory. The hippocampus processes longer-term and episodic memories. And the amygdala processes emotional memories. When the neurons in these regions become damaged by cytotoxicity—producing the beta-amyloid oligomers, plaque and tau tangles—the ability for the brain to connect sensory transmissions with memories is interfered with.

As discussed earlier, those neurons that make up these regions can become damaged by cytotoxicity—producing neural tangles and plaque. But how is this effecting brain transmissions?

Let's say that you receive a call on your cell phone and the voice on the other side is garbled, then the line is dropped. You can assume one of three things: You can assume the cell phone is broken—not that great an assumption if the phone was working earlier. Or you can assume that the cell towers in the area all went down, and aren't operating. This may also not be a great assumption if other cell phone users are able to make calls from the area.

Or you can assume there are mountains or other forms of interference that are blocking your phone from a clear transmission from the cell tower. This last possibility is probably the most likely, given the durability of most cell phones and cell phone towers.

But cell towers do go down sometimes. Perhaps we're talking about 50 years from now—at a time when many cell phone towers are getting old and obsolete. At that time, it might be more likely that a cell tower has gone down. Or perhaps there has been lightning in the area, and cell towers are getting hit by lightning strikes.

We can correlate brain transmissions with cell phone transmissions. These both occur using waveform technology as we discussed earlier. If there is some interference caused by a mountain or other barrier, cell phone transmissions won't get through.

We might compare a cell tower to a neuron because these are responsible for transmitting information, just as neurons are. Should neurons become damaged, the processing of information will also be damaged.

That would likely damage transmissions. Such a lightning strike might even damage the tower completely to the point where nothing was being transmitted.

We can liken the cell tower to a neuron. If a neuron is damaged, it cannot transmit those transmissions that are traveling through the brain.

In the brain, if there is a buildup of beta-amyloid or other damage to neurons typically used to transmit information, the information will not be transmitted correctly. If there is sensory data being transmitted, say through the optic nerve, perhaps some amyloid damage between the optic nerve, the frontal cortex and the hippocampal neurons will prevent the sensory information from being processed within the hippocampus and consolidated into memories.

Our brains have so many neurons that one damaged neuron won't usually make that big a difference, as the brain will simply redirect transmissions through other neurons. This would be like the cell phone call going through an optional cell tower to get to the other user.

But if too many of these neurons become damaged, then the transmission becomes irreparably damaged. And signals just don't get to travel around the brain as they normally might.

This is particularly the case with the limbic system, because this is where waveform transmissions are directed to be stored for later use. Our memories are contained within special neurons that store these waveform combinations, within the cortices, the frontal lobe, hippocampus, amygdala and elsewhere in the limbic system.

When this damage occurs in the brain, the personality still exists, and is unaffected. In the cell tower analogy above, the person trying to make a cell phone call is still there. They simply cannot communicate with others through the cell phone.

Using these relationships, we can understand how an Alzheimer's patient has difficulty communicating and relating with others. But what about memories? How does Alzheimer's disease affect memories and the mind in general? For this, we have to dig deeper into just what the mind is, and what memories are in relation to that.

Chapter Eleven

Where is the Mind?

Western science has been struggling with the location and definition of the mind for thousands of years. The Greek physician Galen of Pergamon (129-210 BC) struggled with the then-accepted cardiocentric theory—which proposed that the seat of the mind is in the heart. Galen produced a number of anatomical experiments with vivisection, illustrating the difference between the central nervous system and the arterial system.

Despite some intense debate among the Stoics and others following Galen's experiments, there was increasing acceptance that the central nervous system played an integral role in the mind's processes. Yet from these ancient times to the modern day, researchers are still speculating and debating on the precise location of the mind.

The planarian worm (*Dugesia dorotocephala*) was Dr. James McConnell's favorite lab subject for his learning and conditioning studies began in 1955. In one test, Dr. McConnell subjected a group of planaria to bright light followed by a mild electric shock. The shock would make the worms curl up in pain. This light-and-shock sequence was repeated hundreds of times for reinforcement. Eventually the worms would immediately curl up once the light was turned on, with or without a shock. This illustrated not only the worms' conscious attempts to avoid pain (a concept avoided by science), but also their ability to remember the circumstances surrounding the pain. Where were these memories stored?

The planaria worm has a tiny brain and central nervous system. However, these worms have an incredible ability to reproduce immediately upon being cut or sliced. This is commonly referred to as regeneration. Not all sliced worms regenerate on both ends. Most will at least regenerate at the tail end. Many amphibians also have this ability—they will typically regenerate a limb following its amputation.

The planarian worm however, can be cut in half and each half will develop into a physically complete organism. This is thought to occur through a regeneration of the head on the tail side of the split. Each side then will develop a full body, tail and head. Each will also retain their own memory.

In order to test for the location of memory, Dr. McConnell sliced the planarians into two pieces, in the middle of the body, between the head and tail. Assuming memory was stored in the head end where the central nervous system is, the head side regeneration should remember the light-shock training and curl up, while the tail-sided regeneration would not remember the shock treatment.

Not so fast. Contrary to this assumption, both regenerated worm halves remembered the training, and in many cases the tail-generated worms remembered the training better than the brain-side worm did. This research theoretically indicated that memory was not necessarily stored in the brain (McConnell *et al.* 1960).

This research underscores some of the studies referenced earlier, showing continuing memory and cognition despite partial brain removal or damage to loci known for particular functions. In Mishkin (1978) and Mumby *et al.* (1992), for example, surgical removal of the amygdala and hippocampus resulted either in minor memory impairment or none at all. Vargha-Khadem and Polkey (1992) reviewed multiple studies of hemidecortication—the removal of at least half of the brain. Full cognitive recovery following hemidecortication resulted in more than 80% of all subjects.

Magnetic imaging of human patients following brain damage have confirmed the movement of mental functions from one part of the brain to the other. This has resulted in the theory of brain plasticity, as discussed earlier. It is not difficult to logically conclude that if mental function moves from one part of the brain to another, the mind must have a composition separate from the brain tissues. Truly, this composition has continued to baffle researchers.

MRI imaging can certainly locate electromagnetic activity correlated to cognition, memory and decision-making—the executive activities—within the brain. Electromagnetic activity may also indicate active regions and pathways during particular thought activity. Yet the precise location and composition of the mind and memory has remained mysterious.

The brain is not restricted to the gray matter within the skull. This gray region of the brain is composed of the right and left hemispheres of the cerebrum, the cerebellum, and the brain stem—composed of the midbrain, the pons and medulla.

The brain also includes the spinal column and spinal nerves. It would thus be more accurate to describe the brain as the central nervous system or the neural network, which expands to the peripheral nervous system located throughout the body. The spinal column and spinal nerve system serve as a bridge between the lower activity centers and the higher and more subtle waveform translation centers of the brain. From the spinal column radiates various waveforms that stimulate organ activity. These direct pathways from the spine drive the autonomic systems and the programmed response centers throughout the central nervous system.

The virtual link between the senses, the brain and the mind lies hidden within the waveform interference patterns guided by the personality through the limbic system and imaging cortices. The inner personality's executive processes are generated through the prefrontal cortex and translated through the thalamus, hypothalamus and hippocampal complex to their respective loci.

These areas are to be considered the interbrain. Using a network of subtle and gross conduits, they negotiate the information between the senses and the subtle mind. They also bridge the feedback of the mind's instructions and the initiation of brain and motor function. For this reason, many physicians attribute the amygdala as being the seat of emotion, although removal of it does not prevent emotion to be exhibited.

Why is this? It is because emotion arises from the unseen inner personality. The limbic system provides an insertion point for emotions to guide and steer the processes of prioritization. However, a surgeon still would not find any emotion within a surgically removed limbic organ.

The neural network is a system of interconnected neurons. Connecting different parts of the anatomy are nerve tracts. Nerve tracts are armored passageways that protect neurons and accelerate wave transmissions. These tracts might be compared to a household network of wire conduits protecting the wires and circuitry. When electricity must travel through underground wires, heavy-duty conduit piping will be used as shielding. These pipe tubes protect the wires from the decomposing elements of the soil. It also protects the local environment from electricity running through the wiring.

Nerve tracts serve similar purposes within the body. They provide the sheathing allowing pulsed waveforms to channel throughout the body and interact with multiple waveforms moving via nerves, ion channels and other messenger systems. As they interact, informational messages are created in the form of interference patterns.

Some of the nerve cells among the CNS are specific to particular types of waveforms. Sensory nerves function altogether differently from motor nerves, for example. However, many CNS nerve tracts contain both sensory and motor fibers. A motor nerve radiates nerve impulses from the CNS out to the muscle and organ tissue cells. These motor nerves stimulate specific activity—thus they transmit specific instructional waveforms. Sensory nerves typically transmit in the other direction, carrying information waves from the various organs, tissues and sense organs into the CNS for processing.

The intentional consciousness of the personality are translated through the mind into physiological instructions. Once translated, these intentions will stimulate both the motor cortex and the thalamus and hypothalamus. The thalamus regulates or adjusts thermogenesis, which controls the body's heat levels, providing a foundation for metabolic activity. Meanwhile the hypothalamus negotiates the sympathetic and parasympathetic activities of the body's autonomic system through the stimulation of the pituitary gland.

Via the hypothalamus, the mind autonomically dictates control to regulate the functions of the body's metabolic activities through the pathways of the endocrine system. Through the vehicle of the motor cortex, the mind stimulates physical activity. We can thus conclude from these basic physiological cascades—confirmed by many years of research—that the physical interface or conduit between the mind and the physical body is located in the frontal lobe and limbic system. This might be compared to the magnetic heads that 'read' the polarity states recorded onto a computer's hard disks.

Mapping the Mind

Research using active EEG, MEG, MRI and PET imagery has produced the hypothesis by many researchers that the mind is composed of a collection of electromagnetic signals.

This began with the mapping of the brain by Dr. Wilder Penfield, as discussed earlier. Dr. Penfield was able to associate memories and responses to particular brain regions, resulting in a map of the cortices and their potential functions. Dr. Lashley also confirmed much of this mapping system.

The problem became, however, that these functions can move from cortex to cortex, and neuron to neuron when needed. This plasticity requires a different understanding than particular nerve centers being responsible for certain functions.

Then came Dr. Karl Pribran's research on memory and engrams. Dr. Pribran found that when nerves and brain parts were removed or severed, cognition continued. When the optic nerve was severed, an animal could still perceive an image in detail. This led to Dr. Pribran's conclusion that perception and cognition were deeper than the anatomy.

Wave interference patterns became the subject of research, especially in mapping memories. Dr. Pribran, Dr. David Bohm and Dr. Dennis Gabor arrived at the understanding that cognition and memory were related to the mechanics of wave transmission. Using Fourier analysis—in which sine wave function is calculated with action, the holonomic brain model of cognitive function was developed. This used the Gabor function, which described the holographic nature of light and perception.

This indicates the existence of an inner personality—deeper than the mind, who is the observer of the mind and the user of the brain. Let's prove this out as we investigate the mind's subtle net further.

When we examine some of the expansive research done in the field of brainwaves, we see how both brain function and the mind are closely related to rhythmic wave mechanics. The electroencephalogram measures the voltage potential differences among different regions of the brain. These voltage differences result in a wave formation, which can range in wavelength, frequency and amplitude among a collection of neurons. These brainwaves are not single units in themselves. They are surges of collective interference patterns created by the billions of reflecting waves of billions of neurons, cells and the various other waveforms large and small moving through the body.

Delta waves cycle from one to three hertz, and tend to predominate during NREM (non-rapid eye movement) sleep, and some meditation. During this type of sleep, dreaming is minimal and the body is often in motion. Delta waves tend to resonate more actively in the frontal cortex. Delta waves correlate with an increase in the production and circulation of growth hormone. One of growth hormone's more important attributes within the body is its ability to advance the healing and regeneration process.

Theta waves cycle at four to seven hertz and dominate during mid-stage sleeping. Theta waves are more elusive, but seem to most active during memory retrieval and consolidation during sleep, and become more active in creative endeavors and behavior modification during waking hours. The hippocampus appears to actively accommodate and transduce these waves. Observations have noted peak hippocampus activity during predominantly theta wave periods. The hippocampus is associated with spatial recognition and short-term memory consolidation.

Alpha waves will cycle at eight to thirteen cycles per second, and are dominant during light sleep and dreaming, as well as some meditation states. Alpha waves are seen dominant during memorization tasks, especially those related to words, persons and visual impressions.

They tend to be most prominent at the back of the skull and towards the side of the body most favored by the organism. The earth's predominating waveforms cycle in the alpha range. This is called the Schumann resonance, discovered by Dr. Winfried Otto Schumann in 1952. The earth has several Schumann Resonance nodes, including the alpha level eight hertz (rounded), fourteen hertz, twenty hertz, twenty-six hertz, thirty-two hertz, thirty-nine hertz and forty-five hertz. The harmonic here is approximately six to eight hertz. Audio testing has concluded that listening to an eighth hertz beat will increase alpha brainwave levels. This essentially establishes a harmonic between the body's wave activity and the earth's.

Beta waves will cycle at fourteen to thirty hertz and are dominant during active, waking consciousness. These waves tend to be prominent towards the front of the brain on the side predominating during that activity. Beta waves reflect a state of focused attention and activity. A lack of beta waves during waking hours—or lower frequency beta waves—tends to occur with a lack of focus or concentration. On the other hand, as the brainwave levels increase toward the higher range of beta and into the gamma range at over thirty cycles per second, a higher level of focus and concentration occurs.

Gamma waves are higher frequency brain waves, and are often referred to as high-frequency beta waves. Gamma waves predominate during intense problem solving and focused learning. Gamma waves cycle at thirty to sixty hertz. Recent research has determined that gamma waves will be synchronized and coded by phase within the visual cortex. This phase shifting creates a coherence mechanism—a sorting process where gamma waves with the same phases are segregated and commingled. The resulting sorting process allows the gamma waves to interfere and provide associations of particular thoughts, images or impressions of sensual information.

High gamma waves cycle from sixty to two hundred hertz, and have only become obvious to researchers using more sensitive equipment. These brainwaves are seen during the most intense cognitive functions. The slower waves of theta, delta and alpha tend to resonate with distinct physical attributes. The high gamma waves tend to relate to higher states, and tend to be more diverse in their connection points and locations around the regions of the central nervous system. In one study of eight subjects, for example, high gamma brainwave activity increased during the practice of pranayama—a method of concentrated meditative breath control (Vialatte *et al.* 2008).

Another type of brainwaves were found using sensitive microelectrodes. These have been termed ripples. Ripples are high frequency oscillations that appear to be generated in the hippocampus. They have been observed oscillating with the negative portion of slower brainwaves. Ripples appear to transduce through the medial temporal lobe, notably between the hippocampus and the rhinal cortex—a region associated with the processing of explicit memory recall. Explicit memory includes active intentional recall during conscious cognition. In other words, ripples appear to function as informational waveform 'bites' used to access recent, conscious memories and instructions. It is part of our active information biocommunication system.

The discovery of ripples augments our position that EEG research has tended to oversimplify the role of brain waveforms that oscillate through the various neurons. The brain's mapping has focused on larger regions of the brain. There are still intra-neuronal networks that function on a more subtle basis. For example, a central pivoting exchange factor of the brain's networking system includes the pyramidal neuron networks. Pyramidal neurons lie within the cortex regions of the brain. Regions more dense with pyramidal neurons are often collectively referred to as the neocortex. Here their densities can be as high as 75%.

Researchers have estimated the total number of pyramidal neurons in the brain to be in the neighborhood of fifteen to twenty billion. These specialized neurons crystallize and transduce waveform signals between the cortices and the rest of the central nervous system. Some of these signals have different frequency attributes. They appear to transduce through the polar gateway systems of ion channels.

These are not unlike the on-off states of computer machine code, except there is typically more than one type of on-off state among each gateway, to allow for feedback loops. Another, more dimensional description of this transduction is called signal coupling. This is when multiple waveforms are "coupled" to create a unique pattern. We might refer to this as a multiple wave interference model.

Research has clocked the brain's activity has speeds of between 1/1000 and 10/1000 of a second, which would convert to 100-1000 meters/second. As these frequencies relate to the wave nature of the electrical activity of the brain, they also imply that there is a wave function to the mechanics of the mind. The fact that the frequency increases as our mind becomes more active indicates that higher activity exerts a greater wave speed.

Certainly if we consider how instantaneous reactions and thoughts move around the body, we are talking not only about speed. We are dealing with a network broadcasting system allowing for nearly instantaneous communication. Not that this communication system is not linear as well; it is linear yet still global: concurrently spreading into the vast territories of organs, tissues and muscles.

Allopathic medical science considers all of this activity moving through the nervous system to be electricity. Yes, electricity is involved, but even electricity is conducted in electromagnetic waves.

We would rather compare this biocommunication process to the network access of a website to billions of browsers connected on the internet. This certainly requires an information technology quite a bit more complicated than a home electricity circuit. This type of technology utilizes a mechanism of simultaneous information data coherence.

One example of how multiple waveform coherence works is the potassium channels—discovered several decades ago. Potassium channels are specialized proteins found in brain neurons, which regulate the voltage moving between neurons around the brain. As we look closer at these channels, we find they oscillate between gateway states, regulating ionic electrical pulses. These channels provide just one of the conduits for transmitting information.

As we examine the instructional pathways connecting neurons together with the physical activity of the body, we can conclude these circuits crystallize and broadcast complex waveforms, disseminating conscious intention from one part of the body throughout various regions of the anatomy.

These pathways for waveform broadcasting from one part of the brain to another appear to be necessary for the mind to develop complete images. Multiple researchers have confirmed that neurons of the visual cortex do not readily pick the full spectrum of frequencies necessary to form a complete image of what we perceive. The ramification of this is significant, simply because we typically assume that what we perceive is "out there" in the physical domain. We assume that we are receiving a complete picture.

Russian scientist Dr. Nikolai Bernstein performed film studies on human perception for several decades in the mid-twentieth century, illustrating that human movement could be translated into wave patterns using Fourier calculations. This is illustrated as we watch television or a movie. When we perceive movement on the TV or movie screen, we are not actually seeing any movement. We are merely seeing a series of still pictures flashed in sequence faster than we can consciously notice. Between the flashed images is a significant dead space or dark image. Our minds fill in the blanks and create the illusion of movement.

The work of neuroscientist Dr. Russell DeValois focused on this element of visual perception over the past several of decades. His research papers documented how the mind integrates batches of visual inputs such as color and motion. His years of groundbreaking research culminated in a 1990 compendium Spatial Vision, co-authored with his wife Kathleen— also a professor in the subject.

Dr. DeValois' memorial quoted him describing his lifetime's work in visual perception as:

> "... the physiological and anatomical organization underlying visual perception. In particular, how wavelength information is analyzed and encoded, the contribution of wavelength and luminance information to spatial vision, and how spatial information is analyzed and encoded in the visual nervous system."

In one study performed by Dr. DeValois at the University of California at Berkeley, the responses of cats and monkeys were analyzed while responding to visual checkerboard patterns. Rather than responding to the patterns themselves, the animals responded to the interference patterns created by the complementary aspects of the design, consistent with Fourier-calculated interference waves.

The work of Dr. Fergus Campbell at Cambridge University has confirmed that the human cerebral cortex picks up particular frequencies and not others. The cerebral component neurons are 'tuned' to specific wavelengths and frequencies. Dr. Pribran also confirmed this in his sometimes-cruel studies on cats and monkeys.

During these tests, it became apparent that combinations of waves of particular frequencies were being received, processed and converted into perceived images as they were combined with internally created waveforms. These internal waveforms are drawn from memory through a hierarchical cortical mapping sorting process.

In the 1970s, Dr. Benjamin Libet began researching decision-making and brain electrical response at the University of California at San Francisco. His goal was to explore a concept first introduced by Luder Deeke and Hans Kurnhuber called bereitschafts-potential—which translates to readiness potential.

In Dr. Libet's studies, human volunteers hooked up to an electroencephalograph were told to perform activities such as button pressing or finger flicking. Dr. Libet's research compared three points in time: When the subject consciously made the decision to press the button; when the button was pressed; and when brainwaves indicated an instruction from the motor cortex was made using the EEG.

As expected, the conscious decision preceded the button pushing by an average of about 200 milliseconds (or 150 milliseconds considering a 50 msec margin of error). Surprisingly, however, the brainwaves associated with the instruction to press the bottom actually preceded the subject's conscious decision to take the action. Stunned by these results, Dr. Libet and others spent several years confirming the results. Several scientific articles documented the findings (Libet et al. 1983; Libet 1985).

These results indicated that the action somehow was not originating from the conscious mind, but must be coming from a deeper source. Still, as Dr. Libet wrote in 2003, the gap between the conscious mind and the physical act gives the conscious mind an ability to "block or veto the process, resulting in no motor act." This, Dr. Libet said, is confirmed by the common experience of consciously blocking urges incompatible with social acceptability.

In 2004—more than two decades after his groundbreaking discovery—Dr. Libet proposed a theory based on his and others' research in this area. He called this the conscious mental field theory. This theory proposed the mind is a sphere of activity bridging the various rhythmic pulsing of physical nerve cells with the subjective conscious experience. He described this subjective experience as an outgrowth of the various pulses, a sort of gathering or convergence of various inputs.

A neuron is made up of a cell body with a nucleus, and two types of nerve fibers that extend outward from the cell body. The fibers include dendrites, which conduct informational waveforms into the neural cell body. Axons, on the other hand, project waveforms outward, away from the cell body. Most neurons have multiple dendrites that spider outward making several connections.

Sensory nerves typically have only one dendrite, however. Sensory nerves are also typically longer—sometimes measuring up to a meter in length. Dendrites act as receptors. They are tuned into the pulsed waveform messages that pass from neuron to neuron. They carry this rhythmic information into the neuron cell body where it may be translated or even transmuted before being conducted or broadcasted. In some cases, the neuron may simply conduct and amplify the waveform.

In addition to specialized sensory neurons referred to as afferent nerves, there are also motor neurons, which are usually referred to as efferent neurons. The efferent or motor neurons are designed to carry instructional waveforms outward through the central nervous system to specific skeletal or organ cells.

In these locations, these cells respond as instructed by the information provided by these waveform interference patterns. We note this because a single waveform does not necessarily contain enough information to drive a complex motor process. It takes a waveform combination to affect these specialized cells. Some are stimulated into metabolism responses, secretions, or contractions. Because they are stimulated by the efferent neurons, these cells are called effectors.

The intentional personality ultimately stimulates the effector neurons through the facilities offered by the neural network. The neural network generally has three basic types of processes: The first is to receive and translate afferent sensory waveforms from the senses and environment. The second is to project instructional waveform combinations outward through the appropriate neural tracts. The third process of the neural net is to prioritize, sort and catalog memories and various autonomic programs.

The brain grows and develops in the body from a tubular canal called the neural tube. The entire brain is made up of billions of neurons. These are networked into bundles of groupings, which include nerve tracts, gyri, fissures, sulci and cerebrum lobes. These groupings of specialized neurons work conjunctively to accomplish specialized tasks, while transmitting information back and forth through neural superhighways. The locations of these nerve groupings will be common.

Most nerve functions thus have location plasticity, as we've discussed. Plasticity is the ability of the organism to move or reorganize the location or processes involved in accomplishing particular tasks. In other words, should one location not be able to function, the organism will relocate the function to another region of the brain.

The personality primarily utilizes the brain's functions through the frontal cortex. Here the various waveforms provided by the senses and the body's feedback are observed by the personality. The personality utilizes a command center called the prefrontal cortex to respond to these images. This is located towards the front of the brain, behind and on top of the forehead, almost the precise position described by Ayurveda as the region between the sixth and seventh chakra regions—the *soma* chakra.

Indeed this region provides a gateway for the personality to not only observe the condition of the body and the environment, but also submit executive orders in response. For these reasons, researchers have determined that the frontal lobes are stimulated during the processing of decisions related to right and wrong, the prioritization of consequences, and logical thinking. Through the prefrontal region, the personality expresses personality and submits executive orders.

The motor cortex lies just behind the frontal cortex as we comb back over the head. It normally resides within a band of neural grey matter (neuron cells) that wrap around the top of the head onto the two sides. Here physical instructions from the frontal cortex begin their transduction towards execution. Within the motor cortex reside specialized networks of neurons, each network coordinated with specific types of motor activity. The premotor region contains billions of specialized mirroring neurons, which mirror and sort the executive decisions transmitted from the frontal cortex. Behind the premotor cortex is the primary motor cortex.

This region contains specialized neurons that are able to broadcast specific neural waveforms out through the neural network for specific parts of the body. One section will govern the toes, while another will govern the feet, and so on. This organized vertical arrangement of specialized motor neurons is also referred to as the homunculus motor region, because each location is connected to specific body locations.

Behind the region of the motor cortex neurons is another set of regions grouped into what is called the sensory cortex. This region has several individual cortices, and spreads from the top of the head (parietal lobe) through the back of the head (occipital lobe) and along the sides (temporal lobe). Among these lobes lie the visual cortex, the auditory cortex, the olfactory cortex, the postcentral gyrus, and the gustatory cortex.

In these respective regions, the various incoming sensory waveforms are translated and processed. The first three cortices—the visual, auditory and olfactory—are self-explanatory, being the centers that process waveforms of seeing, hearing and smelling, respectively. The postcentral gyrus processes the sensory waveforms of touch and balance, while the gustatory cortex processes taste waveforms from the tongue. Into each sensory cortex, specialized neural tracts conduct in and blend waveforms from the sense organs. The interference patterns of these waveforms blend together to provide an image screen of sorts for the personality to observe.

The critical limbic system is positioned inside these cortex regions, towards the center of the brain. The limbic system is made up of the thalamus, the hypothalamus, the hippocampus, the cingulates, the fomix and the amygdala. Each of these has a slightly different function, but together they translate waveform data from the body in to be processed for memory and observance by the personality. The limbic system's role is to prioritize and sort information according to crystallized neural programming.

The hypothalamus and thalamus are the central translation system for waveforms traveling between the brain and the rest of the body. They also stimulate endocrine release of hormones and neurotransmitters, and translate incoming communications from around the body. The cingulates are programmed to govern the autonomic systems such as the heartbeat, breathing, hunger, and so on.

The amygdala on the other hand, provides a gateway to the lower chakra regions according to Ayurveda. These channel the personality's focus upon survival into fear and anger into the information processing. The hippocampus sorts and prioritizes all this information for memory storage. The fomix channels the waveform information from the hippocampus through a circuitry of memory processing (called the Papex circuit), which we will examine in detail. Together the limbic system provides a translation and staging service for waveform information.

We might compare the limbic system to a computer's operating system. The software might be stored in a particular location within the computer. Nevertheless, its programming instructions govern information translation, assembly, prioritization, storage, and transmission out to processing among peripheral devices and specialized programs.

The brain receives several types of input. The first is called exteroception, which means information gathered by the five basic senses of hearing, taste, smell, vision and touch. Interoception is the reception of signals received by the internal neurons, such as pain and other internal responses. The third reception type is proprioception, which is the internal feedback mechanism gauging coordinated movements, balance and motor efficiency—often referred to as kinesthesia.

Meanwhile equilibrioception is the feedback of motor balance information, which is coordinated with waveforms passing through the vestibular system. Nociception is the reception of pain signals that accompany a threat of damage to tissues or cells. Finally, thermoception is the sensing of heat or coldness within the body. Other interoceptions include the sense of time, the esophageal senses and others. A few other sensations have been proposed, though most could also be considered a subset of interoception.

Each of these types of signals is associated with a particular region of the brain—though most interact in one respect or another within the limbic system and its components. For example, proprioception appears to resonate at the cerebellum. Thermoception resonates with thermoceptor cells in the hypothalamus. Nociception is thought to biocommunicate through the anterior cingulated gyrus (part of the cingulates).

As waveforms are stepped up through neural tracts toward the brain, the waveforms are boosted or converted by neural gateways into waveform configurations that can be managed by the limbic system. It is through the limbic system that various cortex regions are fed interoception from around the body.

Programming sequences drive autonomic responses from the cortices primarily via the limbic system as well. As waveforms travel through the limbic system, the amygdala—channeling survival concerns of the personality—is able to interact and alter these waveforms on their route to the particular cortex. This emotional interference system also works in reverse. Even if a particular decision is being channeled from the motor cortex to initiate a particular response in the body, the amygdala can alter or influence that instructional waveform as it moves back through the limbic system on its way out to stimulate particular motor nerve centers and endocrine responses (initiated primarily through the hypothalamus-pituitary pathway). In this way, motor responses may be exaggerated or muted through fear responses or other emotional responses.

Research has demonstrated an ionic channel based electrochemical beta-adrenergic modulation (Strange and Dolan 2006) facility within the amygdala. This modulation process requires a sophisticated level of waveform collaboration between the sensual inputs coming from the cortices and those arising from the mind web. As mentioned, the amygdala sorts images or impressions with an emotional or fearful perspective, which provides a sorting and priority criteria to the information. Research has concluded that by pegging information with emotional criteria, greater memory recall is established as compared to images without emotional tags (Dolcos *et al.* 2006).

This blending and transduction system could be compared to the internet or worldwide web. The internet or 'web' accomplishes a peer-accepted platform for the convergence of a variety of information gateways—or website portals. The convergence of all these website portals through the internet platform allows a particular user with a computer to choose to view any of the information portals.

On the internet, the computer operator can choose to view a sorted compilation of websites through a search engine. The search terms are of course decided by the computer operator. In the case of the mind's web, the viewer is the personality, and the gateways are the various types of pathways for waveform information being received and retained by the billions of brain cells.

The limbic system offers to the personality a platform where these information waves can be sorted and compiled. The personality uses the sorting facility of the mind to program the search terms and the priorities for search compilation. In acquisition mode, once a search string is established, the limbic system coordinates a search through the standing waves of the various neuron gateways to locate information with similar waveform specifications.

The hippocampus is a central locator and search center to the mind's web. We might compare it to the placement of information throughout a hard disk, or even the assembly of information by search engine spiders. Located on each side of the brain in the temporal lobe, information from the senses and the body are converted by the hippocampus through a complex staging process. As was first published in a 1957 report by Scoville and Milner and later confirmed by Squire *et al.* (1991) along with other researchers, when the hippocampus becomes damaged, the first symptom is typically disorientation, memory acquisition loss, and recall deficiency. This is also evidenced in cases of encephalitis, where the hippocampus does not receive enough oxygen. When the hippocampus is damaged, new memories cannot be retained or recalled.

Within the hippocampus is an intricate pathway called the Papex circuit for electromagnetic rhythms, which can be likened to the cochlear passageway that stages and converts air pressure waves into electromagnetic nerve pulses. In the hippocampal pathway, waveforms from the cortical field (entohinal cortex, perihinal cortex, cerebral cortex, and so on), the subcortical field (amygdala, broca, claustrum, substantia innominata, and so on) mix with pulses from the thalamus and hypothalamus.

These pulses are channeled through the perforant path consisting of three regions of the dentate gyrus. The signals pass through the CA3 and

CA1 regions and on to the subiculum and parahippocampal gyrus. Here, between the subiculum and the parahippocampal gyrus, information in the form of interference waveform patterns is processed and translated to higher frequency waveforms—and broadcast into the neural net for storage or processing.

In all, this circuit vets, tags and prioritizes information, preparing it to be cataloged. The various regions of the brain are also identified during this circuitry, which also identifies potential storage locations for information. In this way, the various neural networks of the different regions of the brain are mapped for waveform information storage and further processing.

In the pathway for visual impressions, for example, waveform combinations of different frequencies strike the retina and pass through the LGM to the visual cortex. Here in the cortex, waveforms drawn from memory through the amygdala are combined with internal stimuli waveforms and the LGM waveform data to create impression waveform interference patterns.

These interference patterns create the specific information images for the personality to see. We might compare this with creating an image by blending light rays of different colors and shapes onto a dark screen. Alone each light ray does not create much of an image, but together the different rays and colors can create a more complete image on the screen.

The images the personality observes within the cortex are thus altered by context and history. The waveforms from the amygdala and memory alter the interference patterns. This accounts for the expression that we 'see what we want to see.' The interference patterns from these different sources eventually deliver convincing impressions to the hippocampus. Because the cortex combines all these waveforms together, the waveform information is forever altered. This creates the reality that each of us actually perceives a slightly different world around us.

In order to attempt to 'standardize' our perception, the personality will seek confirmation from others. Information is thus gathered from others and the different forms of media. This creates a feedback loop between the amygdala, the hippocampus, and the cortices to constantly adjust our perception of reality towards the apparent perception of others. This is an intentional process because the personality is constantly seeking affirmation from others in our never-ending quest for love and fulfillment.

Mapped brain regions also sort and translate incoming waveforms from the hippocampus. These are ultimately governed and coordinated by the prefrontal cortex. The intentions of the personality stimulate a form of waveform programming mechanism that modulates neuron channels for particular waveform biocommunications. This creates a sorting system among those programmed neurons.

The ion channel gateway states, neurotransmitter fluid content, and even genetic structures within the neuron may be manipulated by the executive initiatives programmed by the mind—under the intentions of the personality. Many pre-programmed responses are crystallized within our static DNA. Still, neurons accommodate the executive authority of the inner personality, expressed and translated through the prefrontal cortex and communicated via messenger pathways.

In the limbic system, waveforms from all over the body are converged and translated together with remodeled waves from the sensory cortices and the various feedback centers throughout the body. After translation, the limbic system coordinates instructions out to the body, together with a reflective broadcasting of waveform signals to the frontal cortex for executive review.

Should the personality respond to these inputs, executive waves are fed back to the body through the limbic system and the motor cortex. Here again the limbic system is acting as a transfer station, stimulating the release of various hormones through the hypothalamus and pituitary gland, which cascade through the various glands of the endocrine system. This provides the feedback pathway of executive instruction that Dr. Libet's research illustrated, allowing conscious decisions to take place after (programmed) responsive nerve impulses are detected.

Ultimately, it is the inner personality—utilizing the various equipment of the brain—who initiates executive action. Once converted through the prefrontal and frontal cortices, this is accomplished directly through executive stimulation of the motor cortex and limbic system. This is like a car driver who sets up the proper cruise control speed, then removes his foot from the gas pedal after the cruise control button is pressed.

The cruise control will maintain the speed of the car by accelerating up hills and decelerating down hills automatically. However, should the driver decide to change speeds, avert running into the car ahead, or even stop the car, the driver can immediately take over the gas pedal and control the car's speed directly. In the same way, the personality is driving the vehicle of the body, through both autonomic programming and executive control.

Most autonomic functions can be manipulated directly should the personality consciously intend to change them. In some cases, this takes practice, as biofeedback research illustrates. This conscious insertion of executive command can be initiated even during an autonomic response, just as the car driver can hit the gas pedal at any time to change the car's speed while it is running on cruise control.

As waveform messages from sensory nerves combine with physiology feedback and enter the brain's mapping network through the limbic system, they can be observed by the personality on the interference 'screens' of a particular cortex or a combination of cortices. (The personality can also manipulate, prioritize and distort these incoming physiological waveforms through the amygdala, however.) As they blend in the cortex, the personality is able to review the waveforms and if need be, respond with intention. By this time, however, the programming already in place to process the particular situation is also ready to respond.

Should a conscious 'executive' decision be made by the personality, instructional waveforms are initiated through the prefrontal cortex. These are channeled through the motor cortex, which formats the waveforms for the hypothalamus. The hypothalamus in turn transduces these waveforms into physical response through the endocrine system and central nervous system. These instructional messengers may also contain a stop order to override whatever other instructions may already be in place.

Autonomic responses are established through subconscious intentions and a subsequent programming of key web hubs by the mind. Most of these intentions are related to the survival of the body, translated from the personality's fear of dying. This fear becomes translated into various scenarios that stimulate the programming features of mind. The programming waveforms stimulated by the mind are stored in neurons just as memories are, in the form of standing waves, crystallized by ionic molecular polarity and bonding sequences. Some autonomic programs are more permanently 'wired' into the standing waveforms that make up DNA bonds. These 'hard-wired' programs ultimately are passed on to the body's successors through the DNA.

These 'coded' standing waveforms with neurons are activated by certain types of waveforms incoming through sensory nerves and from interoception translated through the hypothalamus and thalamus. As information moves through this network, the neural programming indirectly relays the personality's ultimate intentions of keeping the body alive with specific autonomic responses. The information will also be stepped up to the mind's web for viewing through the cortices. When we burn our finger, our autonomic programming will immediately respond by pulling the hand away. The personality will also be able to view the incoming information separately, and initiate a separate, conscious response, such as tending to the injury or turning off the flame.

The personality's recognition of information within the frontal cortex (or mind screen) is called cognition. In humans and primates, the central interface or bridge between the incoming impulse pathways of the nervous system and executive control is located in the dorsolateral prefrontal cortex (Otani 2002). It is here waveforms are examined, responded to and their responses relayed onto the motor cortex.

Simultaneously, goal-directed intentions from the personality stimulate the broadcast of waveform messages back into the neural net through the frontal cortex. Instructive waveforms are simultaneously pulsed through the hypothalamus, the specific regions of the motor cortex, and then the lower chakras. These instructive waveforms together stimulate the various elemental channels to respond. In other words, the body is not shocked or jerked into motion solely from pulses moving out from the brain.

There are several pathways of activity initiated during a full-body response. The body's endocrine systems are stimulated. The body's heat-producing centers are stimulated. The body's insulin and energy releasing centers are stimulated. The body's pacemaker, vasomotor, perfusive and respirative functions all are simultaneously stimulated into immediate response. How else could the body react so instantaneously and thoroughly from head to toe following an intentional decision? We certainly have to characterize the chemical binding process as too cumbersome to exclusively provide these broadcasting mechanisms.

The connection between the cognitive functions of higher decision-making and the mind screen web are illustrated by the size of the frontal lobe cortex areas of the brain in more evolved organisms. Behavioral studies with animals and humans have also confirmed that complex executive functions with goal-directed behavior, language and higher cognition in general is associated with a larger, more developed prefrontal cortex (Fuster 2002).

This cascade of messengers is also regulated by the activities of the pineal gland, which coordinate with the rhythmic SCN cells to secrete melatonin. Melatonin triggers a cascading pathway to slow metabolism, leading to sleep and cell repair. Melatonin levels are balanced by other metabolic messengers stimulated through other command cascades. Examples of these are cortisol and the thyroid hormones.

All of these physical components of the brain and messenger systems are within the perimeter of the mind. The brain is a physical transfer and conversion mechanism. The mind is a holographic echoing mechanism utilizing interference patterns and standing waveforms. The mind sorts and governs, resonating with specific neurons to convert memories and data from waveform interference. The mind is a screening device spread throughout the nervous system, yet centralized within the brain. The mind translates the feedback from these central points, and outputs the echoed intentions arising from the intentional personality. The mind is quite simply the operating system software and programming utility utilized by the personality. The brain is the physical utility used by the mind to translate the code into physical activity and memory.

In 2005, Dr. Jim Tucker, a professor at the University of Virginia, compared the mind's relationship with the brain and body to a television set. Dr. Tucker explained that while the TV signal is translated through the television set, the signal of television programming originates from a remote location. In the same way, Dr. Tucker explained, the mind is not the brain, but rather, he insisted, the signals of the mind are transmitted through the brain.

Neurological research headed up by Dr. Robert Knight from the University of California at Berkeley (Krämer *et al.* 2011) illustrated that brainwaves allow different regions of the brain to appear to communicate using combinations of alpha, beta, gamma and theta waves. According to this and related research, the synchronization or coupling effect of these various waves—together with their timing and frequency—transmit specific information. We can certainly compare the television and television programs,—or the computer and computer software—to the brain and the mind. However, the transfer of the information occurs in precisely the same fashion in all of these cases: Through waveform interference pattern transmission.

As they harmonize with the intentional direction of the personality, coherent interference patterns are created: These are thoughts. As the mapping system converts instructions from the personality through the mind, they are connected indirectly to the rest of the body through the various neurochemical messengers and associated waveform biocommunications. In combination, the mix of neurochemical messengers such as hormones and neurotransmitters provide a feedback and response system, keeping the mindscreen in touch with the rest of the body.

For example, nerve pathways from our right arm, elbow, and wrist will travel through the CNS to the upper left hemisphere of the cerebellum—in an area usually referred to as the primary motor region. Meanwhile the sensations from the fingers of our right hand will be received by a lower left side of this region. Our right ankle will travel to an area of the brain further up the left side of this motor area, nearest to the sagittal sutures—the division between the hemispheres.

The pathways for these messages exist through channels of nerve cells bridged by neurotransmitter fluids, microtubules and ion channels, which accelerate complex messages from the body's remote areas. As the various cranial nerves connect these different brain regions to particular parts of the body, the brain wave channels resonate with certain nerve-ending receptors to facilitate the passage of feedback and response messages. This is comparable to a two-way radio antenna receiving and sending broadcast messages.

This coupling of waveform interference may provide a foundation for an adequate explanation for psi. Parapsychologists such as Dr. Stanley Krippner, and Dr. Michael Persinger have established a magnetic field link with extrasensory perception and dreaming after demonstrating that biomagnetic field changes from solar storms and electrical storms interrupt extrasensory perception.

Here telepathics were able to better influence the dreaming of nearby and remote sleepers with geographic visualizations during decreased solar storm activity (Persinger and Krippner, 1989). Both Dr. Persinger and Dr. Krippner independently and with others repeatedly demonstrated geomagnetic effects in dream and psi studies. This indicates the waveform nature of thoughts and dreams—and the similarity between the composition of thoughts and geomagnetic fields.

We find a similar channeling and messaging system with sense perception: Each sensory organ or sensory area of the body will be stimulated by waveform inputs from our environment. These sensations are translated into pulsed waveforms, which conduct through nerve pathways, accelerated by particular neurotransmitters and ion channels toward particular areas of the brain. Upon reaching these brain regions, the sensory pulses are translated into brainwaves, which collide and interact with the various other brainwaves bouncing through the CNS. Coherent interaction among these brainwaves provides a projection observable by the personality.

As to the geomagnetic influence upon the brain, mind and thoughts, Dr. Persinger (1989) was able to demonstrate that the earth's geomagnetic condition affected temporal lobe activity. Further investigations have demonstrated that geomagnetic activity also affected melatonin release from the pineal gland. This illustrates that there is a resonance—or harmonic effect—between the external waveforms surrounding our bodies and those waveforms generated through self-direction. The interference patterns created by magnetic and sensory inputs coalesce to influence the mind's imaging systems—ultimately influencing the personality's decisions.

The complex exchange of instantaneous waveform pulses moving through the body is nothing short of astounding. Some estimate that over six trillion waveform messages per minute are fired through the nervous system alone—not including the higher frequency microtubule pulses, the various hormonal messaging broadcasts, the intercellular biocommunication and the intracellular network. These waveforms pulsing through the physical layers are all sorted for priority and projected through the mind to be imaged by the personality.

Research has illustrated that the left side of the brain is associated with the thoughts relating to logic, language, and mathematics. Meanwhile the right side of the brain has been associated with art, fantasy, and music. Further to this point of specialization, certain regions appear to associate with certain mental skills and particular types of memories. Auditory communication, for example, is associated with the temporal lobe, while written motor skills have been linked with the motor cortex of the frontal lobe. Visual interaction usually utilizes the occipital lobe.

Recent neurological research has confirmed that each of these brain functions also run concurrent with particular types of brainwaves. We also know a hierarchy of waveforms is slated to each thought-type. The slower waves like delta and theta tend to accompany sleep and introspection, while faster waves like beta and gamma waves tend to accompany sensual cognition and information transfer.

Without consciousness, organic matter will not develop, grow, or re-produce. Organic matter does not exhibit emotion or mental program-ming without consciousness being involved. Once consciousness leaves an organism, the body will no longer exhibit growth, fear, emotion, or any type of optional responsiveness.

The hard drive of the mind's memory web has both a subjective and selective tendency. We can see this should we gather various opinions from people. While a group of people may receive the same information through the senses, a variety of perceptions and conclusions will be made by each. Even though the mind may meticulously gather and web together its incoming information, the unique personality can shape and prioritize this information through intention.

We know from various research and practical experience that the mind tends to select and choose information as it is being organized and prepared for storage. Research illustrates that the visual cortex will shape and direct spatial visual information as it is being gathered through signal-ing mechanisms. This process has been termed retino-cortical mapping (Johnston 1986).

Yes, this is complex. But are all of these processes operating by them-selves? Are they operating at random? Certainly not. Or are they operating on automatic? Certainly not any of these. The system is far too complex for them to be random, automatic or autonomic.

Rather, the entire process of the brain and central nervous system would be impossible without a conscious operator combined with a power supply to drive the sorting operations of the mind, utilizing the components of the brain. At the end of the day, the personality is the operator. The mind is the software and the brain is the CPU. The body is the hardware.

The developed frontal lobe cortex enables the personality to command a greater volume of switchboard control and the ability to specify intention through a complex mental capacity. We also note that all highly evolved organisms also have advanced backbones and high-energy entry-points to carry out full-body chakra responses. As for less evolved organisms, we still find key neural points that transduce that personality's intentions, albeit less complexly.

Chapter Twelve

Memory and the Subconscious

The concepts as proposed by Dr. Janet and Dr. Freud not much more than a century ago included the notion of a subconscious mind. The basis for their conclusions was the use of hypnosis. Under hypnosis, their patients demonstrated an awareness of past behavior and information seemingly unavailable to their conscious minds during their normal awakened states. Like Dr. Stevenson's research over the past few decades, their hypnosis research also demonstrated the possibility of past lives, which they considered unexplainable.

Because our conscious minds appear not to be aware of the subtle memories and programming mechanisms utilized by the mind, the concept of a subconscious mind appeared to adequately explain these phenomena. We must question this assumption, however. What is this mysterious subconsciousness? Why can a person who is brought under trance—which is simply a state of suggestion and trust—suddenly be able to recall things that are not otherwise recalled? How does the programming of the mind otherwise operate beneath the awareness of the conscious mind? Furthermore, what is dreaming? How can these be otherwise explained without the theory of the subconscious mind?

The empirical understanding of the existence of the inner personality adequately explains this theoretical subconsciousness seamlessly. It is precisely the positioning of the inner personality—the operator—within the body that creates the ability of the mind to submit to the suggestion of hypnosis. The personality simply makes a determination to submit to suggestion, and the body and mind follow.

It is the partial shielding or cloaking of the inner personality by the veil of misidentification that is responsible for the mysterious nature of the inner personality. Furthermore, it is the permanence of the inner personality throughout the changing physical body that allows one to be able to recall previous lives under hypnosis.

The relationship between visual pictures, imagination and memory can also be explained within the context of the inner personality as the intentional viewer. The mind's holographic pictures are constructed by the combination of the retinal cells, the optic nerve, the LGM, and the visual cortex. We might refer to this as an intentional process called focus. Through conscious intent, the personality can also stimulate the mind to construct internal pictures. We can aptly refer to this as imagination. Through a combination of focus and imagination, intentional pictures are constructed within the mind.

When attached to an intentional picture or image, incoming information can be sorted and stored onto to the neural net. When we connect information with images—including any sensual input such as sound or touch—we are effectively multiplying the number of references within that data. We might compare this with how many search engine spiders prioritize web pages. These bots will travel the net and tabulate the various cross referencing of websites—and to some extent ranking by intra-website referrals This is because the personality tells the mind to prioritize by interest: The more intentional screenings, the higher its priority ranking.

As a result, our retrievable memories of the past are usually connected to events we observed visually, through imagination, or through biofeedback information. We would adequately term these sense perceptions as impressions. By capturing focused sounds, smells, touch, or visual impressions on a focused basis, we are effectively increasing the number of impressions that data are attached to.

An example of this attachment between focused impression and raw data is how a song will reconnect us back to a precise time and place of our historical past. Because the song became connected to our intention during this time in our lives, the song will stimulate the recall of vivid memories of those times—sometimes even details otherwise long forgotten.

This can work with pictures just as well. We may see a particular picture and be reminded of the time, place and details surrounding the moment when that picture was taken. The images in the picture stimulated the retrieval of the memories just as the song did.

Why does the memory work better when connected to mental impressions? What is it about a picture, song, or funny story that enables us to retrieve vivid memories?

As we examine the research of dementia and memory loss, we see a substantial amount of evidence connecting the loss of memory with the loss of function among particular regions of the brain or nerve cells. As we have discussed, we have also observed these same regions involved in a constant exchange and echoing of waveform signals during memory storage and recall.

A lighting-fast interactive mirroring system allows different regions to check and crosscheck information. This crosschecking allows our minds to validate, confirm, and store information. It also increases the number of impressions the connected data has logged. As the information waves interfere, they form a unique webbing of interactivity, much as if we were to throw several stones into a small pond. Assuming each wave contains unique information and a specific history, the crossing and interaction of multiple waves creates a rich multi-layered view of the history of the stone throws.

This is analogous to how a television screen converts various colors, forms, and sounds onto the viewing screen and speakers to image the original broadcast. As information is broadcast into the antenna or cable input, it is also flashed upon the screen.

In a beautiful symphony of homuncular holography, humans have invented and assembled televisions, computers and programs to precisely reflect the functionality of our own human mental programming and web. This simply confirms that our mental and physical programming stems from an intention personality. Computers and televisions are simply reflections of our own mental-physical systems.

The use of television and computers are strictly intentional. In the same way, the source of the intentional ability to save and retrieve particular memories is a function of a living, conscious being. We could entertain a programming feature allowing every input to be equally prioritized and accessed. A driving force of intention is still required. We cannot train a dead rat to do tricks. Neither can we expect a dead human to remember names by shouting those names into the ears of the dead body.

All the brain regions and brain cells may still be intact in a newly deceased dead body. Yet there is no mind web because there is no intention, and there is no priority or organization of the remaining waveforms because the personality has left.

Outside the physical issues and the back-and-forth process of checking and crosschecking between the mind and the neural network lies the conscious intent of the personality driving the process of the mind's information processing software.

The personality within ultimately drives the extent of the memory saved and retrieved. In other words, while we can typically remember many interesting things about our life and retrieve them quite easily without much effort, we have to make a conscious effort to remember details that are less important to us. If we want to remember details taught in a science class for example, we have to make a concerted effort to repeatedly focus on the information in order to retain it and repeat it later.

Simply listening to the lecture and hearing the information once typically does not allow the attachment and recall of massive amounts of unimportant details onto the mind's memory web. We might want good grades, but we may not be interested in the information itself. We do not have any emotional attachment to it.

We will have to listen to it, read about it, write it down and then maybe read about it again in hopes that we will somehow connect enough emotion to the information to remember it. If we are able to utilize some of the methods mentioned above—relating the details to unique pictures and funny stories—our ability to remember these details will be better. The remembrance is occurring because the personality is connecting emotional intention to the information.

For this same reason, we tend to better remember details about the things that interest us the most. For example, we often see men and boys able to remember the batting averages of their favorite baseball players yet unable to remember the latest economic statistics—even though they saw both on the same television news show.

Here the details of intended hobbies and personal missions are placed in a higher priority. We have focused greater intention upon them. As our minds check and crosscheck information—as research indicates is occurring during sleep—the focus is on the areas synchronizing with the intentions of the personality.

This is illustrated by a study published in 2005 (Lindstrom *et al.*) concluding that a positive relationship existed between acquiring later-in-life Alzheimer's disease and increased television viewing among middle-aged adults. 135 elderly Alzheimer's cases and 331 healthy (control) subjects were interviewed and classified for television viewing duration during their mid-life years. The results found for each hour per day of mid-life television viewing, Alzheimer's occurrence increased 1.3 times.

Conversely, intellectually stimulating activities and social activities were associated with lower Alzheimer's rates. The study's authors concluded that social engagement with others somehow better utilized the neurons at risk of dementia-related disorders.

While watching television, the personality's focus becomes increasingly tied to the virtual illusions of the tele-scripted drama, as opposed to the variegated living world around us. These adults presumably reach for their escape from the world by watching television because they prefer to unfocus their attention on the living world. (This assumes fictional dramas, not news and documentary programs reflecting reality.) The living world provides too many problems or difficulties to solve.

Conversely, social activities engage the personality's attention onto the real lives and problems of the world. This requires further emotional involvement from the personality. Life requires us to prioritize the mass of incoming information.

This stresses the neural mechanisms—keeping them better exercised. The real world also stimulates the personality to utilize the tools of the mind to solve the problems of the physical world. The research has indeed confirmed that mental exercise creates better cognition and a more resilient memory.

In the case of television watchers, the personality's lack of focus and work on real world problems leads to a slow degeneration of biocommunication pathways. Like unused muscles, the neurons are under-utilized. They receive less circulation, less detoxification, less interaction and less activity.

This all leads to the slow degeneration of those cells, opening them up to DNA damage and the production of deranged secretase enzymes that produce beta-amyloid oligomers. In the overall picture, however, it is the propensity of the inner personality to escape from reality that under-utilizes the brain's biocommunication equipment. Does this mean the personality wills or intends the Alzheimer's scenario? Not directly, but just as a sedentary lifestyle perpetuates an inability to adequately move and exercise, the propensity to escape certain physical realities perpetuates an inability to utilize regions of the brain that focus on physical realities.

It has long been held by sleep researchers who have measured the brain's electrical activity during sleep that the higher electrical activity from individual brain neurons indicated the neurons were reassembling and sorting the information received during the day.

The neurons were theoretically processing this information into long-term memory. This is referred to as consolidation. This theory however has recently been challenged by memory researchers who have noticed the limbic system and interference processes appear to be the focal point of the higher electrical activity.

As Dr. John Wixted, professor of Psychology at the University of California at San Diego proposed in 2005, the evidence seems to point to interference mechanics created by activities such as sleep. The process of sleep apparently provokes priorities or images that interfere with the consolidation process of memories.

We would contend this is caused by those initial memories not being well-enough synchronized by and to the intentions of the personality. For this reason, not all the recent memory is eliminated during sleep. The memories considered more critical to the personality are retained. Otherwise, how could we remember those things we consider dear (beyond a day) and forget the other details?

Where do the memory waveform interference patterns go as intention distances them—lowering their relative priority? Where do the waveforms not imaged by the mind go? Do they still exist somewhere? Are they hiding within this subconscious mind?

We contend first, that there is no such thing as a subconscious mind. The conscious mind is a mapping and screening mechanism driven by the personality. It is conscious because it is driven by consciousness. The personality, however, is of another nature: The personality is composed of consciousness. Waveform interference patterns continue to exist in the larger realm of consciousness.

However, the bridle of misidentification confines the personality to those interference patterns intentionally collected and translated by the limbic system, and projected by the mind. The brain and mind are simply tools for intention.

This might be comparable to a person going to a lecture and choosing to write down notes on the lecture, even though the person could certainly just listen to the lecture and remember the interesting parts of the lecture. The uninteresting data will likely remain outside the memory web because the personality is not interested in it.

This also means that the mind mechanism is limited by and focused onto the intentions of the personality. Therefore, the mind will sometimes alter or ignore inputs that do not fit with the intentions of the personality. As a result, the personality will not want to maintain a memory that might conflict with its attempts to enjoy the physical world. Most traumas are erased from the "conscious" awareness of the mind simply because the personality does not want to face those painful experiences.

However, if the inner personality does not learn and grow from the experience, the self cannot release its focus upon the trauma. As a result, the waveform interference patterns of the trauma event continue to be linked to the emotions of the personality—which forces the memory to be retained and linked to those emotions. Linked with these emotions, the memory is prioritized near the top of the standing wave hierarchy, forcing the personality to continue to face that memory until it is resolved.

It is only when the trauma has been resolved by the personality that the emotion can be removed from the memory. When the emotional link is removed from the memory, it becomes a worthless detail to the personality, and the mind eventually consolidates it and reprioritizes it downward. Over time, the reprioritization routine of the mind's programming releases the details and the memory is gradually downgraded within the memory net.

The question becomes; how does the personality resolve the trauma? This is accomplished through growth and learning. The personality must determine why the event happened. The personality must forgive the person who we might be holding responsible.

The personality must come to an understanding regarding the event and the people involved. The personality must learn from the event what was supposed to be learned. As soon as this takes place, the personality can detach from the event and move on. This is often communicated by the expression: "What do I need to learn from this experience?" If we do not know, we will probably continue to hold onto it.

Reprioritization or consolidation does not eliminate the event. It still exists in waveform interference pattern form. However, ones mental memory of an event is inseparable from intent. As long as there is intent to remember it—or an emotion connected to it—the waveform will be accessible. This might be compared again to the internet. While so many websites might be out there—some even communicating hatred or violence—we choose to only surf the websites we are interested in. We will ignore those others, and even though they may still be there and possibly even accessible, the web surfer will probably not even be aware of their existence.

Although the mind and its programming are set up based upon the intentions of the personality, the mind is still different from the personality. The mind has its own design, and sometimes the mind can get out of control of the personality. As the mind develops its programming, it can take us to places that ultimately we do not want to be. It can be carried away with the directives we have given it.

The main directive the personality gives the mind is to figure out ways to achieve physical pleasure. The mind begins to concoct various scenarios for physical enjoyment. Sometimes these scenarios will cross the line of decency or morality. The personality is clearly aware of these lines. However, the mind will also produce—should the personality be open to them—various justifications for the activity to appeal to the morality of the personality.

We will then be faced with a moral decision on whether to do something or not. As this decision is being made, the mind will continue to throw justifications for the activity on the screen for the personality to review. Here is where the evolution of the personality becomes critical. Should the personality's level of growth be such that we do not understand the consequences of an activity, or should the personality's growth not be tempered with the intelligence that physical pleasure will not deliver fulfillment, then the prospect of physical enjoyment may outweigh the consequences of the activity.

Many times nature designs consequences that force a choice between our own pleasure and our relationships. This forces us to consider whether our own pleasure is more important to us than our relationships with others. This conflict between the personality's desire for pleasure and the desire to unselfishly love is a constant struggle for the personality.

The Memory Net

Neurologists divide memory into short-term and long-term processes. Long-term memory is further divided into three types: Episodic—when memories are unique to the time and place; semantic—when memories involve concepts or learning; and procedural—when memories revolve around skills. Episodic memories relate to events that happened in the past, or people we knew from the past. Semantic memories relate more to concept understanding. Procedural memories relate to remembering how to ride a bike, write or use a telephone.

Interestingly, memory loss of one type will not typically accompany the loss of another type. Thus in many amnesia cases, long-term memory may appear erased while short-term memory is retained. The person may forget older events yet continue to remember what just happened.

Furthermore, all too frequently one type of long-term memory may be lost while another type may be retained. For example, a person may suffer the loss of their episodic memory—forgetting their name, family, school history, phone number, birth date and other personal details or events of the past. At the same time they may remember how to write, drive, talk on the phone and even retain concepts such as how economic markets work.

Often a particular trauma or event may cause the forgetfulness of either what happened just before the event, or what happened just after the event. The former case is referred to as retrograde amnesia—a loss of memory just prior to a trauma. The latter is referred to as anterograde amnesia—a loss of memory just after a trauma. Both may also occur. The causes of these types of forgetfulness are considered quite mysterious. This is because memory has been miscalculated.

There are other types of memory loss. Many are unconnected to any particular event, while others follow injury to particular brain regions or involve trauma. Trauma-associated amnesia may or may not involve physical injury. It may follow a head injury or automobile accident. Traumatic amnesia may also follow a witnessing of a traumatic event, or may involve abuse.

Rape is an example of traumatic amnesia involving abuse. Psychogenic or dissociative fugue is another type of memory loss, which also may occur following a trauma, and may result in a person re-identifying him- or herself as someone else, and even taking an unexpected trip to a place previously unknown. Other events that can cause memory loss include alcohol and drug related blackouts, and Wernicke-Korsakoff's, which is thought to be caused by thiamin deficiency.

A more common type of amnesia involves the loss of memory of a particular event. This may be the forgetting of certain childhood events, for example. Forgetting certain events may also be referred to as traumatic memory loss. Many of us forget events in the distant past that were not necessarily traumatic as well. It is not unusual for us to forget our younger childhood events. We also may recall something without remembering how we knew it—called source amnesia.

The frontal and medial temporal lobe is considered the seat of long-term and episodic memories—based on EGG and magnetic resonance scans. Within the medial temporal lobe we find the hippocampus, and the neocortical regions called the perirhinal, parahippocampal, and the entorhinal.

Even so, researchers have observed numerous instances where memories are retained when specific regions of the brain thought to control a particular type of memory are removed or incapacitated. This often occurred in hemicortication surgeries—a frequent treatment of childhood epilepsy for many years. In most cases, episodic memories were retained even through the brain regions thought to be involved were removed. We must therefore question the assumption that memories are specific to particular neurons. Yet we still need to address the fact that many memory losses occur following brain damage to particular locations. What is going on here?

The first clue is that most of these cases are specific to short-term memory loss. Long-term memories remain a mystery. In one study (Piolino et al. 2006), thirteen patients with early stage dementia, ten patients with semantic dementia and fifteen patients with frontotemporal dementia were compared to assess the connection between memory loss and damage to the medial temporal lobe.

One of the central areas of focus in this study was the autobiographical amnesia of episodic memories, or the lack of ability to acquire or remember events of ones past. The results of this study concluded no consistency between memory loss and frontal lobe impairment. In some cases, short-term memories were difficult to acquire as a whole, and in other cases, the memory acquisition depended upon the details and importance of the event.

In many cases, long-term "remote" memories were retained and preserved while short-term details and events were not. This led the study authors to support a newer theory called the multiple trace theory, which says that memory acquisition occurs through more than one physical mechanism, and can be stored in multiple locations.

In a similar study (Matuszewski et al. 2006) on autobiographical episodic memory loss among frontotemporal dementia patients, near learning abilities with semantic memories revealed a shifting executive function with multiple processes. As for other possible models of memory acquisition, several studies have indicated that the hippocampus complex was significantly involved in the storage and recall of recent memories, but not for older memories. Other research has offered evidence that the hippocampal complex is responsible for autobiographical episodic memory and special memory, but the storage of other types of memory was shifted to other locations (Nadel and Moscovitch 1997).

In a 2002 report (Nester *et al.*) published in *Neuropsychologia* on autobiographical memories among semantic dementia patients, the preservation of recent memories and the loss of remote memories supported the trace theory of memory retention and acquisition.

Episodic autobiographical memory is also damaged from the earliest stages of Alzheimer's disease. Yes, it is true that episodic autobiographical memory tends to decrease as we age. But it is also linked to the trace memory relationships.

In 2016, researchers from Italy's University of Vergata (De Simone *et al.*) studied the episodic autobiographical memories of Alzheimer's patients together with healthy people. They found that both utilized trace memorization to reclaim their episodic autobiographical memories, even though the Alzheimer's patients' episodic autobiographical memories were damaged. They stated:

> *"Our findings provide new evidence that the combined action of both age of memory and retrieval frequency could provide a valuable framework for predicting patterns of episodic autobiographical memory loss, at least in early Alzheimer's patients. In line with the Multiple Trace Theory, we speculated that retrieval frequency protects episodic trace recall against hippocampal damage by reinforcing the neural representation of personal context-rich memories, which consequently are easier to access and recall."*

These studies indicate that memory storage and retrieval is a process driven by the personality within, rather than simply a product of neural chemistry.

We can logically compare memories to data stored on a computer's hard drive. However, modern science has yet to locate the program, the language nor the methods used to categorize, place and retain memories.

This is because modern science does not understand the most basic understandings of living biology. Again, we first must know who the driver of the vehicle of the body is. From there we must understand the means for the operation of the vehicle.

Just as a car's driver uses the wheel, the clutch and the gas pedal to move the car, the driver of the body also utilizes particular equipment to drive the body. The reality is, the mind is the software of the brain, and the brain assembles information as programmed by the mind. The personality dictates the functioning of the mind through conscious intention: desire.

This was clearly exposed in a study of memory-challenged patients with different brain disorders (Thomas-Anterion 2000). Twelve Alzheimer's patients and twelve frontotemporal dementia patients with functionally similar semantic memory, logical memory and retrograde memory test scores were studied for antegrade verbal memory and frontal lobe activity.

Despite similar memory acquisition scores and types of memory loss, physiological brain function occurred in different locations among the subjects. This illustrated flexibility in brain region utilization, quite similar to practical daily living: Should we be unable to pick up something with one hand, we will quickly adjust and pick up the item with the other hand. In the same way, the personality, using the utility of the mind, can often accomplish the same purpose using different neurons, cortices and/ or limbic components.

Should the intent to remember exist, memory can be retained using a variety of external physical mechanisms as well. Humans have indeed resorted to various tools to replace or augment memory function for thousands of years. For example, a person may retain memories within a diary to assist in the recall of particular thoughts, emotions and events. Projects or objectives may be recorded onto daily planners, or onto digital voice recorders for later recall.

Most students and businesspeople carry notebooks to every class and meeting to assist with the retention and recall of lectures and discussions. These external memory devices replace or augment limited memorization abilities. They also illustrate an intention to remember.

The memory experiments by Dr. Wilder Penfield at the Montreal Neurological Institute in the 1970s clearly illustrated that memories typically accompanied emotions and intentions. When Dr. Penfield's weak electrical currents excited locations within the brain, the subject would recall historical facts associated with past experiences. Their recollections included songs connected to feelings from the past, aromas connected to experiences, people connected to personal relationships, and events connected to other emotional events.

Dry information such as what score a person received twenty years ago on a test or sporting event might seem like raw data, but even this data are connected to personal intentions to win or receive a good score. Without an emotional, intentional attachment, the ability to recall that event subsides as the personality's intention to remember it weakens.

What this tells us is that memory is impossible without emotion or consciousness. Memory studies have shown that when a person is emotionally involved in a particular incident or detail, the recall rate of that incident or detail is significantly higher. Furthermore, as the event converts to longer-term memory, if it has no emotional attachment, it is typically sorted out during our consolidation process—which typically takes place as we sleep. In order to remember trivial details, those subjects who connect the detail to a colorful, emotional or funny association will dramatically increase the likelihood of recalling it later.

Certainly, without consciousness there would be no need for memory or recall. We might think that a robot must have a memory in order to store its programming information. However, we also know that no robot would be built without an original conscious intention. Without consciousness, there would be no purpose for a robot. The robot, then, is simply a surrogate of a conscious person's purpose and intention. This is precisely what the physical body is.

From these points, we can logically conclude that the inner personality utilizes the physical elements of the brain for memory retention and recall, but only by utilizing the programming of the mind. This also means that damage to the hardware may also destroy the organism's ability to recall and apply those memories. Memorization and recall may be shifted to a variety of brain regions and even external tools. The hardware is still necessary, however. This is because memories are waveform interference patterns linked to emotion.

Yes, the waveforms are crystallized within groups of resonating neurons. However, the memories will not be retrievable without conscious intention. Should those brain cells become damaged, those memories may become difficult to retrieve. The retrieval difficulty is due to a drop in the link between the inner personality and those interference patterns. The standing waveforms may still be there, but the emotional tie to those waveform patterns will be severed.

This is not to say the personality has no memory without the body. This is clearly evidenced by near death experiences and past life regression research. The personality has the ability to recall events without the tools of the brain's neurons. The real question is whether once the personality has moved on from a particular body; does the personality retain any real intent to remember events related to the petty details of that former body's history? Without the body's existence, what good would remembering these details be to us? Memories may provide interesting conversation or perhaps pathological interest (as Drs. Freud and Janet might have), but have little application to the personality's emotional situation once the body has decomposed.

We can just imagine how confusing life would be if we each could harken back at will to the different physical bodies we have lived within. We would be simply remembering the traumatic events leading to the death of that body, along with various details that would serve us only with regrets and the missing of loved ones who are probably still around us in different bodies anyway (as loved ones and family members often transmigrate together). Currently it is difficult to remember all the names, dates, appointments and other details of this life, let alone past ones. Imagine the overload if we could mix memories of different lifetimes together at will.

Consistent with many of the ancient sciences, the personality has another identity transcendental to this physical dimension. This identity has the ability to retain and remember everything in the past and present, assuming the personality is not locked up within the confines of the false identification within a physical body. Just as a dark movie theatre blocks our ability to see what is going on around us as we focus upon a movie, our absorption into our mind and present physical body buries our ability to recall events of previous lifetimes.

Because memories are part of the personality's learning process, we still intuitively draw upon the learning experiences of previous lifetimes without the mind being involved in the memory of that lifetime. We will elaborate on this innate ability to retain and learn from the past as we discuss the "subconsciousness" later.

The personality might have the ultimate ability to learn and grow from the events that take place here. The waveform patterns crystallized by brain neurons linked to emotions are what we might call virtual memories, or more accurately, holographic memories. In other words, the memorized details we associate with emotional intentions are related to the accommodation of our desires. We remember the type of information that we feel will contribute to our enjoyment of our body the most. This takes place on several levels, but it is certainly tied to our intention to accomplish happiness within the physical world.

The sensual information we absorb with our senses is transmitted via waveform mechanics. Our senses convert waveforms from one medium into waveforms that can travel within the medium of the neural biology. As these waveform pulses are stepped into higher frequency waveforms, they are transmitted through the various neural pathways, including the microtubules, as we have discussed. These waveforms come together within our cortices to create coherent interference patterns, which tie together with the brainwaves arising from our limbic system. Together these interference patterns create networks of standing waveform patterns that bond molecule and ion sequences within our neurons. They accumulate to create a web of networked waveforms.

This might be compared to looking at a pond after many stones have been tossed into it. The confluence of intersecting and interfering ripples contain the data that reveal the original event to an intelligent observer.

The interference patterns reveal whether a single stone or multiple stones were thrown in. They may reveal how large the stones were, how long ago they were thrown in and how far apart the stones were thrown in.

Even one of the stones' waves, ripped up by interference patterns, can be followed back to the original stone throws, because they have each become interconnected through the medium of the pond. In this way, the ripples and waves of the stone throws are all interconnected into a web of waveforms.

In the case of the mental web, we are speaking of a convergence of millions of sensory, neural and brain waveforms all interacting within the system. This wave interaction keeps each memory associated with various other events and memories. This interactive pattern might also be compared to that of a spider's web—weaved and linked with silk strands interlaced into a sturdy net. One strand alone will not hold much. Networked together, they are strong. In the same way, our holographic memory retention is based upon a linking of emotions with sensory images, all wrapped together by the intention to succeed and enjoy the current physical body.

As some strands become older or less important, they gradually become pushed further away from the priority strands that are tied to the current events now central to our current goals. These older memories might still available in the grand web of interlocking waveforms. However, they become increasingly difficult for us to recall, as they fade from our intentional priorities.

For this reason, we find it fairly easy to replace actual memories with forged memories. The forged memories are inserted through emotional intention. This intention holds the forged memories in place, and after awhile the mind sees no difference between the forged and the real memories.

The reason tumors in the hippocampus have been known to cause amnesia is because the hippocampus is a conversion tool used by the mind to transmute event waveform combinations from one type to another. The ability of the limbic system to translate impulses into the memory web map and also access that map—translating the webbed memories back into physical recall—has been damaged. In the same way, if we got cancer of the vocal cords, we would not be able to convert our thoughts into words. Losing the conversion tool does not bode well for that activity.

The bridge between the physical waveforms of the neural net and the subtle mapping of those rhythms has been broken. As research has indicated, should another part of the limbic system be available for web building and should the intent remain, the personality may still be able to shift that function elsewhere, though it will be difficult. It is easier to shift cortex functions because there are several cortex regions situated around the brain, each having similarly structured neurons.

We can compare the mapping technology of the memory web or net to the tracking location system of a computer hard drive memory disk. The computer hardware is compared to the limbic system, which coordinates the mapping and retrieval of particular memory waveforms. The hippocampus, hypothalamus and amygdala work together with the rest of the limbic system to coordinate the storage and retrieval of particular informational waveforms. These are of course fed in from the senses along with feedback from the body, converted, and then escorted through the particular neurotransmitter messenger relays.

Together this sorted information is both sent to memory and projected in the frontal cortex for the personality to view. Together these waveforms create a harmonic coherence, because the events are strung together by our emotional intent. Our intentions are thus inserted into the sorting process of the limbic system. The waveform synchronization is finally projected upon the mind screen web for the personality's direct interaction.

The personality's feedback from this viewing becomes tied together historically using the formatting and storage mechanisms of the hippocampus and prefrontal cortex. This reformatting sorts specific types of waveform patterns to resonate with other historical information, tying them together within the particular region of the brain that resonates with that wave format.

Each memory waveform or set of interference waveforms is held in resonance and crystallized within a region of neural cell molecules. Protein crystal semiconductors provide the platform for these waveform combinations to be retained in standing waves. Though this statement might deceive us into thinking the memories are contained in the neuron chemistry, this is immediately refutable. Research has illustrated that when we sleep, the mind quietly shuffles and reprioritizes the memory banks, aligning them with the personality's current objectives. Less important memories are shuffled out, while memories considered more critical to the personality are retained. The rejected memories are discarded, yet those neurons remain, albeit with newly crystallized waveform interference patterns.

The Self and Memory

The above evidence indicates the existence of an inner personality, separate from the mind and the brain. This and only this can explain the fact that each of us can observe what is going on in the mind. Who is the observer of the mind? How can someone observe their thoughts—and even edit or change them—if there wasn't a personality separate from those thoughts?

This of course is why one can say, "I changed my mind."

Then there is memory. The reality is that we are not our memories. We can know this by being able to observe our memories.

For example, we might hear a song from decades ago and suddenly we will be observing our memories of that time. This ability to observe our memories means our memories are separate from us.

This is also why a person can forget things and still be the same person.

Let's say this again: A person might forget their family members. Or they might forget what they did yesterday. But they are still the same person. It wasn't as if someone snuck in to their bedroom and stole the person within away. The personality is still there. They simply are not able to—for whatever reason—to access certain types of memories—due to a transmission problem within their brains.

If we can accept this point—of a personality within who is separate from the body, the brain and the mind, then all the puzzle pieces of this topic of Alzheimer's disease will begins to fall into place.

Remember the research above about the babies born without brains? How about people whose brain regions died from stroke, or those who had half their brain removed. So many of these people continued to function normally despite losing critical regions of their brains—or not even having brains.

These along with the other evidence discussed above indicates the existence of a personality who is aloof from the brain and the mind—someone who utilizes these just as a computer operator would operate the software and hardware of a computer.

What is this personality made of, you ask? Frankly, the personality's composition must be spirit—that dimension not perceivable by the eyes and the senses. When this invisible personality leaves the body at the time of death, the body becomes lifeless. This is the difference between a dead body and a living body. Right after death, the body contains all the cells, organs, tissues, fluids and chemicals that were in the living body. The difference was the personality left the body—making it lifeless.

While it is alive, the personality is operating the body much as a computer operator operates a computer.

But just imagine sitting at your computer where all the metals within the circuit boards have become rusty. Say you have been using your computer outside in an area high in humidity: The humidity will begin to rust the metals within the computer. Soon the computer circuit boards will begin dropping transmissions due to the rust.

As a result, you might type in a command into the computer's keyboard, and the computer simply doesn't respond. Suddenly you can't get the computer to do what you want it to.

You will probably also find that the computer's software begins malfunctioning. It is not that the software program that was loaded into the computer is faulty. But because the circuit boards are unable to process the machine language, the software cannot properly instruct the hardware operations in the rusty computer.

This analogy of the rusty computer actually serves multiple purposes. The evidence and tools we lay out in the next chapter will illustrate that a process in the body called oxidation—and the resulting oxidation stress— is a process that is very similar to the process that metals go through when they begin to rust.

But just as an intelligent computer operator can take some practical steps to prevent the rust, and even take steps to remove some of the rust in the computer, the personality within can take practical steps to help prevent Alzheimer's disease and even use some practical tools to possibly slow or even turn around the progression.

But greater than this is the hope and understanding the science of this section communicates for those with developing Alzheimer's or those family members of Alzheimer's patients.

This hope and understanding communicates that while the brain of an Alzheimer's patient may be damaged; their facilities to communicate may be interfered with; their ability to retain and recall physical memories may be partially blocked: the person is still there.

The same personality who was there when the brain operated effectively is still there within that body. The same person who loved and still loves; who cared and still cares; who laughed and still laughs within: is still there.

We must see this person within. We must see the spiritual force and the spiritual sense of our person. This includes the element of spiritual love that remains with the personality forever, even after the brain dies and the personality leaves the body.

References and Bibliography

Abdou AM, Higashiguchi S, Horie K, Kim M, Hatta H, Yokogoshi H. Relaxation and immunity enhancement effects of gamma-aminobutyric acid GABA). Biofactors. 2006;26(3):201-8.

Abner EL, Dennis BC, Mathews MJ, Mendiondo MS, Caban-Holt A, Kryscio RJ, Schmitt FA; PREADViSE Investigators, Crowley JJ; SELECT Investigators. Practice effects in a longitudinal, multi-center Alzheimer's disease prevention clinical trial. Trials. 2012 Nov 20;13:217. doi: 10.1186/1745-6215-13-217.

Abou-Seif MA. Blood antioxidant status and urine sulfate and thiocyanate levels in smokers. J Biochem Toxicol. 1996;11(3):133-138.

Ackerman D. A Natural History of the Senses. New York: Vintage, 1991.

Ackermann RT, Mulrow CD, Ramirez G, Gardner CD, Morbidoni L, Lawrence VA. Garlic shows promise for improving some cardiovascular risk factors. Arch Intern Med. 2001 Mar 26;161(6):813-24.

Agarwal SK, Singh SS, Verma S. Antifungal principle of sesquiterpene lactones from Anamirta cocculus. Indian Drugs. 1999;36:754-5.

Aggarwal BB, Harikumar KB. Potential therapeutic effects of curcumin, the anti-inflammatory agent, against neurodegenerative, cardiovascular, pulmonary, metabolic, autoimmune and neoplastic diseases. Int J Biochem Cell Biol. 2009 Jan;41(1):40-59.

Aggarwal BB, Sung B. Pharmacological basis for the role of curcumin in chronic diseases: an age-old spice with modern targets. Trends Pharmacol Sci. 2009 Feb;30(2):85-94.

Ahmed ME, Javed H, Khan MM, Vaibhav K, Ahmad A, Khan A, Tabassum R, Islam F, Safhi MM, Islam F. Attenuation of oxidative damage-associated cognitive decline by Withania somnifera in rat model of streptozotocin-induced cognitive impairment. Protoplasma. 2013 Jan 23.

Ahn YJ, Park SJ, Woo H, Lee HE, Kim HJ, Kwon G, Gao Q, Jang DS, Ryu JH. Effects of allantoin on cognitive function and hippocampal neurogenesis. Food Chem Toxicol. 2014 Feb;64:210-6. doi: 10.1016/j.fct.2013.11.033.

Ahrberg K, Dresler M, Niedermaier S, Steiger A, Genzel L. The interaction between sleep quality and academic performance. J Psychiatr Res. 2012 Dec;46(12):1618-22.

Airola P. How to Get Well. Phoenix, AZ: Health Plus, 1974.

Aisen PS, Egelko S, Andrews H, Diaz-Arrastia R, Weiner M, DeCarli C, Jagust W, Miller JW, Green R, Bell K, Sano M. A pilot study of vitamins to lower plasma homocysteine levels in Alzheimer disease. Am J Geriatr Psychiatry. 2003 Mar-Apr;11(2):246-9.

Aisen PS, Petersen RC, Donohue MC, Gamst A, Raman R, Thomas RG, et al. Clinical core of the alzheimer's disease neuroimaging initiative: progress and plans. Alzheimers Dement 2010;6:239-46.

Aisen PS, Schneider LS, Sano M, Diaz-Arrastia R, van Dyck CH, Weiner MF, Bottiglieri T, Jin S, Stokes KT, Thomas RG, Thal LJ; Alzheimer Disease Cooperative Study. High-dose B vitamin supplementation and cognitive decline in Alzheimer disease: a randomized controlled trial. JAMA. 2008 Oct 15;300(15):1774-83. doi: 10.1001/jama.300.15.1774.

Aissa J, Harran H, Rabeau M, Boucherie S, Brouilhet H, Benveniste J. Tissue levels of histamine, PAF-acether and lysopaf-acether in carrageenan-induced granuloma in rats. Int Arch Allergy Immunol. 1996 Jun;110(2):182-6.

Aissa J, Jurgens P, Litime M, Béhar I, Benveniste J. Electronic transmission of the cholinergic signal. FASEB Jnl. 1995;9: A683.

Aissa J, Litime M, Attias E, Allal A, Benveniste J. Transfer of molecular signals via electronic circuitry. FASEB Jnl. 1993;7: A602.

Aissa J, Litime MH, Attis E., Benveniste J. Molecular signalling at high dilution or by means of electronic circuitry. J Immunol. 1993;150:A146.

Aissa J, Nathan N, Arnoux B, Benveniste J. Biochemical and cellular effects of heparin-protamine injection in rabbits are partially inhibited by a PAF-acether receptor antagonist. Eur J Pharmacol. 1996 Apr 29;302(1-3):123-8.

Aizenstein HJ, Nebes RD, Saxton JA, Price JC, Mathis CA, Tsopelas ND, et al. Frequent amyloid deposition without significant cognitive impairment among the elderly. Arch Neurol 2008;65:1509-17.

Aizenstein HJ, Nebes RD, Saxton JA, Price JC, Mathis CA, Tsopelas ND, Ziolko SK, James JA, Snitz BE, Houck PR, Bi W, Cohen AD, Lopresti BJ, DeKosky ST, Halligan EM, Klunk WE. Frequent amyloid deposition without significant cognitive impairment among the elderly. Arch Neurol. 2008 Nov;65(11):1509-17. doi: 10.1001/archneur.65.11.1509.

Alam A, Shaikh S, Ahmad SS, Shakil S, Rizvi Smd, Shakil S, Imran M, Tabrez S, Kamal MA. Molecular Interaction of Human Brain Acetylcholinesterase with a Natural Inhibitor Huperzine-B: An Enzoinformatics Approach. CNS Neurol Disord Drug Targets. 2013 Sep 19.

Alam N, Hossain M, Mottalib MA, Sulaiman SA, Gan SH, Khalil MI. Methanolic extracts of Withania somnifera leaves, fruits and roots possess antioxidant properties and antibacterial activities. BMC Complement Altern Med. 2012 Oct 7;12:175.

Albarracin SL, Stab B, Casas Z, Sutachan JJ, Samudio I, Gonzalez J, Gonzalo L, Capani F, Morales L, Barreto GE. Effects of natural antioxidants in neurodegenerative disease. Nutr Neurosci. 2012 Jan;15(1):1-9.

Albrechtsen O. The influence of small atmospheric ions on human well-being and mental performance. Intern. J. of Biometeorology. 1978;22(4): 249-262.

247

Alcalay RN, Gu Y, Mejia-Santana H, Cote L, Marder KS, Scarmeas N. The association between Mediterranean diet adherence and Parkinson's disease. Mov Disord. 2012 May;27(6):771-4.

Alcántar-Aguirre FC, Chagolla A, Tiessen A, Délano JP, González de la Vara LE. ATP produced by oxidative phosphorylation is channeled toward hexokinase bound to mitochondrial porin (VDAC) in beetroots (Beta vulgaris). Planta. 2013 Mar 17.

Alexandre P, Darmanyan D, Yushen G, Jenks W, Burel L, Eloy D, Jardon P. Quenching of Singlet Oxygen by Oxygen- and Sulfur-Centered Radicals: Evidence for Energy Transfer to Peroxyl Radicals in Solution. J. Am. Chem. Soc., 120 (2), 396 -403, 1998.

Alexandrov PN, Dua P, Hill JM, Bhattacharjee S, Zhao Y, Lukiw WJ. microRNA (miRNA) speciation in Alzheimer's disease (AD) cerebrospinal fluid (CSF) and extracellular fluid (ECF). Int J Biochem Mol Biol. 2012;3(4):365-73.

Alhola P, Polo-Kantola P. Sleep deprivation: Impact on cognitive performance. Neuropsychiatr Dis Treat. 2007;3(5):553-67.

Allais G, Bussone G, De Lorenzo C, Castagnoli Gabellari I, Zonca M, Mana O, Borgogno P, Acuto G, Benedetto C. Naproxen sodium in short-term prophylaxis of pure menstrual migraine: pathophysiological and clinical considerations. Neurol Sci. 2007 May;28 Suppl 2:S225-8.

Allen KV, Frier BM, Strachan MW. The relationship between type 2 diabetes and cognitive dysfunction: longitudinal studies and their methodological limitations. Eur. J. Pharmacol. 2004 490:169–175. doi:10.1016/j.ejphar.2004.02.054

Allen SJ, Okoko B, Martinez E, Gregorio G, Dans LF. Probiotics for treating infectious diarrhea. The Cochrane Library. 2004;3. Chichester, UK: John Wiley & Sons, Ltd.

Alleva R, Tomasetti M, Bompadre S, Littarru GP. Oxidation of LDL and their subfractions: kinetic aspects and CoQ10 content. Mol Aspects Med. 1997;18 Suppl:S105-12.

Amassian VE, Cracco RQ, Maccabee PJ. A sense of movement elicited in paralyzed distal arm by focal magnetic coil stimulation of human motor cortex. Brain Res. 1989 Feb 13;479(2):355-60.

American Conference of Governmental Industrial Hygienists. Threshold limit values for chemical substances and physical agents in the work environment. Cincinnati, OH: ACGIH, 1986.

American Dietetic Association; Dietitians of Canada. Position of the American Dietetic Association and Dietitians of Canada: vegetarian diets. Can J Diet Pract Res. 2003 Summer;64(2):62-81.

Ammon HP. Boswellic acids (components of frankincense) as the active principle in treatment of chronic inflammatory diseases. Wien Med Wochenschr. 2002;152(15-16):373-8.

Ammon HP. Boswellic acids in chronic inflammatory diseases. Planta Med. 2006 Oct;72(12):1100-16.

Ammor MS, Michaelidis C, Nychas GJ. Insights into the role of quorum sensing in food spoilage. J Food Prot. 2008 Jul;71(7):1510-25.

Anand P, Thomas SG, Kunnumakkara AB, Sundaram C, Harikumar KB, Sung B, Tharakan ST, Misra K, Priyadarsini IK, Rajasekharan KN, Aggarwal BB. Biological activities of curcumin and its analogues (Congeners) made by man and Mother Nature. Biochem Pharmacol. 2008 Dec 1;76(11):1590-611.

Anderson JL, May HT, Horne BD, Bair TL, Hall NL, Carlquist JF, Lappé DL, Muhlestein JB; Intermountain Heart Collaborative (IHC) Study Group. Relation of vitamin D deficiency to cardiovascular risk factors, disease status, and incident events in a general healthcare population. Am J Cardiol. 2010 Oct 1;106(7):963-8.

Anderson JW, Baird P, Davis RH Jr, Ferreri S, Knudtson M, Koraym A, Waters V, Williams CL. Health benefits of dietary fiber. Nutr Rev. 2009 Apr;67(4):188-205.

Anderson M., Grissom C. Increasing the Heavy Atom Effect of Xenon by Adsorption to Zeolites: Photolysis of 2,3-Diazabicyclo[2.2.2]oct-2-ene. J. Am. Chem. Soc. 1996;118:9552-9556.

Anderson RC, Anderson JH. Acute toxic effects of fragrance products. Arch Environ Health. 1998 Mar-Apr;53(2):138-46.

Anderson RC, Anderson JH. Toxic effects of air freshener emissions. Arch Environ Health. 1997 Nov-Dec;52(6):433-41.

Anderson SD, Charlton B, Weiler JM, Nichols S, Spector SL, Pearlman DS; A305 Study Group. Comparison of mannitol and methacholine to predict exercise-induced bronchoconstriction and a clinical diagnosis of asthma. Respir Res. 2009 Jan 23;10:4.

Andoh T, Zhang Q, Yamamoto T, Tayama M, Hattori M, Tanaka K, Kuraishi Y. Inhibitory Effects of the Methanol Extract of Ganoderma lucidum on Mosquito Allergy-Induced Itch-Associated Responses in Mice. J Pharmacol Sci. 2010 Oct 8.

André C, André F, Colin L. Effect of allergen ingestion challenge with and without cromoglycate cover on intestinal permeability in atopic dermatitis, urticaria and other symptoms of food allergy. Allergy. 1989;44 Suppl 9:47-51.

André C. Food allergy. Objective diagnosis and test of therapeutic efficacy by measuring intestinal permeability. Presse Med. 1986 Jan 25;15(3):105-8.

Andre F, Andre C, Feknous M, Colin L, Cavagna S. Digestive permeability to different-sized molecules and to sodium cromoglycate in food allergy. Allergy Proc. 1991 Sep-Oct;12(5):293-8.

Andreasen N, Hesse C, Davidsson P, Minthon L, Wallin A, Winblad B, et al. Cerebrospinal fluid beta-amyloid(1-42) in Alzheimer disease: differences between early- and late-onset Alzheimer disease and stability during the course of disease. Arch Neurol 1999;56:673-80.

Andrews RC, Cooper AR, Montgomery AA, Norcross AJ, Peters TJ, Sharp DJ, Jackson N, Fitzsimons K, Bright J, Coulman K, England CY, Gorton J, McLenaghan A, Paxton E, Polet A, Thompson C, Dayan CM. Diet or diet plus physical activity versus usual care in patients with newly diagnosed type 2 diabetes: the Early ACTID randomised controlled trial. Lancet. 2011 Jul 9;378(9786):129-39.

Angeli JP, Ribeiro LR, Bellini MF, Mantovani. Anti-clastogenic effect of beta-glucan extracted from barley towards chemically induced DNA damage in rodent cells. Hum Exp Toxicol. 2006 Jun;25(6):319-24.

Anim-Nyame N, Sooranna SR, Johnson MR, Gamble J, Steer PJ. Garlic supplementation increases peripheral blood flow: a role for interleukin-6? J Nutr Biochem. 2004 Jan;15(1):30-6.

Annweiler C, Fantino B, Parot-Schinkel E, Thiery S, Gautier J, Beauchet O. Alzheimer's disease--input of vitamin D with mEmantine assay (AD-IDEA trial): study protocol for a randomized controlled trial. Trials. 2011 Oct 20;12:230. doi: 10.1186/1745-6215-12-230.

Annweiler C, Schott AM, Berrut G, Chauviré V, Le Gall D, Inzitari M, Beauchet O. Vitamin D and ageing: neurological issues. Neuropsychobiology. 2010 Aug;62(3):139-50.

Annweiler C. Vitamin D in dementia prevention. Ann N Y Acad Sci. 2016 Mar;1367(1):57-63. doi: 10.1111/nyas.13058. Miller BJ, Whisner CM, Johnston CS. Vitamin D Supplementation Appears to Increase Plasma Aβ40 in Vitamin D Insufficient Older Adults: A Pilot Randomized Controlled Trial. J Alzheimers Dis. 2016 Mar 31;52(3):843-7. doi: 10.3233/JAD-150901.

Anonymous. Cimetidine inhibits the hepatic hydroxylation of vitamin D. Nutr Rev. 1985;43:184-5.

Antczak A, Nowak D, Shariati B, Król M, Piasecka G, Kurmanowska Z. Increased hydrogen peroxide and thiobarbituric acid-reactive products in expired breath condensate of asthmatic patients. Eur Respir J. 1997 Jun;10(6):1235-41.

Anwer T, Sharma M, Pillai KK, Khan G. Protective effect of Withania somnifera against oxidative stress and pancreatic beta-cell damage in type 2 diabetic rats. Acta Pol Pharm. 2012 Nov-Dec;69(6):1095-101.

Aoki T, Usuda Y, Miyakoshi H, Tamura K, Herberman RB. Low natural killer syndrome: clinical and immunologic features. Nat Immun Cell Growth Regul. 1987;6(3):116-28.

Apáti P, Houghton PJ, Kite G, Steventon GB, Kéry A. In-vitro effect of flavonoids from Solidago canadensis extract on glutathione S-transferase. J Pharm Pharmacol. 2006 Feb;58(2):251-6.

Appleby PN, Thorogood M, Mann JI, Key TJ. The Oxford Vegetarian Study: an overview. Am J Clin Nutr. 1999 Sep;70(3 Suppl):525S-531S.

Argento A, Tiraferri E, Marzaloni M. Oral anticoagulants and medicinal plants. An emerging interaction. Ann Ital Med Int. 2000 Apr-Jun;15(2):139-43.

Armstrong BK. Absorption of vitamin B12 from the human colon. Am J Clin Nutr. 1968;21:298-9.

Aronne LJ, Thornton-Jones ZD. New targets for obesity pharmacotherapy. Clin Pharmacol Ther. 2007 May;81(5):748-52.

Arterburn LM, Oken HA, Bailey Hall E, Hamersley J, Kuratko CN, Hoffman JP. Algal-oil capsules and cooked salmon: nutritionally equivalent sources of docosahexaenoic acid. J Am Diet Assoc. 2008 Jul;108(7):1204-9.

Arterburn LM, Oken HA, Hoffman JP, Bailey-Hall E, Chung G, Rom D, Hamersley J, McCarthy D. Bioequivalence of Docosahexaenoic acid from different algal oils in capsules and in a DHA-fortified food. Lipids. 2007 Nov;42(11):1011-24.

Ashaye A, Gaziano J, Djoussé L. Red meat consumption and risk of heart failure in male physicians. Nutr Metab Cardiovasc Dis. 2010 Jul 30.

Ashour OM, Abdel-Naim AB, Abdallah HM, Nagy AA, Mohamadin AM, Abdel-Sattar EA. Evaluation of the potential cardioprotective activity of some Saudi plants against doxorubicin toxicity. Z Naturforsch C. 2012 May-Jun;67(5-6):297-307.

Ashrafi K, Chang FY, Watts JL, Fraser AG, Kamath RS, Ahringer J, Ruvkun G. Genome-wide RNAi analysis of Caenorhabditis elegans fat regulatory genes. Nature. 2003 Jan 16;421(6920):268-72.

Asimov I. The Chemicals of Life. New York: Signet, 1954.

Askeland D. The Science and Engineering of Materials. Boston: PWS, 1994.

Aso E, Ferrer I. CB2 Cannabinoid Receptor As Potential Target against Alzheimer's Disease. Front Neurosci. 2016 May 31;10:243. doi: 10.3389/fnins.2016.00243.

Aspect A, Grangier P, Roger G. Experimental Realization of Einstein-Podolsky-Rosen-Bohm Gedankenexperiment: A New Violation of Bell's Inequalities. Physical Review Letters. 1982;49(2): 91-94.

Ataie-Jafari A, Larijani B, Alavi Majd H, Tahbaz F. Cholesterol-lowering effect of probiotic yogurt in comparison with ordinary yogurt in mildly to moderately hypercholesterolemic subjects. Ann Nutr Metab. 2009;54(1):22-7.

Aton SJ, Colwell CS, Harmar AJ, Waschek J, Herzog ED. Vasoactive intestinal polypeptide mediates circadian rhythmicity and synchrony in mammalian clock neurons. Nat Neurosci. 2005 Apr;8(4):476-83.

Atsumi T, Tonosaki K. Smelling lavender and rosemary increases free radical scavenging activity and decreases cortisol level in saliva. Psychiatry Res. 2007 Feb 28;150(1):89-96.

Avanzini G, Lopez L, Koelsch S, Majno M. The Neurosciences and Music II: From Perception to Performance. Annals of the New York Academy of Sciences. 2006 Mar;1060.

Aymard JP, Aymard B, Netter P, Bannwarth B, Trechot P, Streiff F. Haematological adverse effects of histamine H2-receptor antagonists. Med Toxicol Adverse Drug Exp. 1988 Nov-Dec;3(6):430-48.

Bach E. Bach Flower Remedies. New Canaan, CN: Keats, 1997.

Bach E. Heal Thyself. Saffron Walden: CW Daniel, 1931-2003.

Bachmann KA, Sullivan TJ, Jauregui L, Reese J, Miller K, Levine L. Drug interactions of H2-receptor antagonists. Scand J Gastroenterol Suppl. 1994;206:14-9.

Backster C. Primary Perception: Biocommunication with Plants, Living Foods, and Human Cells. Anza, CA: White Rose Millennium Press, 2003.

Bacskai BJ, Frosch MP, Freeman SH, Raymond SB, Augustinack JC, Johnson KA, et al. Molecular imaging with Pittsburgh Compound B confirmed at autopsy: a case report. Arch Neurol 2007;64:431-4.

Bader J. The relative power of SNPs and haplotype as genetic markers for association tests. Pharmacogenomics. 2001;2:11-24.

Bae GS, Kim MS, Jung WS, Seo SW, Yun SW, Kim SG, Park RK, Kim EC, Song HJ, Park SJ. Inhibition of lipopolysaccharide-induced inflammatory responses by piperine. Eur J Pharmacol. 2010 Sep 10;642(1-3):154-62.

Bai H, Yu P, Yu M. Effect of electroacununcture on sex hormone levels in patients with Sjogren's syndrome. Zhen Ci Yan Jiu. 2007;32(3):203-6.

Baitharu I, Jain V, Deep SN, Hota KB, Hota SK, Prasad D, Ilavazhagan G. Withania somnifera root extract ameliorates hypobaric hypoxia induced memory impairment in rats. J Ethnopharmacol. 2013 Jan 30;145(2):431-41.

Baker DW. An introduction to the theory and practice of German electroacupuncture and accompanying medications. Am J Acupunct. 1984;12:327-332.

Baker DW. An introduction to the theory and practice of German electroacupuncture and accompanying medications. Am J Acupunct. 1984;12:327-332.

Baker SM. Detoxification and Healing. Chicago: Contemporary Books, 2004.

Balch P, Balch J. Prescription for Nutritional Healing. New York: Avery, 2000.

Ball IJ, Shoker J, Miles JN. Odour-based context reinstatement effects with indirect measures of memory: the curious case of rosemary. Br J Psychol. 2010 Nov;101(Pt 4):655-78. doi: 10.1348/000712609X479663.

Ballentine R. Diet & Nutrition: A holistic approach. Honesdale, PA: Himalayan Int., 1978.

Ballentine RM. Radical Healing. New York: Harmony Books, 1999.

Balliett M, Burke JR. Changes in anthropometric measurements, body composition, blood pressure, lipid profile, and testosterone in patients participating in a low-energy dietary intervention. J Chiropr Med. 2013 Mar;12(1):3-14. doi: 10.1016/j.jcm.2012.11.003.

Banno N, Akihisa T, Yasukawa K, Tokuda H, Tabata K, Nakamura Y, Nishimura R, Kimura Y, Suzuki T. Anti-inflammatory activities of the triterpene acids from the resin of Boswellia carteri. J Ethnopharmacol. 2006 Sep 19;107(2):249-53.

Banyo T. The role of electrical neuromodulation in the therapy of chronic lower urinary tract dysfunction. Ideggyogy Sz. 2003 Jan 20;56(1-2):68-71.

Barak Y, Levine J, Glasman A, Elizur A, Belmaker RH. Inositol treatment of Alzheimer's disease: a double blind, cross-over placebo controlled trial. Prog Neuropsychopharmacol Biol Psychiatry. 1996 May;20(4):729-35.

Baranauskas G, Nistri A. Sensitization of pain pathways in the spinal cord: cellular mechanisms. Prog Neurobiol. 1998 Feb;54(3):349-65.

Barbagallo G, Barbagallo M, Giordano M, Meli M, Panzarasa R. alpha-Glycerophosphocholine in the mental recovery of cerebral ischemic attacks. An Italian multicenter clinical trial. Ann N Y Acad Sci. 1994 Jun 30;717:253-69.

Barber CF. The use of music and colour theory as a behaviour modifier. Br J Nurs. 1999 Apr 8-21;8(7):443-8.

Barker A. Scientific Method in Ptolemy's Harmonics. Cambridge: Cambridge University Press, 2000.

Barreto Pde S, Demougeot L, Pillard F, Lapeyre-Mestre M, Rolland Y. Exercise training for managing behavioral and psychological symptoms in people with dementia: A systematic review and meta-analysis. Ageing Res Rev. 2015 Nov;24(Pt B):274-85. doi: 10.1016/j.arr.2015.09.001.

Barron M. Light exposure, melatonin secretion, and menstrual cycle parameters: an integrative review. Biol Res Nurs. 2007 Jul;9(1):49-69.

Bastide M, Doucet-Jaboeuf M, Daurat V. Activity and chronopharmacology of very low doses of physiological immune inducers. Immun Today. 1985;6: 234-235.

Bastide M. Immunological examples on ultra high dilution research. In: Endler P, Schulte J (eds.): Ultra High Dilution. Physiology and Physics. Dordrech: Kluwer Academic Publishers, 1994:27-34.

Basu A, Devaraj S, Jialal I. Dietary factors that promote or retard inflammation. Arterioscler Thromb Vasc Biol. 2006 May;26(5):995-1001.

Basu A, Du M, Leyva MJ, Sanchez K, Betts NM, Wu M, Aston CE, Lyons TJ. Blueberries decrease cardiovascular risk factors in obese men and women with metabolic syndrome. J Nutr. 2010 Sep;140(9):1582-7. doi: 10.3945/jn.110.124701.

Bates DW, Cullen DJ, Laird N, Petersen LA, Small SD, Servi D, Laffel G, Sweitzer BJ, Shea BF, Hallisey R, et al. Incidence of adverse drug events and potential adverse drug events. Implications for prevention. ADE Prevention Study Group. JAMA. 1995 Jul 5;274(1):29-34.

Batmanghelidj F. Neurotransmitter histamine: an alternative view point, Science in Medicine Simplified. Falls Church, VA: Foundation for the Simple in Medicine, 1990.

Batmanghelidj F. Pain: a need for paradigm change. Anticancer Res. 1987 Sep-Oct;7(5B):971-89.

Beaulieu A, Fessele K. Agent Orange: management of patients exposed in Vietnam. Clin J Oncol Nurs. 2003 May-Jun;7(3):320-3.

Beauvais F, Bidet B, Descours B, Hieblot C, Burtin C, Benveniste J. Regulation of human basophil activation. I. Dissociation of cationic dye binding from histamine release in activated human basophils. J Allergy Clin Immunol. 1991 May;87(5):1020-8.

Beauvais F, Burtin C, Benveniste J. Voltage-dependent ion channels on human basophils: do they exist? Immunol Lett. 1995 May;46(1-2):81-3.

REFERENCES AND BIBLIOGRAPHY

Beauvais F, Echasserieau K, Burtin C, Benveniste J. Regulation of human basophil activation; the role of Na+ and Ca2+ in IL-3-induced potentiation of IgE-mediated histamine release from human basophils. Clin Exp Immunol. 1994 Jan;95(1):191-4.

Beauvais F, Shimahara T, Inoue I, Hieblot C, Burtin C, Benveniste J. Regulation of human basophil activation. II. Histamine release is potentiated by K+ efflux and inhibited by Na+ influx.. J Immunol. 1992 Jan 1;148(1):149-54.

Becker DJ, French B, Morris PB, Silvent E, Gordon RY. Phytosterols, red yeast rice, and lifestyle changes instead of statins: a randomized, double-blinded, placebo-controlled trial. Am Heart J. 2013 Jul;166(1):187-96. doi:10.1016/j.ahj.2013.03.019.

Becker DJ, Gordon RY, Halbert SC, French B, Morris PB, Rader DJ. Red yeast rice for dyslipidemia in statin-intolerant patients: a randomized trial. Ann Intern Med. 2009 Jun 16;150(12):830-9, W147-9.

Becker KG, Simon RM, Bailey-Wilson JE, Freidlin B, Biddison WE, McFarland HF, Trent JM. Clustering of non-major histocompatibility complex susceptibility candidate loci in human autoimmune diseases. Proc Natl Acad Sci U S A. 1998 Aug 18;95(17):9979-84.

Becker R. Cross Currents. Los Angeles: Jeremy P. Tarcher, 1990.

Becker R. The Body Electric. New York: William Morrow, 1985.

Beckerman H, Becher J, Lankhorst GJ. The effectiveness of vibratory stimulation in anejaculatory men with spinal cord injury. Paraplegia. 1993 Nov;31(11):689-99.

Beddoe AF. Biologic Ionization as Applied to Human Nutrition. Warsaw: Wendell Whitman, 2002.

Beecher GR. Phytonutrients' role in metabolism: effects on resistance to degenerative processes. Nutr Rev. 1999 Sep;57(9 Pt 2):S3-6.

Beeson, C. The moon and plant growth. Nature. 1946;158:572–3.

Belcaro G, Cesarone MR, Errichi S, Zulli C, Errichi BM, Vinciguerra G, Ledda A, Di Renzo A, Stuard S, Dugall M, Pellegrini L, Gizzi G, Ippolito E, Ricci A, Cacchio M, Cipollone G, Ruffini I, Fano F, Hosoi M, Rohdewald P. Variations in C-reactive protein, plasma free radicals and fibrinogen values in patients with osteoarthritis treated with Pycnogenol. Redox Rep. 2008;13(6):271-6.

Bell B, Defouw R. Concerning a lunar modulation of geomagnetic activity. J Geophys Res. 1964;69:3169-3174.

Bell IR, Baldwin CM, Schwartz GE, Illness from low levels of environmental chemicals: relevance to chronic fatigue syndrome and fibromyalgia. Am J Med. 1998;105 (suppl 3A).:74-82. S.

Bellavia A, Larsson SC, Bottai M, Wolk A, Orsini N. Fruit and vegetable consumption and all-cause mortality: a dose-response analysis. Am J Clin Nutr. 2013 Jun 26.

Beloff J. Parapsychology and radical dualism. J Rel & Psych Res. 1985;8, 3-10.

Beltowski J. Hydrogen sulfide in pharmacology and medicine--An update. Pharmacol Rep. 2015 Jun;67(3):647-58. doi: 10.1016/j.pharep.2015.01.005.

Benatuil L, Apitz-Castro R, Romano E. Ajoene inhibits the activation of human endothelial cells induced by porcine cells: implications for xenotransplantation. Xenotransplantation. 2003 Jul;10(4):368-73.

Benatuil L, Apitz-Castro R, Romano E. Ajoene inhibits the activation of human endothelial cells induced by porcine cells: implications for xenotransplantation. Xenotransplantation. 2003 Jul;10(4):368-73.

Benedetti F, Radaelli D, Bernasconi A, Dallaspezia S, Falini A, Scotti G, Lorenzi C, Colombo C, Smeraldi E. Clock genes beyond the clock: CLOCK genotype biases neural correlates of moral valence decision in depressed patients. Genes Brain Behav. 2007 Mar 26.

Bengmark S. Curcumin, an atoxic antioxidant and natural NFkappaB, cyclooxygenase-2, lipooxygenase, and inducible nitric oxide synthase inhibitor: a shield against acute and chronic diseases. JPEN J Parenter Enteral Nutr. 2006 Jan-Feb;30(1):45-51.

Bengmark S. Immunonutrition: role of biosurfactants, fiber, and probiotic bacteria. Nutrition. 1998 Jul-Aug;14(7-8):585-94.

Bennett GJ, Update on the neurophysiology of pain transmission and modulation: focus on the NMDA-receptor. J Pain Symptom Manage. 2000;19 (suppl 1):S.:2-6.

Bennett GJ, Update on the neurophysiology of pain transmission and modulation: focus on the NMDA-receptor. J Pain Symptom Manage. 2000;19 (suppl 1):S.:2-6.

Bennett L, Kersaitis C, Macaulay SL, Münch G, Niedermayer G, Nigro J, Payne M, Sheean P, Vallotton P, Zabaras D, Bird M. Vitamin D2-enriched button mushroom (Agaricus bisporus) improves memory in both wild type and APPswe/PS1dE9 transgenic mice. PLoS One. 2013 Oct 18;8(10):e76362. doi: 10.1371/journal.pone.0076362. eCollection 2013.

Bennett L, Sheean P, Zabaras D, Head R. Heat-stable components of wood ear mushroom, Auricularia polytricha (higher Basidiomycetes), inhibit in vitro activity of beta secretase (BACE1). Int J Med Mushrooms. 2013;15(3):233-49.

Benor D. Healing Research. Volume 1. Munich, Germany: Helix Verlag, 1992.

Bensky D, Gable A, Kaptchuk T (transl.). Chinese Herbal Medicine Materia Medica. Seattle: Eastland Press, 1986.

Benson S, Downey LA, Stough C, Wetherell M, Zangara A, Scholey A. An acute, double-blind, placebo-controlled cross-over study of 320 mg and 640 mg doses of Bacopa monnieri (CDRI 08) on multitasking stress reactivity and mood. Phytother Res. 2014 Apr;28(4):551-9. doi: 10.1002/ptr.5029.

Bentley E. Awareness: Biorhythms, Sleep and Dreaming. London: Routledge, 2000

Berg A, Konig D, Deibert P, Grathwohl D, Berg A, Baumstark MW, Franz IW. Effect of an oat bran enriched diet on the atherogenic lipid profile in patients with an increased coronary heart disease risk. A controlled randomized lifestyle intervention study. Ann Nutr Metab. 2003;47(6):306-11.

Bergner P. The Healing Power of Garlic. Prima Publishing, Rocklin CA 1996.

Berk M, Dodd S, Henry M. Do ambient electromagnetic fields affect behaviour? A demonstration of the relationship between geomagnetic storm activity and suicide. Bioelectromagnetics. 2006 Feb;27(2):151-5.

Berkow R., (Ed.) The Merck Manual of Diagnosis and Therapy. 16th Edition. Rahway, N.J.: Merck Research Labs, 1992.

Berkrot B. Pfizer, J&J scrap Alzheimer's studies as drug fails. Reuters Life. Tue Aug 7, 2012

Berman S, Fein G, Jewett D, Ashford F. Luminance-controlled pupil size affects Landolt C task performance. J Illumin Engng Soc. 1993;22:150-165.

Berman S, Jewett D, Fein G, Saika G, Ashford F. Photopic luminance does not always predict perceived room brightness. Light Resch and Techn. 1990;22:37-41.

Bernardi D, Dini FL, Azzarelli A, Giaconi A, Volterrani C, Lunardi M. Sudden cardiac death rate in an area characterized by high incidence of coronary artery disease and low hardness of drinking water. Angiology. 1995;46:145-149.

Bernstein AM, Sun Q, Hu FB, Stampfer MJ, Manson JE, Willett WC. Major dietary protein sources and risk of coronary heart disease in women. Circulation. 2010 Aug 31;122(9):876-83.

Berntsen S, Kragstrup J, Siersma V, Waldemar G, Waldorff FB. Alcohol consumption and mortality in patients with mild Alzheimer's disease: a prospective cohort study. BMJ Open. 2015 Dec 11;5(12):e007851. doi: 10.1136/bmjopen-2015-007851.

Berr C, Portet F, Carriere I, Akbaraly TN, Feart C, Gourlet V, Combe N, Barberger-Gateau P, Ritchie K. Olive oil and cognition: results from the three-city study. Dement Geriatr Cogn Disord. 2009;28(4):357-64. doi: 10.1159/000253483.

Berridge MJ. Vitamin D, reactive oxygen species and calcium signalling in ageing and disease. Philos Trans R Soc Lond B Biol Sci. 2016 Aug 5;371(1700). pii: 20150434. doi: 10.1098/rstb.2015.0434.

Berteau O and Mulloy B. 2003. Sulfated fucans, fresh perspectives: structures, functions, and biological properties of sulfated fucans and an overview of enzymes active toward this class of polysaccharide. Glycobiology. Jun;13(6):29R-40R.

Bertin G. Spiral Structure in Galaxies: A Density Wave Theory. Cambridge: MIT Press, 1996.

Besednova NN, Somova LM, Guliaev SA, Zaporozhets TS. [Neuroprotective effects of sulfated polysaccharides from seaweed]. Vestn Ross Akad Med Nauk. 2013;(5):52-9.

Bevan R, Young C, Holmes P, Fortunato L, Slack R, Rushton L; British Occupational Cancer Burden Study Group. Occupational cancer in Britain. Gastrointestinal cancers: liver, oesophagus, pancreas and stomach. Br J Cancer. 2012 Jun 19;107 Suppl 1:S33-40. doi: 10.1038/bjc.2012.116.

Bhandari U, Sharma JN, Zafar R. The protective action of ethanolic ginger (Zingiber officinale) extract in cholesterol fed rabbits. J Ethnopharmacol. 1998 Jun;61(2):167-71.

Bharani A, Ganguli A, Mathur LK, Jamra Y, Raman PG. Efficacy of Terminalia arjuna in chronic stable angina: a double-blind, placebo-controlled, crossover study comparing Terminalia arjuna with isosorbide mononitrate. Indian Heart J. 2002 Mar-Apr; 54(2):170-5.

Bharani A, Ganguly A, Bhargava KD. Salutary effect of Terminalia Arjuna in patients with severe refractory heart failure. Int J Cardiol. 1995 May;49(3):191-9.

Bhattacharjee S, Lukiw WJ. Alzheimer's disease and the microbiome. Front Cell Neurosci. 2013 Sep 17;7:153. doi: 10.3389/fncel.2013.00153.

Bialystok E, Craik FI, Freedman M. Bilingualism as a protection against the onset of symptoms of dementia. Neuropsychologia. 2007 Jan 28;45(2):459-64.

Bialystok E, Craik FI, Luk G. Bilingualism: consequences for mind and brain. Trends Cogn Sci. 2012 Apr;16(4):240-50. doi: 10.1016/j.tics.2012.03.001.

Bicíková V, Sosvorová L, Bradác O, Pán M, Bicíková M. Phytoestrogens in menopause: working mechanisms and clinical results in 28 patients. Ceska Gynekol. 2012 Feb;77(1):10-4.

Bidulescu A, Chambless LE, Siega-Riz AM, Zeisel SH, Heiss G. Usual choline and betaine dietary intake and incident coronary heart disease: the Atherosclerosis Risk in Communities (ARIC) study. BMC Cardiovasc Disord. 2007;7:20.

Birks J, Flicker L. Selegiline for Alzheimer's disease. Cochrane Database Syst Rev. 2003;(1):CD000442.

Birks J. Cholinesterase inhibitors for Alzheimer's disease. Cochrane Database Syst Rev. 2006 Jan 25;(1):CD005593.

Bishop B. Pain: its physiology and rationale for management. Part III. Consequences of current concepts of pain mechanisms related to pain management. Phys Ther. 1980 Jan;60(1):24-37.

Bishop, C. Moon influence in lettuce growth. Astrol J. 1977;10(1):13-15.

Bisset N.. Herbal Drugs and Phytopharmaceuticals. Stuttgart: CRC, 1994.

Biswal BM, Sulaiman SA, Ismail HC, Zakaria H, Musa KI. Effect of Withania somnifera (Ashwagandha) on the Development of Chemotherapy-Induced Fatigue and Quality of Life in Breast Cancer Patients. Integr Cancer Ther. 2012 Nov 9.

Bitbol M, Luisi PL. Autopoiesis with or without cognition: defining life at its edge. J R Soc Interface. 2004 Nov 22;1(1):99-107.

Blackmore SJ. Near-death experiences. J R Soc Med. 1996 Feb;89(2):73-6.

Blood AJ, Zatorre RJ, Bermudez P, Evans AC. Emotional responses to pleasant and unpleasant music correlate with activity in paralimbic brain regions. Nat Neurosci. 1999;2:382-7.

Blumenthal M (ed.) The Complete German Commission E Monographs. Boston: Amer Botan Council, 1998.

Blumenthal M, Brinckmann J, Goldberg A (eds). Herbal Medicine: Expanded Commission E Monographs. Newton, MA: Integrative Med., 2000.

Bockemühl, J. Towards a Phenomenology of the Etheric World. New York: Anthroposophical Press, 1985.

REFERENCES AND BIBLIOGRAPHY

Bode C, Bode JC. Effect of alcohol consumption on the gut. Best Pract Res Clin Gastroenterol. 2003 Aug;17(4):575-92.

Bodnar L, Simhan H. The prevalence of preterm birth varies by season of last menstrual period. Am J Obst and Gyn. 2003:195(6);S211-S211.

Boissoneault J, Frazier I, Lewis B, Nixon SJ. Effects of Age and Acute Moderate Alcohol Administration on Electrophysiological Correlates of Working Memory Maintenance. Alcohol Clin Exp Res. 2016 Jul 15. doi: 10.1111/acer.13154.

Boivin DB, Czeisler CA. Resetting of circadian melatonin and cortisol rhythms in humans by ordinary room light. Neuroreport. 1998 Mar 30;9(5):779-82.

Boivin DB, Duffy JF, Kronauer RE, Czeisler CA. Dose-response relationships for resetting of human circadian clock by light. Nature. 1996 Feb 8;379(6565):540-2.

Bonfils P, Halimi P, Malinvaud D. Adrenal suppression and osteoporosis after treatment of nasal polyposis. Acta Otolaryngol. 2006 Dec;126(11):1195-200.

Bongartz D, Hesse A. Selective extraction of quercetin in vegetable drugs and urine by off-line coupling of boronic acid affinity chromatography and high-performance liquid chromatography. J Chromatogr B Biomed Appl. 1995 Nov 17;673(2):223-30.

Borchers AT, Hackman RM, Keen CL, Stern JS, Gershwin ME. Complementary medicine: a review of immunomodulatory effects of Chinese herbal medicines. Am J Clin Nutr. 1997 Dec;66(6):1303-12.

Borets VM, Lis MA, Pyrochkin VM, Kishkovich VP, Butkevich ND. Therapeutic efficacy of pantothenic acid preparations in ischemic heart disease patients. Vopr Pitan. 1987 Mar-Apr;(2):15-7.

Bose J. Response in the Living and Non-Living. New York: Longmans, Green & Co., 1902.

Bottorff JL. The use and meaning of touch in caring for patients with cancer. Oncol Nurs Forum. 1993 Nov-Dec;20(10):1531-8.

Bourgine P, Stewart J. Autopoiesis and cognition. Artif Life. 2004 Summer;10(3):327-45.

Bowler PJ. The Eclipse of Darwinism: Antievolutionary Theories in the Decades Around 1900. Baltimore: Johns Hopkins, 1983.

Boyce R, Glasgow SD, Williams S, Adamantidis A. Causal evidence for the role of REM sleep theta rhythm in contextual memory consolidation. Science. 2016 May 13;352(6287):812-6. doi: 10.1126/science.aad5252.

Bradette-Hébert ME, Legault J, Lavoie S, Pichette A. A new labdane diterpene from the flowers of Solidago canadensis. Chem Pharm Bull. 2008 Jan;56(1):82-4.

Brainard GC, Hanifin JP, Warfield B, Stone MK, James ME, Ayers M, Kubey A, Byrne B, Rollag M. Short-wavelength enrichment of polychromatic light enhances human melatonin suppression potency. J Pineal Res. 2015 Apr;58(3):352-61. doi: 10.1111/jpi.12221.

Brasseur JG, Nicosia MA, Pal A, Miller LS. Function of longitudinal vs circular muscle fibers in esophageal peristalsis, deduced with mathematical modeling. World J Gastroenterol. 2007 Mar 7;13(9):1335-46.

Braude S. First Person Plural: Multiple Personality and the Philosophy of Mind. Landham, MD: Rowman & Littlefield, 1995.

Braunstein G, Labat C, Brunelleschi S, Benveniste J, Marsac J, Brink C. Evidence that the histamine sensitivity and responsiveness of guinea-pig isolated trachea are modulated by epithelial prostaglandin E2 production. Br J Pharmacol. 1988 Sep;95(1):300-8.

Brighenti F, Valtueña S, Pellegrini N, Ardigò D, Del Rio D, Salvatore S, Piatti P, Serafini M, Zavaroni I. Total Antioxidant Capacity of the Diet Is Inversely and Independently Related to Plasma Concentration of High-Sensitivity C-Reactive Protein in Adult Italian Subjects. Br J Nutr. 2005;93(5):619-25.

Brinkhaus B, Witt CM, Jena S, Linde K, Streng A, Hummelsberger J, Irnich D, Hammes M, Pach D, Melchart D, Willich SN. Physician and treatment characteristics in a randomised multicentre trial of acupuncture in patients with osteoarthritis of the knee. Complement Ther Med. 2007 Sep;15(3):180-9.

Britt R. Hole Drilled to Bottom of Earth's Crust, Breakthrough to Mantle Looms. LiveScience. 2005. 07 Apr. http://www.livescience.com/ technology/050407_earth_drill.html. Acc. 2006 Nov.

Britton WB, Bootzin RR. Near-death experiences and the temporal lobe. Psychol Sci. 2004 Apr;15(4):254-8.

Brodeur P. Currents of Death. New York: Simon and Schuster, 1989.

Brody J. Jane Brody's Nutrition Book. New York: WW Norton, 1981.

Brosseau LU, Pelland LU, Casimiro LY, Robinson VI, Tugwell PE, Wells GE. Electrical stimulation for the treatment of rheumatoid arthritis. Cochrane Database Syst Rev. 2002;(2):CD003687.

Brown V. The Amateur Naturalists Handbook. Englewood Cliffs, NJ: Prentice-Hall, 1980.

Brown, F. & Chow, C.S. Lunar-correlated variations in water uptake by bean seeds. Biolog Bull. 1973;145:265-278.

Brown, F. The rhythmic nature of animals and plants. Cycles. 1960 Apr:81-92.

Brown, J. Stimulation-produced analgesia: acupuncture, TENS and alternative techniques. Anaesthesia &intensive care medicine. 2005 Feb;6(2):45-47.

Browne J. Developmental Care - Considerations for Touch and Massage in the Neonatal Intensive Care Unit. Neonatatal Network. 2000 Feb;19(1).

Brownstein D. Salt: Your Way to Health. West Bloomfield, MI: Medical Alternatives, 2006.

Brummer RJ, Geerling BJ, Stockbrugger RW. Initial and chronic gastric acid inhibition by lansoprazole and omeprazole in relation to meal administration. Dig Dis Sci. 1997;42:2132-7.

Bruneton J. Pharmacognosy, Phytochemistry, Medicinal Plants. Paris: Lavoisier, 1995.

Buck L, Axel R. A novel multigene family may encode odorant receptors: A molecule basis for odor recognition. Cell. 1991;65(April 5):175-187.

253

Buckley NA, Whyte IM, Dawson AH. There are days ... and moons. Self-poisoning is not lunacy. Med J Aust. 1993 Dec 6-20;159(11-12):786-9.

Budzianowski J. Coumarins, caffeoyltartaric acids and their artifactual methyl esters from Taraxacum officinale leaves. Planta Med. 1997 Jun;63(3):288.

Buijs RM, Scheer FA, Kreier F, Yi C, Bos N, Goncharuk VD, Kalsbeek A. Organization of circadian functions: interaction with the body. Prog Brain Res. 2006;153:341-60.

Bulsing PJ, Smeets MA, van den Hout MA. Positive Implicit Attitudes toward Odor Words. Chem Senses. 2007 May 7.

Burack MA, Hartlein J, Flores HP, Taylor-Reinwald L, Perlmutter JS, Cairns NJ. In vivo amyloid imaging in autopsy-confirmed Parkinson disease with dementia. Neurology 2010;74:77-84.

Burdge GC, Jones AE, Wootton SA. Eicosapentaenoic and docosapentaenoic acids are the principal products of alpha-linolenic acid metabolism in young men. B J Nutr. 2002 Oct;88(4):355-63.

Burgess JF. Causative Factors in Eczema. Can Med Assoc J. 1930 Feb; 22(2): 207-211.

Burke V, Zhao Y, Lee AH, Hunter E, Spargo RM, Gracey M, Smith RM, Beilin LJ, Puddey IB. Health-related behaviours as predictors of mortality and morbidity in Australian Aborigines. Prev Med. 2007 Feb;44(2):135-42.

Burks W, Jones SM, Berseth CL, Harris C, Sampson HA, Scalabrin DM. Hypoallergenicity and effects on growth and tolerance of a new amino acid-based formula with docosahexaenoic acid and arachidonic acid. J Pediatr. 2008 Aug;153(2):266-71.

Burney PG, Luczynska C, Chinn S, Jarvis D. The European Community Respiratory Health Survey. Eur Respir J. 1994;7: 954-960.

Burnham K, Andersson D. Model Selection and Inference. A Practical Information-Theoretic Approach. New York: Springer, 1998

Burr H, Hovland C. Bio-Electric Potential Gradients in the Chick. Yale Journal of Biology & Medicine. 1937;9:247-258

Burr H, Lane C, Nims L. A Vacuum Tube Microvoltmeter for the Measurement of Bioelectric Phenomena. Yale Journal of Biology & Medicine. 1936;10:65-76.

Burr H, Smith G, Strong L. Bio-electric Properties of Cancer-Resistant and Cancer-Susceptible Mice. American Journal of Cancer. 1938;32:240-248

Burr H. The Fields of Life. New York: Ballantine, 1972.

Buzsaki G. Theta rhythm of navigation: link between path integration and landmark navigation, episodic and semantic memory. Hippocampus. 2005;15(7):827-40.

Caglar E, Kuscu OO, Selvi Kuvvetli S, Kavaloglu Cildir S, Sandalli N, Twetman S. Short-term effect of ice-cream containing Bifidobacterium lactis Bb-12 on the number of salivary mutans streptococci and lactobacilli. Acta Odontol Scand. 2008 Jun;66(3):154-8.

Cahn J, Borzeix MG. Administration of procyanidolic oligomers in rats. Observed effects on changes in the permeability of the blood-brain barrier. Sem Hop. 1983 Jul 7;59(27-28):2031-4.

Cajochen C, Jewett ME, Dijk DJ. Human circadian melatonin rhythm phase delay during a fixed sleep-wake schedule interspersed with nights of sleep deprivation. J Pineal Res. 2003 Oct;35(3):149-57.

Cajochen C, Zeitzer JM, Czeisler CA, Dijk DJ. Dose-response relationship for light intensity and ocular and electroencephalographic correlates of human alertness. Behav Brain Res. 2000 Oct;115(1):75-83.

Calabrese C, Gregory WL, Leo M, Kraemer D, Bone K, Oken B. Effects of a standardized Bacopa monnieri extract on cognitive performance, anxiety, and depression in the elderly: a randomized, double-blind, placebo-controlled trial. J Altern Complement Med. 2008 Jul;14(6):707-13.

Calder PC. Dietary modification of inflammation with lipids. Proc Nutr Soc. 2002 Aug;61(3):345-58.

Calderón-Garcidueñas L, Avila-Ramírez J, Calderón-Garcidueñas A, González-Heredia T, Acuña-Ayala H, Chao CK, Thompson C, Ruiz-Ramos R, Cortés-González V, Martínez-Martínez L, García-Pérez MA, Reis J, Mukherjee PS, Torres-Jardón R, Lachmann I. Cerebrospinal Fluid Biomarkers in Highly Exposed PM2.5 Urbanites: The Risk of Alzheimer's and Parkinson's Diseases in Young Mexico City Residents. J Alzheimers Dis. 2016 Sep 6;54(2):597-613. doi: 10.3233/JAD-160472.

Calderón-Garcidueñas L. Smoking and Cerebral Oxidative Stress and Air Pollution: A Dreadful Equation with Particulate Matter Involved and One More Powerful Reason Not to Smoke Anything! J Alzheimers Dis. 2016 Jul 22;54(1):109-12. doi: 10.3233/JAD-160510.

Callender ST, Spray GH. Latent pernicious anemia. Br J Haematol 1962;8:230-240.

Calvin W. The Handbook of Brain Theory and Neural Networks. Boston: MIT Press, 1995.

Campbell A. The role of aluminum and copper on neuroinflammation and Alzheimer's disease. J Alzheimers Dis. 2006 Nov;10(2-3):165-72.

Campbell TC, Campbell TM. The China Study. Dallas, TX: Benbella Books, 2006.

Campbell WW, Tang M. Protein intake, weight loss, and bone mineral density in postmenopausal women. J Gerontol A Biol Sci Med Sci. 2010 Oct;65(10):1115-22.

Cao G, Alessio HM, Cutler RG. Oxygen-radical absorbance capacity assay for antioxidants. Free Radic Biol Med. 1993 Mar;14(3):303-11.

Capitani D, Yethiraj A, Burnell EE. Memory effects across surfactant mesophases. Langmuir. 2007 Mar 13;23(6):3036-48.

Cara L, Dubois C, Borel P, Armand M, Senft M, Portugal H, Pauli AM, Bernard PM, Lairon D. Effects of oat bran, rice bran, wheat fiber, and wheat germ on postprandial lipemia in healthy adults. Am J Clin Nutr. 1992 Jan;55(1):81-8.

REFERENCES AND BIBLIOGRAPHY

Caramia G. The essential fatty acids omega-6 and omega-3: from their discovery to their use in therapy. Minerva Pediatr. 2008 Apr;60(2):219-33.

Carlsen E, Olsson C, Petersen JH, Andersson AM, Skakkebaek NE. Diurnal rhythm in serum levels of inhibin B in normal men: relation to testicular steroids and gonadotropins. J Clin Endocrinol Metab. 1999 May;84(5):1664-9.

Carlson DL, Hites RA. Polychlorinated biphenyls in salmon and salmon feed: global differences and bioaccumulation. Environ Sci Technol. 2005 Oct 1;39(19):7389-95.

Carpita N. C., Kanabus J., Housley T. L. Linkage structure of fructans and fructan oligomers from Triticum aestivum and Festuca arundinacea leaves. J. Plant Physiol. 1989;134:162-168

Carroll D. The Complete Book of Natural Medicines. New York: Summit, 1980.

Cassidy A, Rimm EB, O'Reilly EJ, Logroscino G, Kay C, Chiuve SE, Rexrode KM. Dietary flavonoids and risk of stroke in women. Stroke. 2012 Apr;43(4):946-51.

Cassileth B, Trevisan C, Gubili J. Complementary therapies for cancer pain. Curr Pain Headache Rep. 2007 Aug;11(4):265-9.

Cavalli-Sforza L, Feldman M. Cultural Transmission and Evolution: A quantitative approach. Princeton: Princeton UP, 1981.

Celec P, Ostatníková D, Hodosy J, Skoknová M, Putz Z, Kúdela M. Infradian rhythmic variations of salivary estradioland progesterone in healthy men. Biol Res. 2006;37(1): 37-44.

Celec P, Ostatníková D, Putz Z, Hodosy J, Burský P, Stárka L, Hampl R, Kúdela M. Circatrigintan Cycle of Salivary Testosterone in Human Male. Biol Rhythm Res. 2003;34(3): 305-315.

Celec P. Analysis of rhythmic variance - ANORVA. A new simple method for detecting rhythms in biological time series. Biol Res. 2004;37:777-782.

Cenacchi T, Bertoldin T, Farina C, Fiori MG, Crepaldi G. Cognitive decline in the elderly: a double-blind, placebo-controlled multicenter study on efficacy of phosphatidylserine administration. Aging (Milano). 1993 Apr;5(2):123-33.

Cengel YA, Heat Transfer: A Practical Approach. Boston: McGraw-Hill, 1998.

Centers for Disease Control and Prevention (CDC). Obesity prevalence among low-income, preschool-aged children—United States, 1998-2008. MMWR Morb Mortal Wkly Rep. 2009 Jul 24;58(28):769-73.

Centers for Disease Control and Prevention (CDC). Vital signs: nonsmokers' exposure to secondhand smoke—United States, 1999-2008. MMWR Morb Mortal Wkly Rep. 2010 Sep 10;59(35):1141-6.

Cereijido M, Contreras RG, Flores-Benítez D, Flores-Maldonado C, Larre I, Ruiz A, Shoshani L. New diseases derived or associated with the tight junction. Arch Med Res. 2007 Jul;38(5):465-78.

Cermak NM, Gibala MJ, van Loon LJ. Nitrate supplementation's improvement of 10-km time-trial performance in trained cyclists. Int J Sport Nutr Exerc Metab. 2012 Feb;22(1):64-71.

Cesarone MR, Belcaro G, Nicolaides AN, Ricci A, Geroulakos G, Ippolito E, Brandolini R, Vinciguerra G, Dugall M, Griffin M, Ruffini I, Acerbi G, Corsi M, Riordan NH, Stuard S, Bavera P, Di Renzo A, Kenyon J, Errichi BM. Prevention of venous thrombosis in long-haul flights with Flite Tabs: the LONFLIT-FLITE randomized, controlled trial. Angiology. 2003 Sep-Oct;54(5):531-9.

Chaitow L. Conquer Pain the Natural Way. San Francisco: Chronicle Books, 2002.

Cham, B. Solasodine glycosides as anti-cancer agents: Pre-clinical and Clinical studies. Asia Pac J Pharmac. 1994;9: 113-118.

Chan A, Paskavitz J, Remington R, Rasmussen S, Shea TB. Efficacy of a vitamin/nutriceutical formulation for early-stage Alzheimer's disease: a 1-year, open-label pilot study with an 16-month caregiver extension. Am J Alzheimers Dis Other Demen. 2008 Dec-2009 Jan;23(6):571-85. doi: 10.1177/1533317508325093.

Chan A, Remington R, Kotyla E, Lepore A, Zemianek J, Shea TB. A vitamin/nutriceutical formulation improves memory and cognitive performance in community-dwelling adults without dementia. J Nutr Health Aging. 2010 Mar;14(3):224-30.

Chandra RK. Effect of vitamin and trace-element supplementation on cognitive function in elderly subjects. Nutrition. 2001 Sep;17(9):709-12. Retraction in: Meguid MM. Nutrition. 2005 Feb;21(2):286.

Chandrasekhar K, Kapoor J, Anishetty S. A prospective, randomized double-blind, placebo-controlled study of safety and efficacy of a high-concentration full-spectrum extract of Ashwagandha root in reducing stress and anxiety in adults. Ind Jnl Psych Med. 2012 34(3): 255-262.

Chaney M, Ross M. Nutrition. New York: Houghton Mifflin, 1971.

Chaney M, Ross M. Nutrition. New York: Houghton Mifflin, 1971.

Chang CH, Chen CY, Chiou JY, Peng RY, Peng CH. Astaxanthine secured apoptotic death of PC12 cells induced by beta-amyloid peptide 25–35: its molecular action targets. J Med Food. 2010;13:548–556. doi: 10.1089/jmf.2009.1291.

Chao A, Thun MJ, Connell CJ, McCullough ML, Jacobs EJ, Flanders WD, Rodriguez C, Sinha R, Calle EE. Meat Consumption and Risk of Colorectal Cancer. JAMA. 2005 January 12: 172-182.

Chapat L, Chemin K, Dubois B, Bourdet-Sicard R, Kaiserlian D. Lactobacillus casei reduces CD8+ T cell-mediated skin inflammation. Eur J Immunol. 2004 Sep;34(9):2520-8.

Chapidze G, Kapanadze S, Dolidze N, Bachutashvili Z, Latsabidze N. Prevention of coronary atherosclerosis by the use of combination therapy with antioxidant coenzyme q10 and statins. Georgian Med News. 2005 Jan;(1):20-5.

Characterization and quantitation of Antioxidant Constituents of Sweet Pepper (Capsicum annuum—Cayenne). J Agric Food Chem. 2004 Jun 16;52(12):3861-9.

Chen CY, Milbury PE, Collins FW, Blumberg JB. Avenanthramides are bioavailable and have antioxidant activity in humans after acute consumption of an enriched mixture from oats. J Nutr. 2007 Jun;137(6):1375-82.

Chen HY, Shi Y, Ng CS, Chan SM, Yung KK, Zhang QL. Auricular acupuncture treatment for insomnia: a systematic review. J Altern Complement Med. 2007 Jul-Aug;13(6):669-76.

Chen L, Huang J, Xue L. [Effect of compound Polygonum multiflorum extract on Alzheimer's disease]. Zhong Nan Da Xue Xue Bao Yi Xue Ban. 2010 Jun;35(6):612-5. doi: 10.3969/j.issn.1672-7347.2010.06.012. Chinese.

Chen MS, Zhang JH, Wang JL, Gao L, Chen XX, Xiao JH. Anti-fibrotic effects of neferine on carbon tetrachloride-induced hepatic fibrosis in mice. Am J Chin Med. 2015;43(2):231-40. doi: 10.1142/S0192415X15500159.

Chen SJ, Chao YL, Chen CY, Chang CM, Wu EC, Wu CS, Yeh HH, Chen CH, Tsai HJ. Prevalence of autoimmune diseases in in-patients with schizophrenia: nationwide population-based study. Br J Psychiatry. 2012 May;200(5):374-80.

Cheng J, Xia X, Rui Y, Zhang Z, Qin L, Han S, Wan Z. The combination of 1α,25dihydroxyvitaminD3 with resveratrol improves neuronal degeneration by regulating endoplasmic reticulum stress, insulin signaling and inhibiting tau hyperphosphorylation in SH-SY5Y cells. Food Chem Toxicol. 2016 Jul;93:32-40. doi: 10.1016/j.fct.2016.04.021.

Chen-Goodspeed M, Cheng Chi Lee. Tumor suppression and circadian function. J Biol Rhythms. 2007 Aug;22(4):291-8.

Chételat G, Villemagne VL, Villain N, Jones G, Ellis KA, Ames D, Martins RN, Masters CL, Rowe CC; AIBL Research Group. Accelerated cortical atrophy in cognitively normal elderly with high β-amyloid deposition. Neurology. 2012 Feb 14;78(7):477-84. doi: 10.1212/WNL.0b013e318246d67a.

Chevallier A. Encyclopedia of Medicinal Plants. New York, NY: DK Publishing; 1996.

Chew EY, Clemons TE, Agrón E, Launer LJ, Grodstein F, Bernstein PS; Age-Related Eye Disease Study 2 (AREDS2) Research Group. Effect of Omega-3 Fatty Acids, Lutein/Zeaxanthin, or Other Nutrient Supplementation on Cognitive Function: The AREDS2 Randomized Clinical Trial. JAMA. 2015 Aug 25;314(8):791-801. doi: 10.1001/jama.2015.9677

Chilton F, Tucker L. Win the War Within. New York: Rodale, 2006.

Chilton FH, Rudel LL, Parks JS, Arm JP, Seeds MC. Mechanisms by which botanical lipids affect inflammatory disorders. Am J Clin Nutr. 2008 Feb;87(2):498S-503S.

Chirkova E. Mathematical methods of detection of biological and heliogeophysical rhythms in the light of developments in modern heliobiology: A platform for discussion. Cybernet Sys. 2000;31(6):903-918.

Chirkova EN, Suslov LS, Avramenko MM, Krivoruchko GE. Monthly and daily biorhythms of amylase in the blood of healthy men and their relation with the rhythms in the external environment. Lab Delo. 1990;(4):40-4.

Choi DW. Glutamate neurotoxicity and diseases of the nervous system. Neuron. 1988;1:623-34.

Chon SH, Yang EJ, Lee T, Song KS. β-Secretase (BACE1) inhibitory and neuroprotective effects of p-terphenyls from Polyozellus multiplex. Food Funct. 2016 Aug 11.

Chong AS, Boussy IA, Jiang XL, Lamas M, Graf LH Jr. CD54/ICAM-1 is acostimulator of NK cell-mediated cytotoxicity. Cell Immunol. 1994 Aug;157(1):92-105.

Chong NW, Codd V, Chan D, Samani NJ. Circadian clock genes cause activation of the human PAI-1 gene promoter with 4G/5G allelic preference. FEBS Lett. 2006 Aug 7;580(18):4469-72.

Christensen AS, Viggers L, Hasselström K, Gregersen S. Effect of fruit restriction on glycemic control in patients with type 2 dia-betes—a randomized trial. Nutr J. 2013 Mar 5;12:29.

Christopher J. School of Natural Healing. Springville UT: Christopher Publ, 1976.

Christophersen, A. G., Jun, H., Jørgensen, K., and Skibsted, L. H. Photobleaching of astaxanthin and canthaxanthin: quantum-yields dependence of solvent, temperature, and wavelength of irradiation in relation to packageing and storage of carotenoid pigmented salmonoids. Z. Lebensm. Unters. Forsch., 1991;192:433-439.

Chu Q, Wang L, Liu GZ. Clinical observation on acupuncture for treatment of diabetic nephropathy. Zhongguo Zhen Jiu. 2007 Jul;27(7):488-90.

Chu YF, Liu RH. Cranberries inhibit LDL oxidation and induce LDL receptor expression in hepatocytes. Life Sci. 2005;77(15):1892-1901.

Churchill G, Doerge R. Empirical threshold values for quantitative trait mapping. Genetics 1994;138:963-971.

Chwirot B, Kowalska M, Plóciennik N, Piwinski M, Michniewicz Z, Chwirot S. Variability of spectra of laser-induced fluorescence of colonic mucosa: Its significance for fluorescence detection of colonic neoplasia. Indian J Exp. Biol. 2003;41(5):500-510.

Chwirot WB, Popp F. White-light-induced luminescence and mitotic activity of yeast cells. Folia Histochemica et Cytobiologica. 1991;29(4):155.

Citro M, Endler PC, Pongratz W, Vinattieri C, Smith CW, Schulte J. Hormone effects by electronic transmission. FASEB J. 1995:Abstract 12161.

Citro M, Smith CW, Scott-Morley A, Pongratz W, Endler PC. Transfer of information from molecules by means of electronic amplification, in P.C. Endler, J. Schulte (eds.): Ultra High Dilution. Physiology and Physics. Dordrecht: Kluwer Academic Publishers. 1994;209-214.

Clark D. The use of electrical current in the treatment of nonunions. Vet Clin North Am Small Anim Pract. 1987 Jul;17(4):793-8.

Cocilovo A. Colored light therapy: overview of its history, theory, recent developments and clinical applications combined with acupuncture. Am J Acupunct. 1999;27(1-2):71-83.

Cohen S, Popp F. Biophoton emission of the human body. J Photochem & Photobio. 1997;B 40:187-189.

Cohen S, Popp F. Low-level luminescence of the human skin. Skin Res Tech. 1997;3:177-180.

REFERENCES AND BIBLIOGRAPHY

Coles JA, Yamane S. Effects of adapting lights on the time course of the receptor potential of the anuran retinal rod. J Physiol. 1975 May;247(1):189-207.

Coll AP, Farooqi IS, O'Rahilly S. The hormonal control of food intake. Cell. 2007 Apr 20;129(2):251-62.

Colquhoun DM, Moores D, Somerset SM, Humphries JA. Comparison of the effects on lipoproteins and apolipoproteins of a diet high in monounsaturated fatty acids, enriched with avocado, and a high-carbohydrate diet. Am J Clin Nutr. 1992 Oct;56(4):671-7.

Conely J. Music and the Military. Air University Review. 1972 Mar-Ap.

Connelly PJ, Prentice NP, Cousland G, Bonham J. A randomised double-blind placebo-controlled trial of folic acid supplementation of cholinesterase inhibitors in Alzheimer's disease. Int J Geriat Psychiatry. 2008 Feb;23(2):155-60.

Conquer JA, Holub BJ. Dietary docosahexaenoic acid as a source of eicosapentaenoic acid in vegetarians and omnivores. Lipids. 1997 Mar;32(3):341-5.

Contreras D, Steriade M. Cellular basis of EEG slow rhythms: a study of dynamic corticothalamic relationships. J Neurosci. 1995 Jan;15(1 Pt 2):604-22.

Cook J, The Therapeutic Use of Music. Nursing Forum. 1981;20:3: 253-66.

Cooper K. The Aerobics Program for Total Well-Being. New York: Evans, 1980.

Corkin S, Amaral DG, González RG, et al: H. M.'s medial temporal lobe lesion: findings from magnetic resonance imaging. J Neurosci. 1997;17:3964-3979.

Corrigan FM, Van Rhijn A, Horrobin DF. Essential fatty acids in Alzheimer's disease. Ann N Y Acad Sci. 1991;640:250-2.

Cotroneo AM, Castagna A, Putignano S, Lacava R, Fantò F, Monteleone F, Rocca F, Malara A, Gareri P. Effectiveness and safety of citicoline in mild vascular cognitive impairment: the IDEALE study. Clin Interv Aging. 2013;8:131-7. doi: 10.2147/CIA.S38420.

Couzy F, Kastenmayer P, Vigo M, Clough J, Munoz-Box R, Barclay DV. Calcium bioavailability from a calcium- and sulfate-rich mineral water, compared with milk, in young adult women. Am J Clin Nutr. 1995 Dec;62(6):1239-44.

Cox CB. Emory-led Study Links Metals to Alzheimer's and Other Neurodegenerative Diseases. Emory Univ Mag. 2007 Aug 10.

Craciunescu CN, Wu R, Zeisel SH. Diethanolamine alters neurogenesis and induces apoptosis in fetal mouse hippocampus. FASEB J. 2006 Aug;20(10):1635-40.

Craft S, Peskind E, Schwartz MW, Schellenberg GD, Raskind M, Porte D Jr. Cerebrospinal fluid and plasma insulin levels in Alzheimer's disease: relationship to severity of dementia and apolipoprotein E genotype. Neurology. 1998 Jan;50(1):164-8.

Crane PK, Gibbons LE, Dams-O'Connor K, Trittschuh E, Leverenz JB, Keene CD, Sonnen J, Montine TJ, Bennett DA, Leurgans S, Schneider JA, Larson EB. Association of Traumatic Brain Injury With Late-Life Neurodegenerative Conditions and Neuropathologic Findings. JAMA Neurol. 2016 Jul 11. doi: 10.1001/jamaneurol.2016.1948.

Crapper DR, Krishnan SS, Dalton AJ. Brain aluminum distribution in Alzheimer's disease and experimental neurofibrillary degeneration. Science. 1973 May 4;180(4085):511-3.

Crawley J. The Biorhythm Book. Boston: Journey Editions, 1996.

Creinin MD, Keverline S, Meyn LA. How regular is regular? An analysis of menstrual cycle regularity. Contraception. 2004 Oct;70(4):289-92.

Crick F. Life Itself: Its Origin and Nature. New York: Simon and Schuster, 1981.

Crofford LJ. Neuroendocrine abnormalities in fibromyalgia and related disorders. Am J Med Sci. 1998;315:359-66.

Crook TH, Tinklenberg J, Yesavage J, Petrie W, Nunzi MG, Massari DC. Effects of phosphatidylserine in age-associated memory impairment. Neurology 1991;41:644-649.

Cross ML. Immune-signalling by orally-delivered probiotic bacteria: effects on common mucosal immunoresponses and protection at distal mucosal sites. Int J Immunopathol Pharmacol. 2004 May-Aug;17(2):127-134.

Cruccu G, Aziz TZ, Garcia-Larrea L, Hansson P, Jensen TS, Lefaucheur JP, Simpson BA, Taylor RS. EFNS guidelines on neurostimulation therapy for neuropathic pain. Eur J Neurol. 2007 Sep;14(9):952-70.

Cummings DE, Overduin J. Gastrointestinal regulation of food intake. J Clin Invest. 2007 Jan;117(1):13-23.

Cummings M. Human Heredity: Principles and Issues. St. Paul, MN: West, 1988.

Curtis LH, Ostbye T, Sendersky V, Hutchison S, Dans PE, Wright A, Woosley RL, Schulman KA. Inappropriate prescribing for elderly Americans in a large outpatient population. Arch Intern Med. 2004 Aug 9-23;164(15):1621-5.

Cuthbert SC, Goodheart GJ Jr. On the reliability and validity of manual muscle testing: a literature review. Chiropr Osteopat. 2007 Mar 6;15:4.

Dalmose A, Bjarkam C, Vuckovic A, Sorensen JC, Hansen J. Electrostimulation: a future treatment option for patients with neurogenic urodynamic disorders? APMIS Suppl. 2003;(109):45-51.

Darrow K. The Renaissance of Physics. New York: Macmillan, 1936.

Das UN. A defect in the activity of Delta6 and Delta5 desaturases may be a factor predisposing to the development of insulin resistance syndrome. Prostagl Leukot Essent Fatty Acids. 2005; May;72(5):343-50.

Davenas E, Beauvais F, Amara J, Oberbaum M, Robinzon B, Miadonna B, Tedeschi A, Pomeranz B, Fortner P, Belon P, Sainte-Laudy J, Poitevin B, Benveniste J. Human basophil degranulation triggered by very dilute antiserum against IgE. Nature. 1988;333: 816-818.

Davidson T. Rhinology: The Collected Writings of Maurice H. Cottle, M.D. San Diego, CA: American Rhinologic Society, 1987.

DaVinci L. (Dickens E. ed.) The Da Vinci Notebooks. London: Profile, 2005.

Davis GE Jr, Lowell WE. Chaotic solar cycles modulate the incidence and severity of mental illness. Med Hypotheses. 2004;62(2):207-14.

Davis GE Jr, Lowell WE. Solar cycles and their relationship to human disease and adaptability. Med Hypotheses. 2006;67(3):447-61.

Davis GE Jr, Lowell WE. The Sun determines human longevity: teratogenic effects of chaotic solar radiation. Med Hypotheses. 2004;63(4):574-81.

de Jager CA, Oulhaj A, Jacoby R, Refsum H, Smith AD. Cognitive and clinical outcomes of homocysteine-lowering B-vitamin treatment in mild cognitive impairment: a randomized controlled trial. Int J Geriatr Psychiatry. 2012 Jun;27(6):592-600. doi: 10.1002/gps.2758.

De Lucca AJ, Bland JM, Vigo CB, Cushion M, Selitrennikoff CP, Peter J, Walsh TJ. CAY-I, a fungicidal saponin from Capsicum sp. fruit. Med Mycol. 2002 Apr;40(2):131-7.

De Simone MS, Fadda L, Perri R, Aloisi M, Caltagirone C, Carlesimo GA. Does retrieval frequency account for the pattern of autobiographical memory loss in early Alzheimer's disease patients? Neuropsychologia. 2016 Jan 8;80:194-200. doi: 10.1016/j.neuropsychologia.2015.11.024.

de Waal H, Stam CJ, Lansbergen MM, Wieggers RL, Kamphuis PJ, Scheltens P, Maestú F, van Straaten EC. The effect of souvenaid on functional brain network organisation in patients with mild Alzheimer's disease: a randomised controlled study. PLoS One. 2014 Jan 27;9(1):e86558. doi: 10.1371/journal.pone.0086558. eCollection 2014.

Dean C. Death by Modern Medicine. Belleville, ON: Matrix Verite-Media, 2005.

Dean E, Mihalasky J, Ostrander S, Schroeder L. Executive ESP. Englewood Cliffs, NJ: Prentice-Hall, 1974.

Dean E. Infrared measurements of healer-treated water. In: Roll W, Beloff J, White R (Eds.): Research in parapsychology 1982. Metuchen, NJ: Scarecrow Press, 1983:100-101.

Deepak M, Sangli GK, Arun PC, Amit A. Quantitative determination of the major saponin mixture bacoside A in Bacopa monnieri by HPLC. Phytochem Anal 2005;16: 24–29.

Defrin R, Ohry A, Blumen N, Urca G. Sensory determinants of thermal pain. Brain. 2002 Mar;125(Pt 3):501-10.

Deitel M. Applications of electrical pacing in the body. Obes Surg. 2004 Sep;14 Suppl 1:S3-8.

Del Bo C, Riso P, Campolo J, Moller P, Loft S, Klimis-Zacas D, Brambilla A, Rizzolo A, Porrini M. A single portion of blueberry (Vaccinium corymbosum L) improves protection against DNA damage but not vascular function in healthy male volunteers. Nutr Res. 2013 Mar;33(3):220-7. doi: 10.1016/j.nutres.2012.12.009.

Del Giudice E, Preparata G, Vitiello G. Water as a free electric dipole laser. Phys Rev Lett. 1988;61:1085-1088.

Del Giudice E. Is the 'memory of water' a physical impossibility?, in P.C. Endler, J. Schulte (eds.): Ultra High Dilution. Physiology and Physics. Dordrecht: Kluwer Academic Publishers, 1994:117-120.

Delcomyn F. Foundations of Neurobiology. New York: W.H. Freeman and Co., 1998.

Dement W, Vaughan C. The Promise of Sleep. New York: Dell, 1999.

Dennett D. Brainstorms: Philosophical Essays on Mind & Psychology. Cambridge: MIT Press., 1980.

Dennett D. Consciousness Explained. London: Little, Brown and Co., 1991.

Depue BE, Banich MT, Curran T. Suppression of emotional and nonemotional content in memory: effects of repetition on cognitive control. Psychol Sci. 2006 May;17(5):441-7.

Dere E, Kart-Teke E, Huston JP, De Souza Silva MA. The case for episodic memory in animals. Neurosci Biobehav Rev. 2006;30(8):1206-24.

Deriemaeker P, Aerenhouts D, De Ridder D, Hebbelinck M, Clarys P. Health aspects, nutrition and physical characteristics in matched samples of institutionalized vegetarian and non-vegetarian elderly (>65yrs). Nutr Metab (Lond). 2011 Jun 14;8(1):37.

Devanand D, Lee J, Luchsinger J, Manly J, Marder K, Mayeux R, Scarmeas N, Schupf N, Stern Y. Lessons from Epidemiologic Research about Risk Factors, Modifiers, and Progression of Late Onset Alzheimer's Disease in New York City at Columbia University Medical Center. J Alzheimers Dis. 2012 Jul 24.

Devaraj TL. Speaking of Ayurvedic Remedies for Common Diseases. New Delhi: Sterling, 1985.

Devirgiliis C, Zalewski PD, Perozzi G, Murgia C. Zinc fluxes and zinc transporter genes in chronic diseases. Mutat Res. 2007 Sep 1;622(1-2):84-93. 2007 Feb 17.

Devulder J, Crombez E, Mortier E. Central pain: an overview. Acta Neurol Belg. 2002 Sep;102(3):97-103.

DeWitt RC, Kudsk KA. The gut's role in metabolism, mucosal barrier function, and gut immunology. Infect Dis Clin North Am. 1999 Jun;13(2):465-81.

Dhond RP, Kettner N, Napadow V. Neuroimaging acupuncture effects in the human brain. J Altern Complement Med. 2007 Jul-Aug;13(6):603-16.

Dimitriadis GD, Raptis SA. Thyroid hormone excess and glucose intolerance. Exp Clin Endocrinol Diabetes. 2001;109 Suppl 2:S225-39.

Dobrowolski J, Ezzahir A, Knapik M. Possibilities of chemiluminescence application in comparative studies of animal and cancer cells with special attention to leucemic blood cells. In: Jezowska-Trzebiatowska, B., et al. (eds.). Photon Emission from Biological Systems. Singapore: World Scientific Publ, 1987:170-183.

Dolcos F, LaBar KS, Cabeza R. Interaction between the amygdala and the medial temporal lobe memory system predicts better memory for emotional events. Neuron. 2004 Jun 10;42(5):855-63.

Domonkos AN, Arnold HL, Odom RB. Andrews' Diseases of the Skin: Clinical Dermatology. 7th ed. Philadelphia, PA

Donato F, Monarca S, Premi S., and Gelatti, U. Drinking water hardness and chronic degenerative diseases. Part III. Tumors, urolithiasis, fetal malformations, deterioration of the cognitive function in the aged and atopic eczema. Ann. Ig. 2003;15:57-70.

REFERENCES AND BIBLIOGRAPHY

Dong MH, Kaunitz JD. Gastroduodenal mucosal defense. Curr Opin Gastroenterol. 2006 Nov;22(6):599-606.

Dooley, M.A. and Hogan S.L. Environmental epidemiology and risk factors for autoimmune disease. Curr Opin Rheum. 2003;15(2):99-103.

D'Orazio N, Ficoneri C, Riccioni G, Conti P, Theoharides TC, Bollea MR. Conjugated linoleic acid: a functional food? Int J Immunopathol Pharmacol. 2003 Sep-Dec;16(3):215-20.

Doré V, Villemagne VL, Bourgeat P, Fripp J, Acosta O, Chetélat G, Zhou L, Martins R, Ellis KA, Masters CL, Ames D, Salvado O, Rowe CC. Cross-sectional and longitudinal analysis of the relationship between Aβ deposition, cortical thickness, and memory in cognitively unimpaired individuals and in Alzheimer disease. JAMA Neurol. 2013 Jul;70(7):903-11.

Dotolo Institute. The Study of Colon Hydrotherapy. Pinellas Park, FL: Dotolo, 2003.

Douaud G, Refsum H, de Jager CA, Jacoby R, Nichols TE, Smith SM, Smith AD. Preventing Alzheimer's disease-related gray matter atrophy by B-vitamin treatment. Proc Natl Acad Sci U S A. 2013 Jun 4;110(23):9523-8.

Downey LA, Kean J, Nemeh F, Lau A, Poll A, Gregory R, Murray M, Rourke J, Patak B, Pase MP, Zangara A, Lomas J, Scholey A, Stough C. An Acute, Double-Blind, Placebo-Controlled Crossover Study of 320 mg and 640 mg Doses of a Special Extract of Bacopa monnieri (CDRI 08) on Sustained Cognitive Performance. Phytother Res. 2012 Dec 19.

Drago V, Babiloni C, Bartrés-Faz D, Caroli A, Bosch B, Hensch T, et al. Disease tracking markers for Alzheimer's disease at the prodromal (MCI) stage. J Alzheimers Dis 2011;26 Suppl 3:159-99.

Drubaix I, Robert L, Maraval M, Robert AM. Synthesis of glycoconjugates by human diseased veins: modulation by procyanidolic oligomers. Int J Exp Pathol. 1997 Apr;78(2):117-21.

Dubrov, A. Human Biorhythms and the Moon. New York: Nova Science Publ., 1996.

Duke J. The Green Pharmacy. New York: St. Martins, 1997.

Duke M. Acupuncture. New York: Pyramid, 1973.

Dunlop KA, Carson DJ, Shields MD. Hypoglycemia due to adrenal suppression secondary to high-dose nebulized corticosteroid. Pediatr Pulmonol. 2002 Jul;34(1):85-6.

Dunne B, Jahn R, Nelson R. Precognitive Remote Perception. Princeton Engineering Anomalies Res Lab Rep. Princeton. 1983 Aug.

Dunstan JA, Roper J, Mitoulas L, Hartmann PE, Simmer K, Prescott SL. The effect of supplementation with fish oil during pregnancy on breast milk immunoglobulin A, soluble CD14, cytokine levels and fatty acid composition. Clin Exp Allergy. 2004 Aug;34(8):1237-42.

Durlach J, Bara M, Guiet-Bara A. Magnesium level in drinking water: its importance in cardiovascular risk. In: Itokawa Y, Durlach J: Magnesium in Health and Disease. London: J.Libbey, 1989:173-182.

Duyckaerts C, Delatour B, Potier MC. Classification and basic pathology of Alzheimer disease. Acta Neuropathol 2009;118:5-36.

Dwivedi S, Agarwal MP. Antianginal and cardioprotective effects of Terminalia arjuna, an indigenous drug, in coronary artery disease. J Assoc Physicians India. 1994 Apr;42(4):287-9.

Dwivedi S, Jauhari R. Beneficial effects of Terminalia arjuna in coronary artery disease. Indian Heart J. 1997 Sep-Oct;49(5):507-10.

Dysken MW, Guarino PD, Vertrees JE, Asthana S, Sano M, Llorente M, Pallaki M, Love S, Schellenberg GD, McCarten JR, Malphurs J, Prieto S, Chen P, Loreck DJ, Carney S, Trapp G, Bakshi RS, Mintzer JE, Heidebrink JL, Vidal-Cardona A, Arroyo LM, Cruz AR, Kowall NW, Chopra MP, Craft S, Thielke S, Turvey CL, Woodman C, Monnell KA, Gordon K, Tomaska J, Vatassery G. Vitamin E and memantine in Alzheimer's disease: clinical trial methods and baseline data. Alzheimers Dement. 2014 Jan;10(1):36-44. doi: 10.1016/j.jalz.2013.01.014.

Dysken MW, Sano M, Asthana S, Vertrees JE, Pallaki M, Llorente M, Love S, Schellenberg GD, McCarten JR, Malphurs J, Prieto S, Chen P, Loreck DJ, Trapp G, Bakshi RS, Mintzer JE, Heidebrink JL, Vidal-Cardona A, Arroyo LM, Cruz AR, Zachariah S, Kowall NW, Chopra MP, Craft S, Thielke S, Turvey CL, Woodman C, Monnell KA, Gordon K, Tomaska J, Segal Y, Peduzzi PN, Guarino PD. Effect of vitamin E and memantine on functional decline in Alzheimer disease: the TEAM-AD VA cooperative randomized trial. JAMA. 2014 Jan 1;311(1):33-44. doi: 10.1001/jama.2013.282834.

Ebbesen F, Agati G, Pratesi R. Phototherapy with turquoise versus blue light. Arch Dis Child Fetal Neonatal Ed. 2003 Sep;88(5):F430-1.

Ebers GC, Kukay K, Bulman DE, Sadovnick AD, Rice G, Anderson C, Armstrong H, Cousin K, Bell RB, Hader W, Paty DW, Hashimoto S, Oger J, Duquette P, Warren S, Gray T, O'Connor P, Nath A, Auty A, Metz L, Francis G, Paulseth JE, Murray TJ, Pryse-Phillips W, Nelson R, Freedman M, Brunet D, Bouchard JP, Hinds D, Risch N. A full genome search in multiple sclerosis. Nat Genet. 1996 Aug;13(4):472-6.

Eccles R. Menthol and related cooling compounds. J Pharm Pharmacol. 1994 Aug;46(8):618-30.

Eden D, Feinstein D. Energy Medicine. New York: Penguin Putnam, 1998.

Edris AE. Pharmaceutical and therapeutic potentials of essential oils and their individual volatile constituents: a review. Phytother Res. 2007 Apr;21(4):308-23.

Edwards B. Drawing on the Right Side of the Brain. Los Angeles, CA: Tarcher, 1979.

Edwards JD, et al. The ACTIVE Study: What We Have Learned and What is Next? APA. July 24, 2016. (PDF)

Edwards R, Ibison M, Jessel-Kenyon J, Taylor R. Light emission from the human body. Comple Med Res. 1989;3(2): 16-19.

Edwards R, Ibison M, Jessel-Kenyon J, Taylor R. Measurements of human bioluminescence. Acup Elect Res, Intl Jnl, 1990;15: 85-94.

Edwards, L. The Vortex of Life, Nature's Patterns in Space and Time. Floris Press, 1993.

Egon G, Chartier-Kastler E, Denys P, Ruffion A. Spinal cord injury patient and Brindley neurostimulation. Prog Urol. 2007 May;17(3):535-9.

Ehling S, Hengel M, and Shibamoto T. Formation of acrylamide from lipids. Adv Exp Med Biol 2005, 561:223-233.

Electromagnetic fields: the biological evidence. Science. 1990;249: 1378-1381.

Electronic Evidence of Auras, Chakras in UCLA Study. Brain/Mind Bulletin. 1978;3:9 Mar 20.

el-Ghazaly M, Nuttall MT, Okpanyi SN, Arens-Corell M. Study of the anti-inflammatory activity of Populus tremula, Solidago virgaurea and Fraxinus excelsior. Arzneimittelforschung. 1992 Mar;42(3):333-6.

Elias S, van Noord P, Peeters P, den Tonkelaar I, Kaaks R, Grobbee D. Menstruation during and after caloric restriction: The 1944-1945 Dutch famine. Fertil Steril. 2007 Jun 1.

Ellingwood F. American Materia Medica, Therapeutics and Pharmacognosy. Portland: Eclectic Medical Publ., 1983.

Elwood PC. Epidemiology and trace elements. Clin Endocrinol Metab. 1985 Aug;14(3):617-28.

Environmental Working Group. Human Toxome Project. 2007. http://www.ewg.org/sites/humantoxome/. Acc. 2007 Sep.

Ercan N, Nuttall FQ, Gannon MC, Lane JT, Burmeister LA, Westphal SA. Plasma glucose and insulin responses to bananas of varying ripeness in persons with noninsulin-dependent diabetes mellitus. J Am Coll Nutr. 1993 Dec;12(6):703-9.

Erdelyi R. MHD waves and oscillations in the solar plasma. Introduction. Philos Transact A Math Phys Eng Sci. 2006 Feb 15;364(1839):289-96.

Ernst E. Frankincense: systematic review. BMJ. 2008 Dec 17;337:a2813.

Ernst E. Herbal remedies for anxiety - a systematic review of controlled clinical trials. Phytomedicine. 2006 Feb;13(3):205-8.

Esch T, Stefano GB. The Neurobiology of Love. Neuro Endocrinol Lett. 2005 Jun;26(3):175-92.

Eschenhagen T, Zimmermann WH. Engineering myocardial tissue. Circ Res. 2005 Dec 9;97(12):1220-31.

Esposito K., Kastorini C.M., Panagiotakos D.B., Giugliano D. Mediterranean diet and weight loss: meta-analysis of randomized controlled trials. Metab Syndr Relat Disord. 2011;9:1—12.

Estruch R, et al. Primary Prevention of Cardiovascular Disease with a Mediterranean Diet. NE Jour. Med. 2013. Jan 25. DOI: 10.1056/NEJMoa1200303

Evans P, Forte D, Jacobs C, Fredhoi C, Aitchison E, Hucklebridge F, Clow A. Cortisol secretory activity in older people in relation to positive and negative well-being. Psychoneuroendocrinology. 2007 Aug 7

Evans P, Forte D, Jacobs C, Fredhoi C, Aitchison E, Hucklebridge F, Clow A. Cortisol secretory activity in older people in relation to positive and negative well-being. Psychoneuroendocrinology. 2007 Aug 7

Everhart JE. Digestive Diseases in the United States. Darby, PA: Diane Pub, 1994.

Ewers M, Sperling RA, Klunk WE, Weiner MW, Hampel H. Neuroimaging markers for the prediction and early diagnosis of Alzheimer's disease dementia. Trends Neurosci 2011;8:430-42.

Exley C. Aluminium and iron, but neither copper nor zinc, are key to the precipitation of beta-sheets of Abeta in senile plaque cores in Alzheimer's disease. J Alzheimers Dis. 2006 Nov;10(2-3):173-7.

Exley C. The toxicity of aluminium in humans. Morphologie. 2016 Jun;100(329):51-5. doi: 10.1016/j.morpho.2015.12.003.

Ezzo JM, Richardson MA, Vickers A, Allen C, Dibble SL, Issell BF, Lao L, Pearl M, Ramirez G, Roscoe J, Shen J, Shivnan JC, Streitberger K, Treish I, Zhang G. Acupuncture-point stimulation for chemotherapy-induced nausea or vomiting. Cochrane Database Syst Rev. 2006 Apr 19;(2):CD002285.

Falcon CT. Happiness and Personal Problems. Lafayette, LA: Sensible Psychology, 1992.

Fallen EL, Kamath MV, Tougas G, Upton A. Afferent vagal modulation. Clinical studies of visceral sensory input. Auton Neurosci. 2001 Jul 20;90(1-2):35-40.

Fan X, Zhang D, Zheng J, Gu N, Ding A, Jia X, Qing H, Jin L, Wan M, Li Q. Preparation and characterization of magnetic nano-particles with radiofrequency-induced hyperthermia for cancer treatment. Sheng Wu Yi Xue Gong Cheng Xue Za Zhi. 2006 Aug;23(4):809-13.

FAO/WHO Expert Committee. Fats and Oils in Human Nutrition. Food and Nutrition Paper. 1994;(57).

Féart C, Pérès K, Samieri C, Letenneur L, Dartigues JF, Barberger-Gateau P. Adherence to a Mediterranean diet and onset of disability in older persons. Eur J Epidemiol. 2011 Sep;26(9):747-56. doi: 10.1007/s10654-011-9611-4.

Fecher LA, Cummings SD, Keefe MJ, Alani RM. Toward a molecular classification of melanoma. J Clin Oncol. 2007 Apr 20;25(12):1606-20.

Fecka I. Qualitative and quantitative determination of hydrolysable tannins and other polyphenols in herbal products from meadowsweet and dog rose. Phytochem Anal. 2009 May;20(3):177-90.

Federal Trade Commission. Lumosity to Pay $2 Million to Settle FTC Deceptive Advertising Charges for Its "Brain Training" Program. Jan 4, 2016.

Fehring RJ, Schneider M, Raviele K. Variability in the phases of the menstrual cycle. J Obstet Gynecol Neonatal Nurs. 2006 May-Jun;35(3):376-84.

Feleszko W, Jaworska J, Rha RD, Steinhausen S, Avagyan A, Jaudszus A, Ahrens B, Groneberg DA, Wahn U, Hamelmann E. Probiotic-induced suppression of allergic sensitization and airway inflammation is associated with an increase of T regulatory-dependent mechanisms in a murine model of asthma. Clin Exp Allergy. 2007 Apr;37(4):498-505.

Felton GE. Fibrinolytic and antithrombotic action of bromelain may eliminate thrombosis in heart patients. Med Hypotheses. 1980 Nov;6(11):1123-33.

Ferrari R, Merli E, Cicchitelli G, Mele D, Fucili A, Ceconi C. Therapeutic effects of L-carnitine and propionyl-L-carnitine on cardiovascular diseases: a review. Ann N Y Acad Sci. 2004 Nov;1033:79-91.

Ferreira LF, Behnke BJ. A toast to health and performance! Beetroot juice lowers blood pressure and the O2 cost of exercise. J Appl Physiol. 2011 Mar;110(3):585-6.

Feskanich D, Willett W, Colditz G. Calcium, vitamin D, milk consumption, and hip fractures: a prospective study among postmenopausal women. Am J Clin Nutr. 2003 Feb;77(2): 504-511.

Fillenbaum GG, Kuchibhatla MN, Hanlon JT, Artz MB, Pieper CF, Schmader KE, Dysken MW, Gray SL. Dementia and Alzheimer's disease in community-dwelling elders taking vitamin C and/or vitamin E. Ann Pharmacother. 2005 Dec;39(12):2009-14.

Filosa A, Valgimigli L, Pedulli GF, Sapone A, Maggio A, Renda D, Scazzone C, Malizia R, Pitrolo L, Lo Pinto C, Borsellino Z, Cuccia L, Capra M, Canistro D, Broccoli M, Soleti A, Paolini M. Quantitative evaluation of oxidative stress status on peripheral blood in beta-thalassaemic patients by means of electron paramagnetic resonance spectroscopy. Br J Haematol. 2005 Oct;131(1):135-40.Nadkarni KM. The Indian Materia Medica. Prakashan Private Ltd., 1908-1989.

Fischer JL, Mihelc EM, Pollok KE, Smith ML. Chemotherapeutic selectivity conferred by selenium: a role for p53-dependent DNA repair. Mol Cancer Ther. 2007 Jan;6(1):355-61.

Fjell AM, Walhovd KB, Fennema-Notestine C, McEvoy LK, Hagler DJ, Holland D, Brewer JB, Dale AM. One-year brain atrophy evident in healthy aging. J Neurosci. 2009 Dec 2;29(48):15223-31.

Flandrin, J, Montanari M(eds.). Food: A Culinary History from Antiquity to the Present. New York: Penguin Books, 1999.

Flicker L, Martins RN, Thomas J, Acres J, Taddei K, Vasikaran SD, Norman P, Jamrozik K, Almeida OP. B-vitamins reduce plasma levels of beta amyloid. Neurobiol Aging. 2008 Feb;29(2):303-5.

Food and Drug Administration, HHS. Food labeling: health claims; soluble dietary fiber from certain foods and coronary heart disease. Interim final rule. Fed Regist. 2002 Oct 2;67(191):61773-83.

Ford AH, Flicker L, Alfonso H, Thomas J, Clarnette R, Martins R, Almeida OP. Vitamins B(12), B(6), and folic acid for cognition in older men. Neurology. 2010 Oct 26;75(17):1540-7. doi: 10.1212/WNL.0b013e3181f962c4. Erratum in: Neurology. 2011 Aug 23;77((8)):804.

Forget-Dubois N, Boivin M, Dionne G, Pierce T, Tremblay RE, Perusse D. A longitudinal twin study of the genetic and environmental etiology of maternal hostile-reactive behavior during infancy and toddlerhood. Infant Behav Dev. 2007 Aug;30(3):453-65.

Foster S, Hobbs C. Medicinal Plants and Herbs. Boston: Houghton Mifflin, 2002.

Fotuhi M, Zandi PP, Hayden KM, Khachaturian AS, Szekely CA, Wengreen H, Munger RG, Norton MC, Tschanz JT, Lyketsos CG, Breitner JC, Welsh-Bohmer K. Better cognitive performance in elderly taking antioxidant vitamins E and C supplements in combination with nonsteroidal anti-inflammatory drugs: the Cache County Study. Alzheimers Dement. 2008 May;4(3):223-7. doi: 10.1016/j.jalz.2008.01.004.

Fox RD, Algoculture. Doctorate Disseration, 1983 Jul.

Fraga CG. Relevance, essentiality and toxicity of trace elements in human health. Mol Aspects Med. 2005 Aug-Oct;26(4-5):235-44.

Frawley D, Lad V. The Yoga of Herbs. Sante Fe: Lotus Press, 1986.

Freeman W. The Physiology of Perception. Sci. Am. 1991 Feb.

Frey A. Electromagnetic field interactions with biological systems. FASEB Jnl. 1993;7: 272-28.

Frick B, Gruber B, Schroecksnadel K, Leblhuber F, Fuchs D. Homocysteine but not neopterin declines in demented patients on B vitamins. J Neural Transm (Vienna). 2006 Nov;113(11):1815-9.

Friend BA, Shahani KM, Long CA, Vaughn LA. The effect of processing and storage on key enzymes, B vitamins, and lipids of mature human milk. Evaluation of fresh samples and effects of freezing and frozen storage. Pediatr Res. 1983 Jan;17(1):61-4.

Frisoni GB, Fox NC, Jack CR, Scheltens P, Thompson PM. The clinical use of structural MRI in Alzheimer disease. Nat Rev Neurol 2010;6:67-77.

Fu XH. Observation on therapeutic effect of acupuncture on early peripheral facial paralysis. Zhongguo Zhen Jiu. 2007 Jul;27(7):494-6.

Fu Y, Hsiao JT, Paxinos G, Halliday GM, Kim WS. ABCA7 Mediates Phagocytic Clearance of Amyloid-β in the Brain. J Alzheimers Dis. 2016 Jul 25.

Fuhrman B, Rosenblat M, Hayek T, Coleman R, Aviram M. Ginger extract consumption reduces plasma cholesterol, inhibits LDL oxidation and attenuates development of atherosclerosis in atherosclerotic, apolipoprotein E-deficient mice. J Nutr. 2000 May;130(5):1124-31.

Fukada Y, Okano T. Circadian clock system in the pineal gland. Mol Neurobiol. 2002 Feb;25(1):19-30.

Fung TT, Schulze M, Manson JE, Willett WC, Hu FB. Dietary patterns, meat intake, and the risk of type 2 diabetes in women. Arch Intern Med. 2004 Nov 8;164(20):2235-40.

Fung TT, Stampfer MJ, Manson JE, Rexrode KM, Willett WC, Hu FB. Prospective study of major dietary patterns and stroke risk in women. Stroke. 2004 Sep;35(9):2014-9.

Fuster JM. Prefrontal neurons in networks of executive memory. Brain Res Bull. 2000 Jul 15;52(5):331-6.

Gabory A, Attig L, Junien C. Sexual dimorphism in environmental epigenetic programming. Mol Cell Endocrinol. 2009 May 25;304(1-2):8-18. 2009 Mar 9.

Gabriel S, Schaffner S, Nguyen H, Moore J, Roy J. The structure of haplotype blocks in the human genome. Science. 2002;296:2225-2229.

Gadad BS, Subramanya PK, Pullabhatla S, Shantharam IS, Rao KS. Curcumin-glucoside, A Novel Synthetic Derivative of Curcumin, Inhibits α-synuclein Oligomer Formation: Relevance to Parkinson's Disease. Curr Pharm Des. 2012 Jan 1.

Galaev, YM. The Measuring of Ether-Drift Velocity and Kinematic Ether Viscosity within Optical Wave Bands. Spacetime & Substance. 2002;3(5): 207-224.

Galasko DR, Peskind E, Clark CM, Quinn JF, Ringman JM, Jicha GA, Cotman C, Cottrell B, Montine TJ, Thomas RG, Aisen P; Alzheimer's Disease Cooperative Study. Antioxidants for Alzheimer disease: a randomized clinical trial with cerebrospinal fluid biomarker measures. Arch Neurol. 2012 Jul;69(7):836-41.

Gambini JP, Velluti RA, Pedemonte M. Hippocampal theta rhythm synchronizes visual neurons in sleep and waking. Brain Res. 2002 Feb 1;926(1-2):137-41.

Gandhi T, Weingart S, Borus J, Seger A, Peterson J, Burdick E, Seger D, Shu K, Federico F, Leape L, Bates D. Adverse drug events in ambulatory care. N Engl J Med. 2003 Apr 17;348(16):1556-64.

Gandy S, Heppner FL. Microglia as dynamic and essential components of the amyloid hypothesis. Neuron. 2013 May 22;78(4):575-7. doi: 10.1016/j.neuron.2013.05.007.

Gandy S, Simon AJ, Steele JW, Lublin AL, Lah JJ, Walker LC, Levey AI, Krafft GA, Levy E, Checler F, Glabe C, Bilker WB, Abel T, Schmeidler J, Ehrlich ME. Days to criterion as an indicator of toxicity associated with human Alzheimer amyloid-beta oligomers. Ann Neurol. 2010 Aug;68(2):220-30. doi: 10.1002/ana.22052.

Garai S, Mahato SB, Ohtani K, Yamasaki K. Dammarane triterpenoid saponins from Bacopa monnieri. Can J Chem 2009;87:1230–1234

Garcia Gomez LJ, Sanchez-Muniz FJ. Review: cardiovascular effect of garlic (Allium sativum). Arch Latinoam Nutr. 2000 Sep;50(3):219-29.

Garcia-Lazaro JA, Ahmed B, Schnupp JW. Tuning to natural stimulus dynamics in primary auditory cortex. Curr Biol. 2006 Feb 7;16(3):264-71.

Gardener S, Gu Y, Rainey-Smith SR, Keogh JB, Clifton PM, Mathieson SL, Taddei K, Mondal A, Ward VK, Scarmeas N, Barnes M, Ellis KA, Head R, Masters CL, Ames D, Macaulay SL, Rowe CC, Szoeke C, Martins RN; AIBL Research Group. Adherence to a Mediterranean diet and Alzheimer's disease risk in an Australian population. Transl Psychiatry. 2012 Oct 2;2:e164. doi: 10.1038/tp.2012.91.

Gardner CD, Fortmann SP, Krauss RM. Association of small low-density lipoprotein particles with the incidence of coronary artery disease in men and women. JAMA. 1996 Sep 18;276(11):875-81.

Gardner CD, Fortmann SP, Krauss RM. Association of small low-density lipoprotein particles with the incidence of coronary artery disease in men and women. JAMA. 1996 Sep 18;276(11):875-81.

Gau SS, Soong WT, Merikangas KR. Correlates of sleep-wake patterns among children and young adolescents in Taiwan. Sleep. 2004 May 1;27(3):512-9.

Gehr P, Im Hof V, Geiser M, Schurch S. The mucociliary system of the lung—role of surfactants. Schweiz Med Wochenschr. 2000 May 13;130(19):691-8.

Geidl W, Pfeifer K. Physical activity and exercise for rehabilitation of type 2 diabetes. Rehabilitation. 2011 Aug;50(4):255-65.

Geissler T, Brandt W, Porzel A, Schlenzig D, Kehlen A, Wessjohann L, Arnold N. Acetylcholinesterase inhibitors from the toadstool Cortinarius infractus. Bioorg Med Chem. 2010 Mar 15;18(6):2173-7. doi: 10.1016/j.bmc.2010.01.074.

George KS, Raghunath N, Bharath MM, Muralidhara. Prophylaxis with Bacopa monnieri attenuates Acrylamide induced neurotoxicity and oxidative damage via elevated antioxidant function. Cent Nerv Syst Agents Med Chem. 2012 Oct 17.

Gerber R. Vibrational Healing. Sante Fe: Bear, 1988.

Ghadioungui P. (transl.) The Ebers Papyrus. Academy of Scientific Research. Cairo, 1987.

Ghayur MN, Gilani AH. Ginger lowers blood pressure through blockade of voltage-dependent calcium Channels acting as a cardiotonic pump activator in mice, rabbit and dogs. J Cardiovasc Pharmacol. 2005 Jan;45(1):74-80.

Gibbons E. Stalking the Healthful Herbs. New York: David McKay, 1966.

Gibson RA. Docosahexaenoic acid (DHA) accumulation is regulated by the polyunsaturated fat content of the diet: Is it synthesis or is it incorporation? Asia Pac J Clin Nutr. 2004;13(Suppl):S78.

Gill HS, Rutherfurd KJ, Cross ML, Gopal PK. Enhancement of immunity in the elderly by dietary supplementation with the probiotic Bifidobacterium lactis HN019. Am J Clin Nutr. 2001 Dec;74(6):833-9.

Gill HS, Rutherfurd KJ, Cross ML. Dietary probiotic supplementation enhances natural killer cell activity in the elderly: an investigation of age-related immunological changes. J Clin Immunol. 2001 Jul;21(4):264-71.

Gionchetti P, Rizzello F, Helwig U, Venturi A, Lammers KM, Brigidi P, Vitali B, Poggioli G, Miglioli M, Campieri M. Prophylaxis of pouchitis onset with probiotic therapy: a double-blind, placebo-controlled trial. Gastroenterology. 2003 May;124:1202-9.

Gironés-Vilaplana A, Valentão P, Moreno DA, Ferreres F, Garcia-Viguera C, Andrade PB. New beverages of lemon juice enriched with the exotic berries Maqui, Açaí, and Blackthorn: bioactive components and in vitro biological properties. J Agric Food Chem. 2012 May 29.

Gisler GC, Diaz J, Duran N. Observations on Blood Plasma Chemiluminescence in Normal Subjects and Cancer Patients. Arq Biol Tecnol. 1983;26(3):345-352.

Gittleman AL. Guess What Came to Dinner. New York: Avery, 2001.

Glover J. The Philosophy of Mind. Oxford University Press, 1976.

Glück U, Gebbers J. Ingested probiotics reduce nasal colonization with pathogenic bacteria (Staphylococcus aureus, Streptococcus pneumoniae, and b-hemolytic streptococci). Am J. Clin. Nutr. 2003;77:517-520.

Goel V, Dolan RJ. The functional anatomy of humor: segregating cognitive and affective components. Nat Neurosci. 2001;4:237-8.

REFERENCES AND BIBLIOGRAPHY

Goff DC Jr, D'Agostino RB Jr, Haffner SM, Otvos JD. Insulin resistance and adiposity influence lipoprotein size and subclass concentrations. Results from the Insulin Resistance Atherosclerosis Study. Metabolism. 2005 Feb;54(2):264-70.

Gohil K, Packer L. Bioflavonoid-Rich Botanical Extracts Show Antioxidant and Gene Regulatory Activity. Ann N Y Acad Sci. 2002;957:70-7.

Goldin BR, Adlercreutz H, Dwyer JT, Swenson L, Warram JH, Gorbach SL. Effect of diet on excretion of estrogens in pre- and postmenopausal women. Cancer Res. 1981 Sep;41(9 Pt 2):3771-3.

Goldin BR, Adlercreutz H, Gorbach SL, Warram JH, Dwyer JT, Swenson L, Woods MN. Estrogen excretion patterns and plasma levels in vegetarian and omnivorous women. N Engl J Med. 1982 Dec 16;307(25):1542-7.

Golimstok A, Rojas JI, Romano M, Zurru MC, Doctorovich D, Cristiano E. Previous adult attention-deficit and hyperactivity disorder symptoms and risk of dementia with Lewy bodies: a case-control study. Eur J Neurol. 2011 Jan;18(1):78-84. doi: 10.1111/j.1468-1331.2010.03064.x.

Golub E. The Limits of Medicine. New York: Times Books, 1994.

Gomes A, Fernandes E, Lima JL. Fluorescence probes used for detection of reactive oxygen species. J Biochem Biophys Methods. 2005 Dec 31;65(2-3):45-80.

Gomez-Abellan P, Hernandez-Morante JJ, Lujan JA, Madrid JA, Garaulet M. Clock genes are implicated in the human metabolic syndrome. Int J Obes. 2007 Jul 24.

Gonzalez CA, Riboli E. Diet and cancer prevention: Contributions from the European Prospective Investigation into Cancer and Nutrition (EPIC) study. Eur J Cancer. 2010 Sep;46(14):2555-62.

González ME, Alarcón B, Carrasco L. Polysaccharides as antiviral agents: antiviral activity of carrageenan. Antimicrob Agents Chemother. 1987 Sep;31(9):1388-93.

Goodman RA, Lochner KA, Thambisetty M, Wingo T, Posner SF, Ling SM. Prevalence of dementia subtypes in U.S. Medicare fee-for-service beneficiaries, 2011-2013. Alzheimers Dement. 2016 May 9. pii: S1552-5260(16)30052-8. doi: 10.1016/j.jalz.2016.04.002.

Gould SJ. Eight Little Piggies. New York: Norton, 1993.

Gould SJ. Wonderful Life: The Burgess Shale and the nature of history. New York: Penguin Books, 1989.

Govindarajan VS, Sathyanarayana MN. Capsicum-production, technology, chemistry, and quality. Part V. Impact on physiology, pharmacology, nutrition, and metabolism; structure, pungency, pain, and desensitization sequences. Crit Rev Food Sci Nutr. 1991;29(6):435-74.

Grad B, Dean E. Independent confirmation of infrared healer effects. In: White R, Broughton R (Eds.): Research in parapsychology 1983. Metuchen, NJ: Scarecrow Press, 1984:81-83.

Grad, B. A telekinetic effect on plant growth: II. Experiments involving treatment of saline in stoppered bottles. Internl J Parapsychol. 1964;6:473-478, 484-488.

Grady D, Herrington D, Bittner V, Blumenthal R, Davidson M, Hlatky M, Hsia J, Hulley S, Herd A, Khan S, Newby LK, Waters D, Vittinghoff E, Wenger N. Cardiovascular disease outcomes during 6.8 years of hormone therapy: Heart and Estrogen/progestin Replacement Study follow-up (HERS II). JAMA. 2002 Jul 3;288(1):49-57.

Grant WB, Holick MF. Benefits and requirements of vitamin D for optimal health: a review. Altern Med Rev. 2005 Jun;10(2):94-111.

Grant WB. Hypothesis—ultraviolet-B irradiance and vitamin D reduce the risk of viral infections and thus their sequelae, including autoimmune diseases and some cancers. Photochem Photobiol. 2008 Mar-Apr;84(2):356-65. 2008 Jan 7.

Grant WB. Using Multicountry Ecological and Observational Studies to Determine Dietary Risk Factors for Alzheimer's Disease. J Am Coll Nutr. 2016 Jul;35(5):476-89. doi: 10.1080/07315724.2016.1161566.

Grasmuller S, Irnich D. Acupuncture in pain therapy. MMW Fortschr Med. 2007 Jun 21;149(25-26):37-9.

Grasso F, Grillo C, Musumeci F, Triglia A, Rodolico G, Cammisuli F, Rinzivillo C, Fragati G, Santuccio A, Rodolico M. Photon emission from normal and tumour human tissues. Experientia. 1992;48:10-13.

Grasso F, Musumeci F, Triglia A, Rodolico G, Cammisuli F, Rinzivillo C, Fragati G, Santuccio A, Rodolico M. In Stanley P, Kricka L (ed). Ultraweak Luminescence from Cancer Tissues. In Bioluminescence and Chemiluminescence - Current Status. New York: J Wiley & Sons. 1991:277-280.

Grasso F, Musumeci F, Triglia A. Yanbastiev M. Borisova, S. Self-irradiation effect on yeast cells. Photochemistry and Photobiology. 1991;54(1):147-149.

Gray H. Anatomy, Descriptive and Surgical. 15th Edition. New York: Random House, 1977.

Gray-Davison F. Ayurvedic Healing. New York: Keats, 2002.

Greger M. Bird Flu: Virus of Our Own Hatching. Mother Earth. 2007 Dec-Jan:103-109.

Griffith HW. Healing Herbs: The Essential Guide. Tucson: Fisher Books, 2000.

Grimm T, Chovanová Z, Muchová J, Sumegová K, Liptáková A, Duracková Z, Högger P. Inhibition of NF-kappaB activation and MMP-9 secretion by plasma of human volunteers after ingestion of maritime pine bark extract (Pycnogenol). J Inflamm (Lond). 2006 Jan 27;3:1.

Grimm T, Schäfer A, Högger P. Antioxidant activity and inhibition of matrix metalloproteinases by metabolites of maritime pine bark extract (pycnogenol). Free Radic Biol Med. 2004 Mar 15;36(6):811-22.

Grimm T, Skrabala R, Chovanová Z, Muchová J, Sumegová K, Liptáková A, Duracková Z, Högger P. Single and multiple dose pharmacokinetics of maritime pine bark extract (pycnogenol) after oral administration to healthy volunteers. BMC Clin Pharmacol. 2006 Aug 3;6:4.

Grimmer T, Tholen S, Yousefi BH, Alexopoulos P, Förschler A, Förstl H, et al. Progression of cerebral amyloid load is associated with the apolipoprotein E ε4 genotype in Alzheimer's disease. Biol Psychiatry 2010;68:879-84.

Grissom C. Magnetic field effects in biology: A survey of possible mechanisms with emphasis on radical pair recombination. Chem. Rev. 1995;95: 3-24.

263

Grobstein P. Directed movement in the frog: motor choice, spatial representation, free will? Neurobiology of motor programme selection. Pergamon Press, 1992.

Grodstein F, O'Brien J, Kang JH, Dushkes R, Cook NR, Okereke O, Manson JE, Glynn RJ, Buring JE, Gaziano M, Sesso HD. Long-term multivitamin supplementation and cognitive function in men: a randomized trial. Ann Intern Med. 2013 Dec 17;159(12):806-14.

Groneberg DA, Wahn U, Hamelmann E. Probiotic-induced suppression of allergic sensitization and airway inflammation is associated with an increase of T regulatory-dependent mechanisms in a murine model of asthma. Clin Exp Allergy. 2007 Apr;37(4):498-505.

Gronfier C, Wright KP Jr, Kronauer RE, Czeisler CA. Entrainment of the human circadian pacemaker to longer-than-24-h days. Proc Natl Acad Sci USA. 2007 May 22;104(21):9081-6.

Groppo FC, Ramacciato JC, Simões RP, Flório FM, Sartoratto A. Antimicrobial activity of garlic, tea tree oil, and chlorhexidine against oral microorganisms. Int Dent J. 2002 Dec;52(6):433-7.

Grosser BI, Monti-Bloch L, Jennings-White C, Berliner DL. Behavioral and electrophysiological effects of androstadienone, a human pheromone. Psychoneuro¬endo¬crin¬ology. 2000 Apr;25(3):289-99.

Grover A, Katiyar SP, Jeyakanthan J, Dubey VK, Sundar D. Blocking Protein kinase C signaling pathway: mechanistic insights into the anti-leishmanial activity of prospective herbal drugs from Withania somnifera. BMC Genomics. 2012;13 Suppl 7:S20.

Grover A, Shandilya A, Agrawal V, Bisaria VS, Sundar D. Computational evidence to inhibition of human acetyl cholinesterase by withanolide a for Alzheimer treatment. J Biomol Struct Dyn. 2012;29(4):651-62.

Grzanna R, Lindmark L, Frondoza CG. Ginger—an herbal medicinal product with broad anti-inflammatory actions. J Med Food. 2005 Summer;8(2):125-32.

Gu Y, Nieves JW, Stern Y, Luchsinger JA, Scarmeas N. Food combination and Alzheimer disease risk: a protective diet. Arch Neurol. 2010 Jun;67(6):699-706.

Gu Y, Scarmeas N. Dietary patterns in Alzheimer's disease and cognitive aging. Curr Alzheimer Res. 2011 Aug;8(5):510-9.

Guajardo-Flores D, Serna-Saldívar SO, Gutiérrez-Uribe JA. Evaluation of the antioxidant and antiproliferative activities of extracted saponins and flavonols from germinated black beans (Phaseolus vulgaris L.). Food Chem. 2013 Nov 15;141(2):1497-503.

Guallar-Castillón P, Rodríguez-Artalejo F, Tormo MJ, Sánchez MJ, Rodríguez L, Quirós JR, Navarro C, Molina E, Martínez C, Marín P, Lopez-Garcia E, Larrañaga N, Huerta JM, Dorronsoro M, Chirlaque MD, Buckland G, Barricarte A, Banegas JR, Arriola L, Ardanaz E, González CA, Moreno-Iribas C. Major dietary patterns and risk of coronary heart disease in middle-aged persons from a Mediterranean country: The EPIC-Spain cohort study. Nutr Metab Cardiovasc Dis. 2010 Aug 11.

Guan JZ, Guan WP, Maeda T, Makino N. Effect of vitamin E administration on the elevated oxygen stress and the telomeric and subtelomeric status in Alzheimer's disease. Gerontology. 2012;58(1):62-9. doi: 10.1159/000327821.

Guarino A, Canani RB, Spagnuolo MI, Albano F, Di Benedetto L. Oral bacterial therapy reduces the duration of symptoms and of viral excretion in children with mild diarrhea. J Pediatr Gastroenterol Nutr. 1997 Nov;25(5):516-9.

Guerin M, Huntley ME, Olaizola M. Haematococcus astaxanthin: applications for human health and nutrition. Trends Biotechnol. 2003 May;21(5):210-6.

Guetin S, Portet F, Picot MC, Defez C, Pose C, Blayac JP, Touchon J. [Impact of music therapy on anxiety and depression for patients with Alzheimer's disease and on the burden felt by the main caregiver (feasibility study)]. Encephale. 2009 Feb;35(1):57-65. doi: 10.1016/j.encep.2007.10.009.

Gundermann KJ, Müller J. Phytodolor—effects and efficacy of a herbal medicine. Wien Med Wochenschr. 2007;157(13-14):343-7.

Guo J. Chronic fatigue syndrome treated by acupuncture and moxibustion in combination with psychological approaches in 310 cases. J Tradit Chin Med. 2007 Jun;27(2):92-5.

Gupta A, Rash GS, Somia NN, Wachowiak MP, Jones J, Desoky A. The motion path of the digits. J Hand Surg. 1998; 23A:1038-1042.

Gupta P, Agarwal AV, Akhtar N, Sangwan RS, Singh SP, Trivedi PK. Cloning and characterization of 2-C-methyl-D-erythritol-4-phosphate pathway genes for isoprenoid biosynthesis from Indian ginseng, Withania somnifera. Protoplasma. 2013 Feb;250(1):285-95.

Gupta R, Singhal S, Goyle A, Sharma VN. Antioxidant and hypocholesterolaemic effects of Terminalia arjuna tree-bark powder: a randomised placebo-controlled trial. J Assoc Physicians India. 2001 Feb;49:231-5.

Gupta YK, Gupta M, Kohli K. Neuroprotective role of melatonin in oxidative stress vulnerable brain. Indian J Physiol Pharmacol. 2003 Oct;47(4):373-86.

Gutmanis J. Hawaiian Herbal Medicine. Waipahu, HI: Island Heritage, 2001.

Guzmán-Vélez E, Tranel D. Does bilingualism contribute to cognitive reserve? Cognitive and neural perspectives. Neuropsychology. 2015 Jan;29(1):139-50. doi: 10.1037/neu0000105.

Haas M, Cooperstein R, Peterson D. Disentangling manual muscle testing and Applied Kinesiology: critique and reinterpretation of a literature review. Chiropr Osteopat. 2007 Aug 23;15:11.

Hadji L, Arnoux B, Benveniste J. Effect of dilute histamine on coronary flow of guinea-pig isolated heart. Inhibition by a magnetic field. FASEB Jnl. 1991;5: A1583.

Hager K, Kenklies M, McAfoose J, Engel J, Münch G. Alpha-lipoic acid as a new treatment option for Alzheimer's disease--a 48 months follow-up analysis. J Neural Transm Suppl. 2007;(72):189-93.

REFERENCES AND BIBLIOGRAPHY

Hagins WA, Penn RD, Yoshikami S. Dark current and photocurrent in retinal rods. Biophys J. 1970 May;10(5):380-412.

Hagins WA, Robinson WE, Yoshikami S. Ionic aspects of excitation in rod outer segments. Ciba Found Symp. 1975;(31):169-89.

Hagins WA, Yoshikami S. Ionic mechanisms in excitation of photoreceptors. Ann N Y Acad Sci. 1975 Dec 30;264:314-25.

Hagins WA, Yoshikami S. Proceedings: A role for Ca2+ in excitation of retinal rods and cones. Exp Eye Res. 1974 Mar;18(3):299-305.

Hagins WA. The visual process: Excitatory mechanisms in the primary receptor cells. Annu Rev Biophys Bioeng. 1972;1:131-58.

Hahm ER, Singh SV. Withaferin A-induced apoptosis in human breast cancer cells is associated with suppression of inhibitor of apoptosis family protein expression. Cancer Lett. 2012 Aug 27.

Haines JL, Ter-Minassian M, Bazyk A, Gusella JF, Kim DJ, Terwedow H, Pericak-Vance MA, Rimmler JB, Haynes CS, Roses AD, Lee A, Shaner B, Menold M, Seboun E, Fitoussi RP, Gartioux C, Reyes C, Ribierre F, Gyapay G, Weissenbach J, Hauser SL, Goodkin DE, Lincoln R, Usuku K, Oksenberg JR, et al. A complete genomic screen for multiple sclerosis underscores a role for the major histocompatability complex. The Multiple Sclerosis Genetics Group. Nat Genet. 1996 Aug;13(4):469-71..

Halliday GM, Agar NS, Barnetson RS, Ananthaswamy HN, Jones AM. UV-A fingerprint mutations in human skin cancer. Photochem Photobiol. 2005 Jan-Feb;81(1):3-8.

Hallmann E, Rembialkowska E. Characterisation of antioxidant compounds in sweet bell pepper (Capsicum annuum L.) under organic and conventional growing systems. J Sci Food Agric. 2012 Feb 24.

Hallmann E. The influence of organic and conventional cultivation systems on the nutritional value and content of bioactive compounds in selected tomato types. J Sci Food Agric. 2012 Feb 20.

Halpern GM, Miller AH. Medicinal Mushrooms: Ancient Remedies for Modern Ailments. New York: M. Evans, 2002.

Halpern S. Tuning the Human Instrument. Palo Alto, CA: Spectrum Research Institute, 1978.

Hamasaki Y, Kobayashi I, Hayasaki R, Zaitu M, Muro E, Yamamoto S, Ichimaru T, Miyazaki S. The Chinese herbal medicine, shinpi-to, inhibits IgE-mediated leukotriene synthesis in rat basophilic leukemia-2H3 cells. J Ethnopharmacol. 1997 Apr;56(2):123-31.

Hamel P. Through Music to the Self: How to Appreciate and Experience Music. Boulder: Shambala, 1979.

Hameroff SR, Penrose R. Conscious events as orchestrated spacetime selections. J Consc Studies. 1996;3(1):36-53.

Hameroff SR, Penrose R. Orchestrated reduction of quantum coherence in brain microtubules: A model for consciousness. In: Hameroff SN, Kaszniak A, Scott AC (eds.): Toward a Science of Consciousness - The First Tucson Discussions and Debates. Cambridge: MIT Press, 1996.

Hameroff SR, Smith, S, Watt.R. Nonlinear electrodynamics in cytoskeletal protein lattices. In: Adey W, Lawrence A (eds.), Nonlinear Electrodynamics in Biological Systems. 1984:567-583.

Hameroff SR, Watt, R. Information processing in microtubules. J Theor Biology. 1982;98:549-561.

Hameroff SR. Coherence in the cytoskeleton: Implications for biological information processing. In: Fröhlich H. (ed.): Biological Coherence and Response to External Stimuli. Springer, Berlin-New York 1988, pp.242-264.

Hameroff SR. Light is heavy: Wave mechanics in proteins - A microtubule hologram model of consciousness. Proceedings 2nd. International Congress on Psychotronic Research. Monte Carlo, 1975:168-169.

Hameroff SR. Ultimate Biocomputing - Biomolecular Consciousness and Nanotechnology. Amsterdam: Elsevier, 1987.

Hameroff, SR. Ch'i: A neural hologram? Microtubules, bioholography and acupuncture. Am J Chin Med. 1974;2(2):163-170.

Hamilton A. Brain Training Reduces Dementia Risk Across 10 Years. American Psychological Association. August 4, 2016.

Hamilton-Miller JM. Probiotics and prebiotics in the elderly. London: Department of Medical Microbiology, Royal Free and University College Medical School, 2004.

Hammond BG, Mayhew DA, Kier LD, Mast RW, Sander WJ. Safety assessment of DHA-rich microalgae from Schizochytrium sp. Regul Toxicol Pharmacol. 2002 Apr;35(2 Pt 1):255-65.

Han SN, Leka LS, Lichtenstein AH, Ausman LM, Meydani SN. Effect of a therapeutic lifestyle change diet on immune functions of moderately hypercholesterolemic humans. J Lipid Res. 2003 Dec;44(12):2304-10.

Handing EP, Andel R, Kadlecova P, Gatz M, Pedersen NL. Midlife Alcohol Consumption and Risk of Dementia Over 43 Years of Follow-Up: A Population-Based Study From the Swedish Twin Registry. J Gerontol A Biol Sci Med Sci. 2015 Oct;70(10):1248-54. doi: 10.1093/gerona/glv038.

Handwerk B. Lobsters Navigate by Magnetism, Study Says. Natl Geogr News. 2003 Jan 6.

Hannoun AB, Nassar AH, Usta IM, Zreik TG, Abu Musa AA. Effect of war on the menstrual cycle. Obstet Gynecol. 2007 Apr;109(4):929-32.

Hans J. The Structure and Dynamics of Waves and Vibrations. New York:.Schocken and Co., 1975.

Hantusch B, Knittelfelder R, Wallmann J, Krieger S, Szalai K, Untersmayr E, Vogel M, Stadler BM, Scheiner O, Boltz-Nitulescu G, Jensen-Jarolim E. Internal images: human anti-idiotypic Fab antibodies mimic the IgE epitopes of grass pollen allergen Phl p 5a. Mol Immunol. 2006 Jul;43(14):2180-7.

Haq IU, Mirza B, Kondratyuk TP, Park EJ, Burns BE, Marler LE, Pezzuto JM. Preliminary evaluation for cancer chemopreventive and cytotoxic potential of naturally growing ethnobotanically selected plants of Pakistan. Pharm Biol. 2012 Nov 8.

265

Hardin P. Transcription regulation within the circadian clock: the E-box and beyond. J Biol Rhythms. 2004 Oct;19(5):348-60.

Hardman RJ, Kennedy G, Macpherson H, Scholey AB, Pipingas A. Adherence to a Mediterranean-Style Diet and Effects on Cognition in Adults: A Qualitative Evaluation and Systematic Review of Longitudinal and Prospective Trials. Front Nutr. 2016 Jul 22;3:22. doi: 10.3389/fnut.2016.00022.

Hardy J, Selkoe DJ. The amyloid hypothesis of Alzheimer's disease: progress and problems on the road to therapeutics. Science 2002;297:353-6.

Harlow HF, Dodsworth RO, Harlow MK. Total social isolation in monkeys. Proc Natl Acad Sci U S A. 1965.

Harlow HF. Development of affection in primates. In Bliss E (ed): Roots of Behavior. New York: Harper, 1962: 157-166.

Harlow HF. Early social deprivation and later behavior in the monkey. In: Abrams A, Gurner H, Tomal J (eds): Unfinished tasks in the behavioral sciences. Baltimore: Williams & Wilkins. 1964: 154-173.

Hauschild M, Theintz G. Severe chronic anemia and endocrine disorders in children. Rev Med Suisse. 2007 Apr 18;3(107):988-91.

Haye-Legrand I, Norel X, Labat C, Benveniste J, Brink C. Antigenic contraction of guinea pig tracheal preparations passively sensitized with monoclonal IgE: pharmacological modulation. Int Arch Allergy Appl Immunol. 1988;87(4):342-8.

Heart Disease. New York State Department of Health. Oct. 2004.

Heath M, Weiler J, Gregory MA, Gill DP, Petrella RJ. A Six-Month Cognitive-Motor and Aerobic Exercise Program Improves Executive Function in Persons with an Objective Cognitive Impairment: A Pilot Investigation Using the Antisaccade Task. J Alzheimers Dis. 2016 Aug 10.

Heckman JD, Ingram AJ, Loyd RD, Luck JV Jr, Mayer PW. Nonunion treatment with pulsed electromagnetic fields. Clin Orthop Relat Res. 1981 Nov-Dec;(161):58-66.

Hectorne KJ, Fransway AF. Diazolidinyl urea: incidence of sensitivity, patterns of cross-reactivity and clinical relevance. Contact Dermatitis. 1994 Jan;30(1):16-9.

Heffernan M, Mather KA, Xu J, Assareh AA, Kochan NA, Reppermund S, Draper B, Trollor JN, Sachdev P, Brodaty H. Alcohol Consumption and Incident Dementia: Evidence from the Sydney Memory and Ageing Study. J Alzheimers Dis. 2016 Mar 29;52(2):529-38. doi: 10.3233/JAD-150537.

Heinrich H. Assessment of non-sinusoidal, pulsed, or intermittent exposure to low frequency electric and magnetic fields. Health Phys. 2007 Jun;92(6):541-6.

Helms JA, Farnham PJ, Segal E, Chang HY. Functional demarcation of active and silent chromatin domains in human HOX loci by noncoding RNAs. Cell. 2007 Jun 29;129(7):1311-23.

Hendel B, Ferreira P. Water & Salt: The Essence of Life. Gaithersburg: Natural Resources, 2003.

Henderson ST, Vogel JL, Barr LJ, Garvin F, Jones JJ, Costantini LC. Study of the ketogenic agent AC-1202 in mild to moderate Alzheimer's disease: a randomized, double-blind, placebo-controlled, multicenter trial. Nutr Metab (Lond). 2009 Aug 10;6:31.

Heo JH, Lee ST, Chu K, Oh MJ, Park HJ, Shim JY, Kim M. An open-label trial of Korean red ginseng as an adjuvant treatment for cognitive impairment in patients with Alzheimer's disease. Eur J Neurol. 2008 Aug;15(8):865-8. doi: 10.1111/j.1468-1331.2008.02157.x.

Heo JH, Lee ST, Chu K, Oh MJ, Park HJ, Shim JY, Kim M. Heat-processed ginseng enhances the cognitive function in patients with moderately severe Alzheimer's disease. Nutr Neurosci. 2012 Nov;15(6):278-82. doi: 10.1179/1476830512Y.0000000027.

Herbert V. Vitamin B12: Plant sources, requirements, and assay. Am J Clin Nutr. 1988;48:852-858.

Hernandez Avila M, Walker AM, Jick H. Use of replacement estrogens and the risk of myocardial infarction. Epidemiology. 1990 Mar;1(2):128-33.

Heusinkveld HJ, Wahle T, Campbell A, Westerink RH, Tran L, Johnston H, Stone V, Cassee FR, Schins RP. Neurodegenerative and neurological disorders by small inhaled particles. Neurotoxicology. 2016 Jul 19;56:94-106. doi: 10.1016/j.neuro.2016.07.007.

Heyers D, Manns M, Luksch H, Güntürkün O, Mouritsen H. A Visual Pathway Links Brain Structures Active during Magnetic Compass Orientation in Migratory Birds. PLoS One. 2007;2(9): e937. 2007.

Hillecke T, Nickel A, Bolay HV. Scientific perspectives on music therapy. Ann N Y Acad Sci. 2005 Dec;1060:271-82.

Hirsch S, Sanchez H, Albala C, de la Maza MP, Barrera G, Leiva L, Bunout D. Colon cancer in Chile before and after the start of the flour fortification program with folic acid. Eur J Gastroenterol Hepatol. 2009 Apr;21(4):436-9.

Ho MW. Assessing Food Quality by Its After-Glow. Inst. Sci in Society. Press release. 2004 May 1.

Ho SE, Ide N, Lau BH. S-allyl cysteine reduces oxidant load in cells involved in the atherogenic process. Phytomedicine. 2001 Jan;8(1):39-46.

Hobbs C. Medicinal Mushrooms. Summertown, TN: Botanica Press, 2003.

Hobbs C. Stress & Natural Healing. Loveland, CO: Interweave Press, 1997.

Hobbs DA, Kaffa N, George TW, Methven L, Lovegrove JA. Blood pressure-lowering effects of beetroot juice and novel beetroot-enriched bread products in normotensive male subjects. Br J Nutr. 2012 Dec 14;108(11):2066-74.

Hoffmann D. Holistic Herbal. London: Thorsons, 1983-2002.

Holick MF. Vitamin D status: measurement, interpretation, and clinical application. Ann Epidemiol. 2009 Feb;19(2):73-8.

REFERENCES AND BIBLIOGRAPHY

Hollfoth K. Effect of color therapy on health and wellbeing: colors are more than just physics. Pflege Z. 2000 Feb;53(2):111-2.

Hollwich F, Dieckhues B. Effect of light on the eye on metabolism and hormones. Klinische Monatsblatter fur Augenheilkunde. 1989;195(5):284-90.

Hollwich F. Hartmann C. Influence of light through the eyes on metabolism and hormones. Ophtalmologie. 1990;4(4):385-9.

Hollwich F. The influence of ocular light perception on metabolism in man and in animal. New York: Springer-Verlag, 1979.

Holmes HC, Burns SP, Michelakakis H, Kordoni V, Bain MD, Chalmers RA, Rafter JE, Iles RA. Choline and L-carnitine as precursors of trimethylamine. Biochem Soc Trans. 1997 Feb;25(1):96S.

Holmquist G. Susumo Ohno left us January 13, 2000, at the age of 71. Cytogenet and Cell Genet. 2000;88:171-172.

Holtrop G, Johnstone AM, Fyfe C, Gratz SW. Diet composition is associated with endogenous formation of N-nitroso compounds in obese men. J Nutr. 2012 Sep;142(9):1652-8.

Hönscheid A, Rink L, Haase H. T-lymphocytes: a target for stimulatory and inhibitory effects of zinc ions. Endocr Metab Immune Disord Drug Targets. 2009 Jun;9(2):132-44.

Hope M. The Psychology of Healing. Longmead UK: Element Books, 1989.

Hoskin M.(ed.). The Cambridge Illustrated History of Astronomy. Cambridge: Cambridge Press, 1997.

Hosny Mansour H, Farouk Hafez H. Protective effect of Withania somnifera against radiation-induced hepatotoxicity in rats. Ecotoxicol Environ Saf. 2012 Jun;80:14-9.

Hosseini S, Pishnamazi S, Sadrzadeh SM, Farid F, Farid R, Watson RR. Pycnogenol((R)) in the Management of Asthma. J Med Food. 2001 Winter;4(4):201-209.

Hou DR, Wang Y, Xue L, Tian Y, Chen K, Song Z, Yang QD. Effect of polygonum multiflorum on the fluidity of the mitochondria membrane and activity of COX in the hippocampus of rats with Abeta 1-40-induced Alzheimer's disease. Zhong Nan Da Xue Xue Bao Yi Xue Ban. 2008 Nov;33(11):987-92.

Hou Q, He WJ, Chen L, Hao HJ, Liu JJ, Dong L, Tong C, Li MR, Zhou ZZ, Han WD, Fu XB. Effects of the Four-Herb Compound ANBP on Wound Healing Promotion in Diabetic Mice. Int J Low Extrem Wounds. 2015 Mar 20. pii: 1534734615575244

Hou Q, He WJ, Hao HJ, Han QW, Chen L, Dong L, Liu JJ, Li X, Zhang YJ, Ma YZ, Han WD, Fu XB. The four-herb Chinese medicine ANBP enhances wound healing and inhibits scar formation via bidirectional regulation of transformation growth factor pathway. PLoS One. 2014 Dec 9;9(12):e112274. doi: 10.1371/journal.pone.0112274.

Howard AL, Robinson M, Smith GJ, Ambrosini GL, Piek JP, Oddy WH. AD/HD is associated with a "Western" dietary pattern in adolescents. J Atten Disord. 2011 Jul;15(5):403-11.

Hoyle F. Evolution from Space. Londong: JM Dent, 1981.

Hu C, Kitts DD. Antioxidant, prooxidant, and cytotoxic activities of solvent-fractionated dandelion (Taraxacum officinale) flower extracts in vitro. J Agric Food Chem. 2003 Jan 1;51(1):301-10.

Hu C, Kitts DD. Dandelion (Taraxacum officinale) flower extract suppresses both reactive oxygen species and nitric oxide and prevents lipid oxidation in vitro. Phytomedicine. 2005 Aug;12(8):588-97.

Hu C, Kitts DD. Luteolin and luteolin-7-O-glucoside from dandelion flower suppress iNOS and COX-2 in RAW264.7 cells. Mol Cell Biochem. 2004 Oct;265(1-2):107-13.

Hu FB, Willett WC. Optimal diets for prevention of coronary heart disease. JAMA. 2002 Nov 27;288(20):2569-78.

Hu X, Wang T, Jin F. Alzheimer's disease and gut microbiota. Sci China Life Sci. 2016 Aug 26.

Hu X, Wu B, Wang P. Displaying of meridian courses travelling over human body surface under natural conditions. Zhen Ci Yan Jiu. 1993;18(2):83-9.

Huang D, Ou B, Prior RL. The chemistry behind antioxidant capacity assays. J Agric Food Chem. 2005 Mar 23;53(6):1841-56.

Huang M, Wang W, Wei S. Investigation on medicinal plant resources of Glycyrrhiza uralensis in China and chemical assessment of its underground part. Zhongguo Zhong Yao Za Zhi. 2010 Apr;35(8):947-52.

Huffman C. Archytas of Tarentum: Pythagorean, philosopher and Mathematician King. Cambridge: Cambridge University Press, 2005.

Hull D. Science as a Process: An evolutionary account of the social and conceptual development of science. Chicago: Univ Chicago Press, 1988.

Human Microbiome Project Consortium. A framework for human microbiome research. Nature. 2012 Jun 13;486(7402):215-21. doi: 10.1038/nature11209.

Hunt V. Infinite Mind: Science of the Human Vibrations of Consciousness. Malibu: Malibu Publ. 2000.

Huntley JD, Gould RL, Liu K, Smith M, Howard RJ. Do cognitive interventions improve general cognition in dementia? A meta-analysis and meta-regression. BMJ Open. 2015 Apr 2;5(4):e005247. doi: 10.1136/bmjopen-2014-005247.

Hur W, Kim SW, Lee YK, Choi JE, Hong SW, Song MJ, Bae SH, Park T, Um SJ, Yoon SK. Oleuropein reduces free fatty acid-induced lipogenesis via lowered extracellular signal-regulated kinase activation in hepatocytes. Nutr Res. 2012 Oct;32(10):778-86.

Hur YM, Rushton JP. Genetic and environmental contributions to prosocial behaviour in 2- to 9-year-old South Korean twins. Biol Lett. 2007 Dec 22;3(6):664-6.

Husby S. Dietary antigens: uptake and humoral immunity in man. APMIS Suppl. 1988;1:1-40.

Hye-Seung J, Sung-Eun K, Mi-Kyung S. 2002. Protective Effect of Soybean Saponins and Major Antioxidants Against Aflatoxin B1-Induced Mutagenicity and DNA-Adduct Formation. Journal of Medicinal Food. Dec, Vol. 5, No. 4 : 235 -240.

Ide N, Lau BH. Garlic compounds minimize intracellular oxidative stress and inhibit nuclear factor-kappa b activation. J Nutr. 2001 Mar;131(3s):1020S-6S.

Igarashi T, Izumi H, Uchiumi T, Nishio K, Arao T, Tanabe M, Uramoto H, Sugio K, Yasumoto K, Sasaguri Y, Wang KY, Otsuji Y, Kohno K. Clock and ATF4 transcription system regulates drug resistance in human cancer cell lines. Oncogene. 2007 Jul 19;26(33):4749-60.

Ihsan-Ul-Haq, Youn UJ, Chai X, Park EJ, Kondratyuk TP, Simmons CJ, Borris RP, Mirza B, Pezzuto JM, Chang LC. Biologically Active Withanolides from Withania coagulans. J Nat Prod. 2013 Jan 25;76(1):22-8.

Iizuka C. at al. Extract of Basidomycetes especially Lentinus edodes, for treatmet of human immunodeficiency virus (HIV). Patent Application by Shokin Kogyo Co. 1990: EP 370,673.

Ikeda Y, Tsuji S, Satoh A, Ishikura M, Shirasawa T, Shimizu T. Protective effects of astaxanthin on 6-hydroxydopamine-induced apoptosis in human neuroblastoma SH-SY5Y cells. J Neurochem. 2008 Dec;107(6):1730-40.

Ikonomov OC, Stoynev AG. Gene expression in suprachiasmatic nucleus and circadian rhythms. Neurosci Biobehav Rev. 1994 Fall;18(3):305-12.

Ikonomovic MD, Klunk WE, Abrahamson EE, Mathis CA, Price JC, Tsopelas ND, et al. Post-mortem correlates of in vivo PiB–PET amyloid imaging in a typical case of Alzheimer's disease. Brain 2008;131:1630-45.

Im KH, Nguyen TK, Choi J, Lee TS. In Vitro Antioxidant, Anti-Diabetes, Anti-Dementia, and Inflammation Inhibitory Effect of Trametes pubescens Fruiting Body Extracts. Molecules. 2016 May 16;21(5). pii: E639. doi: 10.3390/molecules21050639.

Inaba H. INABA Biophoton. Exploratory Research for Advanced Technology. Japan Science and Technology Agency. 1991. http://www.jst.go.jp/erato/project/isf_P/isf_P.html. Acc. 2006 Nov.

Ingelsson M, Fukumoto H, Newell KL, Growdon JH, Hedley-Whyte ET, Frosch MP, et al. Early Abeta accumulation and progressive synaptic loss, gliosis, and tangle formation in AD brain. Neurology. 2004 Mar 23;62(6):925-31.

Innis SM, Hansen JW. Plasma fatty acid responses, metabolic effects, and safety of microalgal and fungal oils rich in arachidonic and docosahexaenoic acids in healthy adults. Am J Clin Nutr. 1996 Aug;64(2):159-67.

International HapMap Consortium. The international HapMap project. Nature. 2003;426:789-794.

Iso-Markku P, Waller K, Vuoksimaa E, Heikkilä K, Rinne J, Kaprio J, Kujala UM. Midlife Physical Activity and Cognition Later in Life: A Prospective Twin Study. J Alzheimers Dis. 2016 Sep 2.

Itokawa Y. Magnesium intake and cardiovascular disease. Clin Calcium. 2005;15(2):154-9.

Ivanchak N, Fletcher K, Jicha GA. Attention-Deficit/Hyperactivity Disorder in Older Adults: Prevalence and Possible Connections to Mild Cognitive Impairment. Current psychiatry reports. 2012;14(5):552-560. doi:10.1007/s11920-012-0305-8.

Ivanovic-Zuvic F, de la Vega R, Ivanovic-Zuvic N, Renteria P. Affective disorders and solar activity. Actas Esp Psiquiatr. 2005 Jan-Feb;33(1):7-12.

Iwase T, Kajimura N, Uchiyama M, Ebisawa T, Yoshimura K, Kamei Y, Shibui K, Kim K, Kudo Y, Katoh M, Watanabe T, Nakajima T, Ozeki Y, Sugishita M, Hori T, Ikeda M, Toyoshima R, Inoue Y, Yamada N, Mishima K, Nomura M, Ozaki N, Okawa M, Takahashi K, Yamauchi T. Mutation screening of the human Clock gene in circadian rhythm sleep disorders. Psychiatry Res. 2002 Mar 15;109(2):121-8.

Jack CR Jr., Wiste HJ, Vemuri P, Weigand SD, Senjem ML, Zeng G, et al. Brain beta-amyloid measures and magnetic resonance imaging atrophy both predict time-to-progression from mild cognitive impairment

Jack CR, Knopman DS, Jagust WJ, Shaw LM, Aisen PS, Weiner MW, et al. Hypothetical model of dynamic biomarkers of the Alzheimer's pathological cascade. Lancet Neurol 2010a;9:119-28.

Jack CR, Lowe VJ, Weigand SD, Wiste HJ, Senjem ML, Knopman DS, et al. Serial PIB and MRI in normal, mild cognitive impairment and Alzheimer's disease: implications for sequence of pathological events in Alzheimer's disease. Brain 2009;132:1355-65.

Jadhav SK, Patel KA, Dholakia BB, Khan BM. Structural characterization of a flavonoid glycosyltransferase from Withania somnifera. Bioinformation. 2012;8(19):943-9. : 10.6026/97320630008943.

Jadoon S, Karim S, Asad MH, Akram MR, Kalsoom Khan A, Malik A, Chen C, Murtaza G. Anti-Aging Potential of Phytoextract Loaded-Pharmaceutical Creams for Human Skin Cell Longevity. Oxid Med Cell Longev. 2015;2015:709628. doi: 10.1155/2015/709628.

Jagetia GC, Aggarwal BB. "Spicing up" of the immune system by curcumin. J Clin Immunol. 2007 Jan;27(1):19-35.

Jagust WJ, Bandy D, Chen K, Foster NL, Landau SM, Mathis CA, Price JC, Reiman EM, Skovronsky D, Koeppe RA; Alzheimer's Disease Neuroimaging Initiative. The Alzheimer's Disease Neuroimaging Initiative positron emission tomography core. Alzheimers Dement. 2010 May;6(3):221-9. doi: 10.1016/j.jalz.2010.03.003.

Jahn R, Dunne, B. Margins of Reality: the Role of Consciousness in the Physical World. New York: Harcourt Brace Jovanovich, 1987.

Janelle KC, Barr SI. Nutrient intakes and eating behavior scores of vegetarian and nonvegetarian women. J Am Diet Assoc. 1995 Feb;95(2):180-6, 189, quiz 187-8.

Janelle KC, Barr SI. Nutrient intakes and eating behavior scores of vegetarian and nonvegetarian women. J Am Diet Assoc. 1995 Feb;95(2):180-6, 189, quiz 187-8.

Janson C, Anto J, Burney P, Chinn S, de Marco R, Heinrich J, Jarvis D, Kuenzli N, Leynaert B, Luczynska C, Neukirch F, Svanes C, Sunyer J, Wjst M; European Community Respiratory Health Survey II. The European Community Respiratory Health Survey: what are the main results so far? European Community Respiratory Health Survey II. Eur Respir J. 2001 Sep;18(3):598-611.

Janssens D, Delaive E, Houbion A, Eliaers F, Remacle J, Michiels C. Effect of venotropic drugs on the respiratory activity of isolated mitochondria and in endothelial cells. Br J Pharmacol. 2000 Aug;130(7):1513-24.

REFERENCES AND BIBLIOGRAPHY

Jarvis DC. Folk Medicine. Greenwich, CN: Fawcett, 1958.

Jauhiainen T, Vapaatalo H, Poussa T, Kyrönpalo S, Rasmussen M, Korpela R. Lactobacillus helveticus fermented milk lowers blood pressure in hypertensive subjects in 24-h ambulatory blood pressure measurement. Am J Hypertens. 2005 Dec;18(12 Pt 1):1600-5.

Jayaprakasam B, Doddaga S, Wang R, Holmes D, Goldfarb J, Li XM. Licorice flavonoids inhibit eotaxin-1 secretion by human fetal lung fibroblasts in vitro. J Agric Food Chem. 2009 Feb 11;57(3):820-5.

Jefferson AL, Gibbons LE, Rentz DM, Carvalho JO, Manly J, Bennett DA, Jones RN. A life course model of cognitive activities, socioeconomic status, education, reading ability, and cognition. J Am Geriatr Soc. 2011 Aug;59(8):1403-11. doi: 10.1111/j.1532-5415.2011.03499.x.

Jenkins DJ, Jones PJ, Lamarche B, Kendall CW, Faulkner D, Cermakova L, Gigleux I, Ramprasath V, de Souza R, Ireland C, Patel D, Srichaikul K, Abdulnour S, Bashyam B, Collier C, Hoshizaki S, Josse RG, Leiter LA, Connelly PW, Frohlich J. Effect of a dietary portfolio of cholesterol-lowering foods given at 2 levels of intensity of dietary advice on serum lipids in hyperlipidemia: a randomized controlled trial. JAMA. 2011 Aug 24;306(8):831-9.

Jensen B. Foods that Heal. Garden City Park, NY: Avery Publ, 1988, 1993.

Jensen B. Nature Has a Remedy. Los Angeles: Keats, 2001.

Jensen HK. The molecular genetic basis and diagnosis of familial hypercholesterolemia in Denmark. Dan Med Bull. 2002 Nov;49(4):318-45.

Jensen R, Lammi-Keefe C, Henderson R, Bush V, Ferris A.M. Effect of dietary intake of n-6 and n-3 fatty acids on the fatty acid composition of human milk in North America. J Pediatr. 1992;120:S87-92.

Jeong JH, Jeong HR, Jo YN, Kim HJ, Shin JH, Heo HJ. Ameliorating effects of aged garlic extracts against Aβ-induced neurotoxicity and cognitive impairment. BMC Complement Altern Med. 2013 Oct 18;13:268. doi: 10.1186/1472-6882-13-268.

Jeong JJ, Woo JY, Kim KA, Han MJ, Kim DH. Lactobacillus pentosus var. plantarum C29 ameliorates age-dependent memory impairment in Fischer 344 rats. Lett Appl Microbiol. 2015 Apr;60(4):307-14. doi: 10.1111/lam.12393.

Jernerén F, Elshorbagy AK, Oulhaj A, Smith SM, Refsum H, Smith AD. Brain atrophy in cognitively impaired elderly: the importance of long-chain ω-3 fatty acids and B vitamin status in a randomized controlled trial. Am J Clin Nutr. 2015 Jul;102(1):215-21. doi: 10.3945/ajcn.114.103283.

Jhon MS. The Water Puzzle and the Hexagonal Key. Uplifting, 2004.

Ji Y, Liu YB, Zheng LY, Zhang XQ. Survey of studies on tissue structures and biological characteristics of channel lines. Zhongguo Zhen Jiu. 2007 Jun;27(6):427-32.

Jiang S, Wang S, Sun Y, Zhang Q. Medicinal properties of Hericium erinaceus and its potential to formulate novel mushroom-based pharmaceuticals. Appl Microbiol Biotechnol. 2014 Sep;98(18):7661-70. doi: 10.1007/s00253-014-5955-5.

Jilani K, Lupescu A, Zbidah M, Shaik N, Lang F. Withaferin A-stimulated Ca2+ entry, ceramide formation and suicidal death of erythrocytes. Toxicol In Vitro. 2013 Feb;27(1):52-8.

Jimbo D, Kimura Y, Taniguchi M, Inoue M, Urakami K. Effect of aromatherapy on patients with Alzheimer's disease. Psychogeriatrics. 2009 Dec;9(4):173-9. doi: 10.1111/j.1479-8301.2009.00299.x.

Jiménez-Jiménez FJ, Molina JA, de Bustos F, Ortí-Pareja M, Benito-León J, Tallón-Barranco A, Gasalla T, Porta J, Arenas J. Serum levels of beta-carotene, alpha-carotene and vitamin A in patients with Alzheimer's disease. Eur J Neurol. 1999 Jul;6(4):495-7.

Jin CN, Zhang TS, Ji LX, Tian YF. Survey of studies on mechanisms of acupuncture and moxibustion in decreasing blood pressure. Zhongguo Zhen Jiu. 2007 Jun;27(6):467-70.

Johansson GK, Ottova L, Gustafsson JA. Shift from a mixed diet to a lactovegetarian diet: influence on some cancer-associated intestinal bacterial enzyme activities. Nutr Cancer. 1990;14(3-4):239-46.

Johansson GK, Ottova L, Gustafsson JA. Shift from a mixed diet to a lactovegetarian diet: influence on some cancer-associated intestinal bacterial enzyme activities. Nutr Cancer. 1990;14(3-4):239-46. PubMed PMID: 2128119.

Johari H. Ayurvedic Massage: Traditional Indian Techniques for Balancing Body and Mind. Rochester, VT: Healing Arts, 1996.

Johari H. Chakras. Rochester, VT: Destiny, 1987.

Johnson KC, Margolis KL, Espeland MA, Colenda CC, Fillit H, Manson JE, Masaki KH, Mouton CP, Prineas R, Robinson JG, Wassertheil-Smoller S; Women's Health Initiative Memory Study and Women's Health Initiative Investigators. A prospective study of the effect of hypertension and baseline blood pressure on cognitive decline and dementia in postmenopausal women: the Women's Health Initiative Memory Study. J Am Geriatr Soc. 2008 Aug;56(8):1449-58. doi: 10.1111/j.1532-5415.2008.01806.x.

Johnson LM. Gitksan medicinal plants—cultural choice and efficacy. J Ethnobiol Ethnomed. 2006 Jun 21;2:29.

Johnston A. A spatial property of the retino-cortical mapping. Spatial Vision. 1986;1(4):319-331.

Johnston RE. Pheromones, the vomeronasal system, and communication. From hormonal responses to individual recognition. Ann N Y Acad Sci. 1998 Nov 30;855:333-48.

Jolliffe N., Archer M. Statistical associations between international coronary heart disease death rates and certain environmental factors. J. Chronic Dis. 1959; 9;636-652,

Jolly CJ. The seed eaters: A new model of hominid differentiation based on a baboon analogy. Man. 1970;5:5—26.

Jones K, Harrison Y. Frontal lobe function, sleep loss and fragmented sleep. Sleep Med Rev. 2001 Dec;5(6):463-475.

Jovanovic-Ignjatic Z, Rakovic D. A review of current research in microwave resonance therapy: novel opportunities in medical treatment. Acupunct Electrother Res. 1999; 24:105-125.

Jovanovic-Ignjatic Z. Microwave Resonant Therapy: Novel Opportunities in Medical Treatment. Acup. & Electro-Therap. Res., The Int. J. 1999;24(2):105-125.

Juergens UR, Dethlefsen U, Steinkamp G, Gillissen A, Repges R, Vetter H. Anti-inflammatory activity of 1.8-cineol (eucalyptol) in bronchial asthma: a double-blind placebo-controlled trial. Respir Med. 2003 Mar;97(3):250-6.

Jukic M, Burcul F, Carev I, Politeo O, Milos M. Screening for acetylcholinesterase inhibition and antioxidant activity of selected plants from Croatia. Nat Prod Res. 2012;26(18):1703-7. doi: 10.1080/14786419.2011.602639.

Julkunen-Tiitto R. A chemotaxonomic survey of phenolics in leaves of northern Salicaceae species. Phytochemistry. 1986;25(3):663-667.

Jung HA, Yokozawa T, Kim BW, Jung JH, Choi JS. Selective inhibition of prenylated flavonoids from Sophora flavescens against BACE1 and cholinesterases. Am J Chin Med. 2010;38(2):415-29.

Jung IH, Jung MA, Kim EJ, Han MJ, Kim DH. Lactobacillus pentosus var. plantarum C29 protects scopolamine-induced memory deficit in mice. J Appl Microbiol. 2012 Dec;113(6):1498-506. doi: 10.1111/j.1365-2672.2012.05437.x.

Jung SY, Jung WS, Jung HK, Lee GH, Cho JH, Cho HW, Choi IY. The mixture of different parts of Nelumbo nucifera and two bioactive components inhibited tyrosinase activity and melanogenesis. J Cosmet Sci. 2014 Nov-Dec;65(6):377-88.

Jung UJ, Lee MK, Jeong KS, Choi MS. The hypoglycemic effects of hesperidin and naringin are partly mediated by hepatic glucose-regulating enzymes in C57BL/KsJ-db/db mice. J Nutr. 2004 Oct;134(10):2499-503.

Jurenka JS. Anti-inflammatory properties of curcumin, a major constituent of Curcuma longa: a review of preclinical and clinical research. Altern Med Rev. 2009 Feb;14(2):141-153.

Juvonen R, Bloigu A, Peitso A, Silvennoinen-Kassinen S, Saikku P, Leinonen M, Hassi J, Harju T. Training improves physical fitness and decreases CRP also in asthmatic conscripts. J Asthma. 2008 Apr;45(3):237-42.

Jyvakorpi SK, Puranen T, Pitkala KH, Suominen MH. Nutritional treatment of aged individuals with Alzheimer disease living at home with their spouses: study protocol for a randomized controlled trial. Trials. 2012 May 24;13:66. doi: 10.1186/1745-6215-13-66.

Kadir A, Almkvist O, Forsberg A, Wall A, Engler H, Långström B, et al. Dynamic changes in PET amyloid and FDG imaging at different stages of Alzheimer's disease. Neurobiol Aging 2012;33:198.e1-14.

Kadir A, Andreasen N, Almkvist O, Wall A, Forsberg A, Engler H, et al. Effect of phenserine treatment on brain functional activity and amyloid in Alzheimer's disease. Ann Neurol 2008;63:621-31.

Kahhak L, Roche A, Dubray C, Arnoux C, Benveniste J. Decrease of ciliary beat frequency by platelet activating factor: protective effect of ketotifen. Inflamm Res. 1996 May;45(5):234-8.

Kähkönen MP, Hopia AI, Vuorela HJ, Rauha JP, Pihlaja K, Kujala TS, Heinonen M. Antioxidant activity of plant extracts containing phenolic compounds. J Agric Food Chem. 1999 Oct;47(10):3954-62.

Kalani A, Bahtiyar G, Sacerdote A. Ashwagandha root in the treatment of non-classical adrenal hyperplasia. BMJ Case Rep. 2012 Sep 17;2012.

Kalmijn S, Launer LJ, Ott A, Witteman JC, Hofman A, Breteler MM. Dietary fat intake and the risk of incident dementia in the Rotterdam Study. Ann of Neurol. 1997;42(5):776-782.

Kalsbeek A, Perreau-Lenz S, Buijs RM. A network of (autonomic) clock outputs. Chronobiol Int. 2006;23(1-2):201-15.

Kamide Y. We reside in the sun's atmosphere. Biomed Pharmacother. 2005 Oct;59 Suppl 1:S1-4.

Kandel E, Siegelbaum S, Schwartz J. Synaptic transmission. Principles of Neural Science. New York: Elsevier, 1991.

Kang Y, Li M, Yan W, Li X, Kang J, Zhang Y. Electroacupuncture alters the expression of genes associated with lipid metabolism and immune reaction in liver of hypercholesterolemia mice. Biotechnol Lett. 2007 Aug 18.

Kapil A, Sharma S. Immunopotentiating compounds from Tinospora cordifolia. J Ethnopharmacol. 1997 Oct;58(2):89-95.

Kaplan A, Mutlu EA, Benson M, Fields JZ, Banan A, Keshavarzian A. Use of herbal preparations in the treatment of oxidant-mediated inflammatory disorders. Complement Ther Med. 2007 Sep;15(3):207-16. 2006 Aug 21.

Kaplan R. The nature of the view from home: psychological benefits. Environ Behav. 2001;33(4):507-42.

Kaplan R. Wilderness perception and psychological benefits: an analysis of a continuing program. Leisure Sci. 1984;6(3):271-90.

Kapoor S. Withania somnifera and its emerging anti-neoplastic effects. Inflammopharmacology. 2012 Dec 8.

Kaptchuk TJ. The placebo effect in alternative medicine: can the performance of a healing ritual have clinical significance? Ann Intern Med. 2002 Jun 4;136(11):817-25.

Karis TE, Jhon MS. Flow-induced anisotropy in the susceptibility of a particle suspension. Proc Natl Acad Sci USA. 1986 Jul;83(14):4973-4977.

Karnstedt J. Ions and Consciousness. Whole Self. 1991 Spring.

Karp A, Kåreholt I, Qiu C, Bellander T, Winblad B, Fratiglioni L. Relation of education and occupation-based socioeconomic status to incident Alzheimer's disease. Am J Epidemiol. 2004 Jan 15;159(2):175-83.

Katagiri M, Satoh A, Tsuji S, Shirasawa T. Effects of astaxanthin-rich Haematococcus pluvialis extract on cognitive function: a randomised, double-blind, placebo-controlled study. J Clin Biochem Nutr. 2012 Sep;51(2):102-7.

Kataoka M, Tsumura H, Kaku N, Torisu T. Toxic effects of povidone-iodine on synovial cell and articular cartilage. Clin Rheumatol. 2006 Sep;25(5):632-8.

Kataria H, Wadhwa R, Kaul SC, Kaur G. Water extract from the leaves of Withania somnifera protect RA differen-tiated C6 and IMR-32 cells against glutamate-induced excitotoxicity. PLoS One. 2012;7(5):e37080.

Kato Y, Kawamoto T, Honda KK. Circadian rhythms in cartilage. Clin Calcium. 2006 May;16(5):838-45.

Kaurav BP, Wanjari MM, Chandekar A, Chauhan NS, Upmanyu N. Influence of Withania somnifera on obsessive compulsive disorder in mice. Asian Pac J Trop Med. 2012 May;5(5):380-4.

REFERENCES AND BIBLIOGRAPHY

Kazlowska K, Hsu T, Hou CC, Yang WC, Tsai GJ. Anti-inflammatory properties of phenolic compounds and crude extract from Porphyra dentata. J Ethnopharmacol. 2010 Mar 2;128(1):123-30.

Keast DR, O'Neil CE, Jones JM. Dried fruit consumption is associated with improved diet quality and reduced obesity in US adults: National Health and Nutrition Examination Survey, 1999-2004. Nutr Res. 2011 Jun;31(6):460-7.

Keenan JM, Goulson M, Shamliyan T, Knutson N, Kolberg L, Curry L. The effects of concentrated barley beta-glucan on blood lipids in a population of hypercholesterolaemic men and women. Br J Nutr. 2007 Jun;97(6):1162-8.

Keil J. New cases in Burma, Thailand, and Turkey: A limited field study replication of some aspects of Ian Stevenson's work. J. Sci. Exploration. 1991;5(1):27-59.

Kekkonen RA, Lummela N, Karjalainen H, Latvala S, Tynkkynen S, Jarvenpaa S, Kautiainen H, Julkunen I, Vapaatalo H, Korpela R. Probiotic intervention has strain-specific anti-inflammatory effects in healthy adults. World J Gastroenterol. 2008 Apr 7;14(13):2029-36.

Kelder P. Ancient Secret of the Fountain of Youth: Book 1. New York: Doubleday, 1998.

Kelley GA, Kelley KS, Tran ZV. Aerobic exercise and lipids and lipoproteins in women: a meta-analysis of randomized controlled trials. J Womens Health. 2004 Dec;13(10):1148-64.

Kelly J, Fulford J, Vanhatalo A, Blackwell JR, French O, Bailey SJ, Gilchrist M, Winyard PG, Jones AM. Effects of short-term dietary nitrate supplementation on blood pressure, O2 uptake kinetics, and muscle and cognitive function in older adults. Am J Physiol Regul Integr Comp Physiol. 2013 Jan 15;304(2):R73-83.

Kelly J, Vanhatalo A, Wilkerson DP, Wylie LJ, Jones AM. Effects of Nitrate on the Power-Duration Relationship for Severe-Intensity Exercise. Med Sci Sports Exerc. 2013 Mar 7

Kelly SA, Summerbell CD, Brynes A, Whittaker V, Frost G. Wholegrain cereals for coronary heart disease. Cochrane Database Syst Rev. 2007 Apr 18;(2):CD005051.

Kelsey NA, Wilkins HM, Linseman DA. Nutraceutical antioxidants as novel neuroprotective agents. Molecules. 2010 Nov 3;15(11):7792-814. doi: 10.3390/molecules15117792.

Kennedy KL, Steidle CP, Letizia TM. Urinary incontinence: the basics. Ostomy Wound Manage. 1995 Aug;41(7):16-8, 20, 22 passim; quiz 33-4.

Keogh JB, Grieger JA, Noakes M, Clifton PM. Flow-Mediated Dilatation Is Impaired by a High-Saturated Fat Diet but Not by a High-Carbohydrate Diet. Arterioscler Thromb Vasc Biol. 2005 Mar 17

Kerckhoffs DA, Brouns F, Hornstra G, Mensink RP. Effects on the human serum lipoprotein profile of beta-glucan, soy protein and isoflavones, plant sterols and stanols, garlic and tocotrienols. J Nutr. 2002 Sep;132(9):2494-505.

Keri RS, Quintanova C, Chaves S, Silva DF, Cardoso SM, Santos MA. New Tacrine Hybrids with Natural-Based Cysteine Derivatives as Multitargeted Drugs for Potential Treatment of Alzheimer's Disease. Chem Biol Drug Des. 2016 Jan;87(1):101-11. doi: 10.1111/cbdd.12633.

Kerr CC, Rennie CJ, Robinson PA. Physiology-based modeling of cortical auditory evoked potentials. Biol Cybern. 2008 Feb;98(2):171-84.

Kesse-Guyot E, Amieva H, Castetbon K, Henegar A, Ferry M, Jeandel C, Hercberg S, Galan P; SU.VI.MAX 2 Research Group. Adherence to nutritional recommendations and subsequent cognitive performance: findings from the prospective Supplementation with Antioxidant Vitamins and Minerals 2 (SU.VI.MAX 2) study. Am J Clin Nutr. 2011 Jan;93(1):200-10. doi: 10.3945/ajcn.2010.29761.

Kesse-Guyot E, Andreeva VA, Jeandel C, Ferry M, Hercberg S, Galan P. A healthy dietary pattern at midlife is associated with subsequent cognitive performance. J Nutr. 2012 May;142(5):909-15.

Keville K, Green M. Aromatherapy: A Complete Guide to the Healing Art. Freedom, CA: Crossing Press, 1995.

Key T, Appleby P, Davey G, Allen N, Spencer E, Travis R. Mortality in British vegetarians: review and preliminary results from EPIC-Oxford. Amer. Jour. Clin. Nutr. Suppl. 2003;78(3): 533S-538S.

Key T, Appleby P, Davey G, Allen N, Spencer E, Travis R. Mortality in British vegetarians: review and preliminary results from EPIC-Oxford. Amer. Jour. Clin. Nutr. Suppl. 2003;78(3): 533S-538S.

Khalil A, Berrougui H, Pawelec G, Fulop T. Impairment of the ABCA1 and SR-BI-mediated cholesterol efflux pathways and HDL anti-inflammatory activity in Alzheimer's disease. Mech Ageing Dev. 2012 Jan;133(1):20-9. doi: 10.1016/j.mad.2011.11.008.

Khan MR, Hu J, Ali GM. Reciprocal loss of CArG-boxes and auxin response elements drives expression divergence of MPF2-Like MADS-box genes controlling calyx inflation. PLoS One. 2012;7(8):e42781.

Khan MR, Hu J, He C. Plant hormones including ethylene are recruited in calyx inflation in Solanaceous plants. J Plant Physiol. 2012 Jul 1;169(10):940-8.

Kiecolt-Glaser JK, Graham JE, Malarkey WB, Porter K, Lemeshow S, Glaser R. Olfactory influences on mood and autonomic, endocrine, and immune function. Psychoneuroendocrinology. 2008 Apr;33(3):328-39.

Kim ES, Weon JB, Yun BR, Lee J, Eom MR, Oh KH, Ma CJ. Cognitive Enhancing and Neuroprotective Effect of the Embryo of the Nelumbo nucifera Seed. Evid Based Complement Alternat Med. 2014;2014:869831. doi: 10.1155/2014/869831.

Kim G, Kim H, Kim KN, Son JI, Kim SY, Tamura T, Chang N. Relationship of cognitive function with B vitamin status, homocysteine, and tissue factor pathway inhibitor in cognitively impaired elderly: a cross-sectional survey. J Alzheimers Dis. 2013;33(3):853-62.

Kim JT, Ren CJ, Fielding GA, Pitti A, Kasumi T, Wajda M, Lebovits A, Bekker A. Treatment with lavender aromatherapy in the post-anesthesia care unit reduces opioid requirements of morbidly obese patients undergoing laparoscopic adjustable gastric banding. Obes Surg. 2007 Jul;17(7):920-5.

271

Kim LS, Waters RF, Burkholder PM. Immunological activity of larch arabinogalactan and Echinacea: a preliminary, randomized, double-blind, placebo-controlled trial. Altern Med Rev. 2002 Apr;7(2):138-49.

Kim MS, Hwang SS, Park EJ, Bae JW. Strict vegetarian diet improves the risk factors associated with metabolic diseases by modulating gut microbiota and reducing intestinal inflammation. Environ Microbiol Rep. 2013 Oct;5(5):765-75. doi: 10.1111/1758-2229.12079.

Kim SJ, Jung JY, Kim HW, Park T. Anti-obesity effects of Juniperus chinensis extract are associated with increased AMP-activated protein kinase expression and phosphorylation in the visceral adipose tissue of rats. Biol Pharm Bull. 2008 Jul;31(7):1415-21.

Kim SY, Moon GS. Photoprotective Effect of Lotus (Nelumbo nucifera Gaertn.) Seed Tea against UVB Irradiation. Prev Nutr Food Sci. 2015 Sep;20(3):162-8. doi: 10.3746/pnf.2015.20.3.162.

Kimata M, Shichijo M, Miura T, Serizawa I, Inagaki N, Nagai H. Effects of luteolin, quercetin and baicalein on immunoglobulin E-mediated mediator release from human cultured mast cells. Clin Exp Allergy. 2000 Apr;30(4):501-8.

Kimura-Kuroda J, Komuta Y, Kuroda Y, Hayashi M, Kawano H. Nicotine-like effects of the neonicotinoid insecticides acetami-prid and imidacloprid on cerebellar neurons from neonatal rats. PLoS One. 2012;7(2):e32432.

Kinoshameg SA, Persinger MA. Suppression of experimental allergic encephalomyelitis in rats by 50-nT, 7-Hz amplitude-modulated nocturnal magnetic fields depends on when after inoculation the fields are applied. J Neulet..2004;08:18.

Kirlian SD, Kirlian V, Photography and Visual Observation by Means of High-Frequency Currents. J Sci Appl Photog. 1963;6(6).

Klatz RM, Goldman RM, Cebula C. Infection Protection. New York: HarperResource, 2002.

Klaus M. Mother and infant: early emotional ties. Pediatrics. 1998 Nov;102(5 Suppl E):1244-6.

Klein E, Smith D, Laxminarayan R. Trends in Hospitalizations and Deaths in the United States Associated with Infections Caused by Staphylococcus aureus and MRSA, 1999-2004. Emerging Infectious Diseases. University of Florida Press Release. 2007 Dec 3.

Klein R, Landau MG. Healing: The Body Betrayed. Minneapolis: DCI:Chronimed, 1992.

Klima H, Haas O, Roschger P. Photon emission from blood cells and its possible role in immune system regulation. In: Jezowska-Trzebiatowska B., et al. (eds.): Photon Emission from Biological Systems. Singapore: World Scientific, 1987:153-169.

Klimova B, Maresova P, Valis M, Hort J, Kuca K. Alzheimer's disease and language impairments: social intervention and medical treatment. Clin Interv Aging. 2015 Aug 27;10:1401-7. doi: 10.2147/CIA.S89714. eCollection 2015.

Kloss J. Back to Eden. Twin Oaks, WI: Lotus Press, 1939-1999.

Klunk WE, Engler H, Nordberg A, Wang Y, Blomqvist G, Holt DP, et al. Imaging brain amyloid in Alzheimer's disease with Pittsburgh compound-B. Ann Neurol 2004;55:306-19.

Kniazeva TA, Kuznetsova LN, Otto MP, Nikiforova TI. Efficacy of chromotherapy in patients with hypertension. Vopr Kurortol Fizioter Lech Fiz Kult. 2006 Jan-Feb;(1):11-3.

Knight EM, Kim SH, Kottwitz JC, Hatami A, Albay R, Suzuki A, Lublin A, Alberini CM, Klein WL, Szabo P, Relkin NR, Ehrlich M, Glabe CG, Gandy S, Steele JW. Effective anti-Alzheimer Aβ therapy involves depletion of specific Aβ oligomer subtypes. Neurol Neuroimmunol Neuroinflamm. 2016 May 10;3(3):e237. doi: 10.1212/NXI.0000000000000237.

Knight EM, Ruiz HH, Kim SH, Harte JC, Hsieh W, Glabe C, Klein WL, Attie AD, Buettner C, Ehrlich ME, Gandy S. Unexpected partial correction of metabolic and behavioral phenotypes of Alzheimer's APP/PSEN1 mice by gene targeting of diabetes/Alzheimer's-related Sorcs1. Acta Neuropathol Commun. 2016 Feb 25;4:16. doi: 10.1186/s40478-016-0282-y.

Kobayashi M, Shoji N, Ohizumi Y. Gingerol, a novel cardiotonic agent, activates the Ca2+-pumping ATPase in skeletal and cardiac sarcoplasmic reticulum. Biochim Biophys Acta. 1987 Sep 18;903(1):96-102.

Koch C. Debunking the Digital Brain. Sci. Am. 1997 Feb.

Koivunen J, Scheinin N, Virta JR, Aalto S, Vahlberg T, Någren K, et al. Amyloid PET imaging in patients with mild cognitive impairment: a 2-year follow-up study. Neurology 2011;76:1085-90.

Koletzko B, Sauerwald U, Keicher U, Saule H, Wawatschek S, Böhles H, Bervoets K, Fleith M, Crozier-Willi G. Fatty acid profiles, antioxidant status, and growth of preterm infants fed diets without or with long-chain polyunsaturated fatty acids. A randomized clinical trial. Eur J Nutr. 2003 Oct;42(5):243-53.

Kollerstrom N, Staudenmaier G. Evidence for Lunar-Sidereal Rhythms in Crop Yield: A Review. Biolog Agri & Hort. 2001;19:247–259

Kollerstrom N, Steffert B. Sex difference in response to stress by lunar month: a pilot study of four years' crisis-call frequency. BMC Psychiatry. 2003 Dec 10;3:20.

Konrath EL, Passos Cdos S, Klein LC Jr, Henriques AT. Alkaloids as a source of potential anticholinesterase inhibitors for the treatment of Alzheimer's disease. J Pharm Pharmacol. 2013 Dec;65(12):1701-25. doi: 10.1111/jphp.12090.

Kontush A, Mann U, Arlt S, Ujeyl A, Lührs C, Müller-Thomsen T, Beisiegel U. Influence of vitamin E and C supplementation on lipoprotein oxidation in patients with Alzheimer's disease. Free Radic Biol Med. 2001 Aug 1;31(3):345-54.

Koo KL, Ammit AJ, Tran VH, Duke CC, Roufogalis BD. Gingerols and related analogues inhibit arachidonic acid-induced human platelet serotonin release and aggregation. Thromb Res. 2001 Sep 1;103(5):387-97.

Koop H, Bachem MG. Serum iron, ferritin, and vitamin B12 during prolonged omeprazole therapy. J Clin Gastroenterol. 1992;14:288-92.

REFERENCES AND BIBLIOGRAPHY

Kostomoiri M, Fragkouli A, Sagnou M, Skaltsounis LA, Pelecanou M, Tsilibary EC, Tauzinia AK. Oleuropein, an Anti-oxidant Polyphenol Constituent of Olive Promotes α-Secretase Cleavage of the Amyloid Precursor Protein (AβPP). Cell Mol Neurobiol. 2012 Oct 7. Koszowski B, Goniewicz M, Czogala J. Alternative methods of nicotine dependence treatment. Przegl Lek. 2005;62(10):1176-9.

Kotani S, Sakaguchi E, Warashina S, Matsukawa N, Ishikura Y, Kiso Y, Sakakibara M, Yoshimoto T, Guo J, Yamashima T. Dietary supplementation of arachidonic and docosahexaenoic acids improves cognitive dysfunction. Neurosci Res. 2006 Oct;56(2):159-64.

Kowalchik C, Hylton W (eds). Rodale's Illustrated Encyclopedia of Herbs. Emmaus, PA: 1987.

Kowalczyk E, Krzesiński P, Kura M, Niedworok J, Kowalski J, Blaszczyk J. Pharmacological effects of flavonoids from Scutellaria baicalensis. Przegl Lek. 2006;63(2):95-6.

Krämer UM, Knight RT, Münte TF. Electrophysiological evidence for different inhibitory mechanisms when stopping or changing a planned response. J Cogn Neurosci. 2011 Sep;23(9):2481-93. doi: 10.1162/jocn.2010.21573.

Krause R, Buhring M, Hopfenmuller W, Holick MF, Sharma AM. Ultraviolet B and blood pressure. Lancet. 1998 Aug 29;352(9129):709-10.

Kräutler B. Colorless Tetrapyrrolic Chlorophyll Catabolites in Ripening Fruit Are Effective Antioxidants. Angewandte Chemie International Edition. 2007;46;8699-8702.

Krebs K. The spiritual aspect of caring—an integral part of health and healing. Nurs Adm Q. 2001 Spring;25(3):55-60.

Kreig M. Black Market Medicine. New York: Bantam, 1968.

Kris-Etherton PM, Pearson TA, Wan Y, Hargrove RL, Moriarty K, Fishell V, Etherton TD. High-monounsaturated Fatty Acid Diets Lower Both Plasma Cholesterol and Triacylglycerol Concentrations. Am J Clin Nutr. 1999;70:1009-15

Krsnich-Shriwise S. Fibromyalgia syndrome: an overview. Phys Ther. 1997;77:68-75.

Kryscio RJ, Abner EL, Schmitt FA, Goodman PJ, Mendiondo M, Caban-Holt A, Dennis BC, Mathews M, Klein EA, Crowley JJ; SELECT Investigators. A randomized controlled Alzheimer's disease prevention trial's evolution into an exposure trial: the PREADViSE Trial. J Nutr Health Aging. 2013 Jan;17(1):72-5. doi: 10.1007/s12603-012-0083-3.

Kubler-Ross E. On Life After Death. Berkeley, CA: Celestial Arts, 1991.

Kubo I, Fujita K, Kubo A, Nihei K, Ogura T. Antibacterial activity of coriander volatile compounds against Salmonella choleraesuis. J Agric Food Chem. 2004 Jun 2;52(11):3329-32.

Kudo Y, Okamura N, Furumoto S, Tashiro M, Furukawa K, Maruyama M, et al. 2-(2-[2-Dimethylaminothiazol-5-yl]ethenyl)-6- (2-[fluoro]ethoxy)benzoxazole: a novel PET agent for in vivo detection of dense amyloid plaques in Alzheimer's disease patients. J Nucleic Med 2007;48:553-61.

Kullo IJ, Ballantyne CM. Conditional risk factors for atherosclerosis. Mayo Clin Proc. 2005 Feb;80(2):219-30.

Kulvinskas V. 1978. Nutritional Evaluation of Sprouts and Grasses. Omango D' Press, Wethersfield, CT.

Kumar A, Panghal S, Mallapur SS, Kumar M, Ram V, Singh BK. Antiinflammatory Activity of Piper longum Fruit Oil. Indian J Pharm Sci. 2009 Jul;71(4):454-6.

Kumar A, Saluja AK, Shah UD, Mayavanshi AV. Pharmacological potential of Albizzia lebbeck: A Review. Pharmacog. 2007 Jan-May; 1(1) 171-174.

Kumar J, Garg G, Sundaramoorthy E, Prasad PV, Karthikeyan G, Ramakrishnan L, Ghosh S, Sengupta S. Vitamin B12 deficiency is associated with coronary artery disease in an Indian population. Clin Chem Lab Med. 2009;47(3):334-8.

Kumar P, Kumar A. Protective effect of hesperidin and naringin against 3-nitropropionic acid induced Huntington's like symptoms in rats: possible role of nitric oxide. Behav Brain Res. 2010 Jan 5;206(1):38-46.

Kumar PU, Adhikari P, Pereira P, Bhat P. Safety and efficacy of Hartone in stable angina pectoris-an open comparative trial. J Assoc Physicians India. 1999 Jul;47(7):685-9.

Kumar S. Dual inhibition of acetylcholinesterase and butyrylcholinesterase enzymes by allicin. Indian J Pharmacol. 2015 Jul-Aug;47(4):444-6. doi: 10.4103/0253-7613.161274.

Kumarihamy M, León F, Pettaway S, Wilson L, Lambert JA, Wang M, Hill C, McCurdy CR, ElSohly MA, Cutler SJ, Muhammad I. In vitro opioid receptor affinity and in vivo behavioral studies of Nelumbo nucifera flower. J Ethnopharmacol. 2015 Aug 7:JEPD15D1341. doi: 10.1016/j.jep.2015.08.006.

Kung HC, Hoyert DL, Xu J, Murphy SL. Deaths: Final Data for 2005. National Vital Statistics Reports. 2008;56(10). http://www.cdc.gov/nchs/data/ nvsr/nvsr56/nvsr56_10.pdf. Accessed: 2008 Jun.

Kuo FF, Kuo JJ. Recent Advances in Acupuncture Research, Institute for Advanced Research in Asian Science and Medicine. Garden City, New York. 1979.

Kuroyanagi M, Murata M, Nakane T, Shirota O, Sekita S, Fuchino H, Shinwari ZK. Leishmanicidal active withanolides from a pakistani medicinal plant, Withania coagulans. Chem Pharm Bull (Tokyo). 2012;60(7):892-7.

Kushwaha S, Roy S, Maity R, Mallick A, Soni VK, Singh PK, Chaurasiya ND, Sangwan RS, Misra-Bhattacharya S, Mandal C. Chemotypical variations in Withania somnifera lead to differentially modulated immune response in BALB/c mice. Vaccine. 2012 Feb 1;30(6):1083-93.

Kuuler R, Ballal S, Laike T Mikellides B, Tonello G. The impact of light and colour on psychological mood: a cross-cultral study of indoor work environments. Ergonomics. 2006 Nov 15;49(14):1496.

Kuznetsova TA, Shevchenko NM, Zviagintseva TN, Besednova NN. Biological activity of fucoidans from brown algae and the prospects of their use in medicine]. Antibiot Khimioter. 2004;49(5):24-30.

Kvamme JM, Wilsgaard T, Florholmen J, Jacobsen BK. Body mass index and disease burden in elderly men and women: the Tromso Study. Eur J Epidemiol. 2010 Mar;25(3):183-93. 2010 Jan 20.

273

Kwang Y, Cha , Daniel P, Wirth J, Lobo R. Does Prayer Influence the Success of in Vitro. Fertilization–Embryo Transfer? Report of a Masked, Randomized Trial. J Reproductive Med. 2001;46(9).

Laaksonen M, Karkkainen M, Outila T, Vanninen T, Ray C, Lamberg-Allardt C. Vitamin D receptor gene BsmI-polymorphism in Finnish premenopausal and postmenopausal women: its association with bone mineral density, markers of bone turnover, and intestinal calcium absorption, with adjustment for lifestyle factors. J Bone Miner Metab. 2002;20(6):383-90.

Lad V. Ayurveda: The Science of Self-Healing. Twin Lakes, WI: Lotus Press.

Lafrenière, G. The material Universe is made purely out of Aether. Matter is made of Waves. 2002. http://www.glafreniere.com/matter.htm. Acc. 2007 June.

Lakin-Thomas PL. Transcriptional feedback oscillators: maybe, maybe not. J Biol Rhythms. 2006 Apr;21(2):83-92.

Lam F, Jr, Tsuei JJ, Zhao Z. Studies on the bioenergetic measurement of acupuncture points for determination of correct dosage of allopathic or homeopathic medicine in the treatment of diabetes mellitus. Am J Acupunct. 1990;18:127-33.

Lambing K. Biophoton Measurement as a Supplement to the Conventional Consideration of Food Quality. In: Popp F, Li K, Gu Q (eds.). Recent Advances in Biophoton Research. Singapore: World Scientific Publ. 1992:393-413.

Landel V, Annweiler C, Millet P, Morello M, Féron F. Vitamin D, Cognition and Alzheimer's Disease: The Therapeutic Benefit is in the D-Tails. J Alzheimers Dis. 2016 May 11;53(2):419-44. doi: 10.3233/JAD-150943.

Landmark K, Reikvam A. Do vitamins C and E protect against the development of carotid stenosis and cardiovascular disease? Tidsskr Nor Laegeforen. 2005 Jan 20;125(2):159-62.

Langballe EM, Ask H, Holmen J, Stordal E, Saltvedt I, Selbæk G, Fikseaunet A, Bergh S, Nafstad P, Tambs K. Alcohol consumption and risk of dementia up to 27 years later in a large, population-based sample: the HUNT study, Norway. Eur J Epidemiol. 2015 Sep;30(9):1049-56. doi: 10.1007/s10654-015-0029-2.

Langhinrichsen-Rohling J, Palarea RE, Cohen J, Rohling ML. Breaking up is hard to do: unwanted pursuit behaviors following the dissolution of a romantic relationship. Violence Vict. 2000 Spring;15(1):73-90.

Lansley KE, Winyard PG, Bailey SJ, Vanhatalo A, Wilkerson DP, Blackwell JR, Gilchrist M, Benjamin N, Jones AM. Acute dietary nitrate supplementation improves cycling time trial performance. Med Sci Sports Exerc. 2011 Jun;43(6):1125-31.

Lappe FM. Diet for a Small Planet. New York: Ballantine, 1971.

Larsson SC, Wolk A. Red and processed meat consumption and risk of pancreatic cancer: meta-analysis of prospective studies. Br J Cancer. 2012 Jan 12.

Last, D, Alsop DC, Abduljalil AM, Marquis RP, de Bazelaire C, Hu K, Cavallerano K, Novak V. Global and regional effects of type 2 diabetes on brain tissue volumes and cerebral vasoreactivity. Diabetes Care. 2007 30:1193–1199. doi:10.2337/dc06-2052

Latour E. Functional electrostimulation and its using in neurorehabilitation. Ortop Traumatol Rehabil. 2006 Dec 29;8(6):593-601.

Lau BH, Riesen SK, Truong KP, Lau EW, Rohdewald P, Barreta RA. Pycnogenol as an adjunct in the management of childhood asthma. J Asthma. 2004;41(8):825-32.

Laura AG, Armas, B, Heaney H, Heaney R. Vitamin D2 Is Much Less Effective than Vitamin D3 in Humans. J Clin Endocr & Metab. 2004;89(11):5387-5391.

LaValle JB. The Cox-2 Connection. Rochester, VT: Healing Arts, 2001.

Lazarou J, Pomeranz BH, Corey PN. Incidence of adverse drug reactions in hospitalized patients: a meta-analysis of prospective studies. JAMA. 1998 Apr.

Lean G. US study links more than 200 diseases to pollution. London Independent. 2004 Nov 14.

Leander M, Cronqvist A, Janson C, Uddenfeldt M, Rask-Andersen A. Health-related quality of life predicts onset of asthma in a longitudinal population study. Respir Med. 2009 Feb;103(2):194-200.

Leape L. Lucian Leape on patient safety in U.S. hospitals. Interview by Peter I Buerhaus. J Nurs Scholarsh. 2004;36(4):366-70.

Leary, PC. Rock as a critical-point system and the inherent implausibility of reliable earthquake prediction. Geophysical Journal International. 1997;131(3):451-466. doi:10.1111/j.1365-246X.1997.

Leblhuber F, Geisler S, Steiner K, Fuchs D, Schütz B. Elevated fecal calprotectin in patients with Alzheimer's dementia indicates leaky gut. J Neural Transm (Vienna). 2015 Sep;122(9):1319-22. doi: 10.1007/s00702-015-1381-9.

Lecheler J, Pfannebecker B, Nguyen DT, Petzold U, Munzel U, Kremer HJ, Maus J. Prevention of exercise-induced asthma by a fixed combination of disodium cromoglycate plus reproterol compared with montelukast in young patients. Arzneimittelforschung. 2008;58(6):303-9.

Leder D. Spooky actions at a distance: physics, psi, and distant healing. J Altern Complement Med. 2005 Oct;11(5):923-30.

Lee DB, Kim DH, Je JY. Antioxidant and Cytoprotective Effects of Lotus (Nelumbo nucifera) Leaves Phenolic Fraction. Prev Nutr Food Sci. 2015 Mar;20(1):22-8. doi: 10.3746/pnf.2015.20.1.22.

Lee E, Haa K, Yook JM, Jin MH, Seo CS, Son KH, Kim HP, Bae KH, Kang SS, Son JK, Chang HW. Anti-asthmatic activity of an ethanol extract from Saururus chinensis. Biol Pharm Bull. 2006 Feb;29(2):211-5.

Lee J, Sehrawat A, Singh SV. Withaferin A causes activation of Notch2 and Notch4 in human breast cancer cells. Breast Cancer Res Treat. 2012 Nov;136(1):45-56.

Lee JH, Noh J, Noh G, Kim HS, Mun SH, Choi WS, Cho S, Lee S. Allergen-specific B cell subset responses in cow's milk allergy of late eczematous reactions in atopic dermatitis. Cell Immunol. 2010;262(1):44-51.

REFERENCES AND BIBLIOGRAPHY

Lee JS, Shukla S, Kim JA, Kim M. Anti-angiogenic effect of Nelumbo nucifera leaf extracts in human umbilical vein endothelial cells with antioxidant potential. PLoS One. 2015 Feb 25;10(2):e0118552. doi: 10.1371/journal.pone.0118552.

Lee ST, Chu K, Sim JY, Heo JH, Kim M. Panax ginseng enhances cognitive performance in Alzheimer disease. Alzheimer Dis Assoc Disord. 2008 Jul-Sep;22(3):222-6. doi: 10.1097/WAD.0b013e31816c92e6.

Lee W, Kim TH, Ku SK, Min KJ, Lee HS, Kwon TK, Bae JS. Barrier protective effects of withaferin A in HMGB1-induced inflammatory responses in both cellular and animal models. Toxicol Appl Pharmacol. 2012 Jul 1;262(1):91-8.

Lee YS, Kim SH, Jung SH, Kim JK, Pan CH, Lim SS. Aldose reductase inhibitory compounds from Glycyrrhiza uralensis. Biol Pharm Bull. 2010;33(5):917-21.

Lefort J, Sedivy P, Desquand S, Randon J, Coeffier E, Maridonneau-Parini I, Floch A, Benveniste J, Vargaftig BB. Pharmacological profile of 48740 R.P., a PAF-acether antagonist. Eur J Pharmacol. 1988 Jun 10;150(3):257-68.

Lehmann B. The vitamin D3 pathway in human skin and its role for regulation of biological processes. Photochem Photobiol. 2005 Nov-Dec;81(6):1246-51.

Leinonen V, Alafuzoff I, Aalto S, Suotunen T, Savolainen S, Någren K, et al. Assessment of beta-amyloid in a frontal cortical brain biopsy specimen and by positron emission tomography with carbon 11-labeled

Leitzmann C. Vegetarian diets: what are the advantages? Forum Nutr. 2005;(57):147-56.

Lennihan B. Homeopathy: natural mind-body healing. J Psychosoc Nurs Ment Health Serv. 2004 Jul;42(7):30-40.

Lewis A. Rescue remedy. Nurs Times. 1999 May 26-Jun 1;95(21):27.

Lewis JE, McDaniel HR, Agronin ME, Loewenstein DA, Riveros J, Mestre R, Martinez M, Colina N, Abreu D, Konefal J, Woolger JM, Ali KH. The effect of an aloe polymannose multinutrient complex on cognitive and immune functioning in Alzheimer's disease. J Alzheimers Dis. 2013;33(2):393-406. doi: 10.3233/JAD-2012-121381.

Lewis WH, Elvin-Lewis MPF. Medical Botany: Plants Affecting Man's Health. New York: Wiley, 1977.

Lewontin R. The Genetic Basis of Evolutionary Change. New York: Columbia Univ Press, 1974.

Leyel CF. Culpeper's English Physician & Complete Herbal. Hollywood, CA: Wilshire, 1971.

Leyva DR, Zahradka P, Ramjiawan B, Guzman R, Aliani M, Pierce GN. The effect of dietary flaxseed on improving symptoms of cardiovascular disease in patients with peripheral artery disease: rationale and design of the FLAX-PAlzheimer's disease randomized controlled trial. Contemp Clin Trials. 2011 Sep;32(5):724-30.

Li H, Karl T, Garner B. Understanding the function of ABCA7 in Alzheimer's disease. Biochem Soc Trans. 2015 Oct;43(5):920-3. doi: 10.1042/BST20150105.

Li KH. Bioluminescence and stimulated coherent radiation. Laser und Elektrooptik 3. 1981:32-35.

Li N, Wang DL, Wang CW, Wu B. Discussion on randomized controlled trials about clinical researches of acupuncture and moxibustion medicine. Zhongguo Zhen Jiu. 2007 Jul;27(7):529-32.

Li QX, Villemagne VL, Doecke JD, Rembach A, Sarros S, Varghese S, McGlade A, Laughton KM, Pertile KK, Fowler CJ, Rumble RL, Trounson BO, Taddei K, Rainey-Smith SR, Laws SM, Robertson JS, Evered LA, Silbert B, Ellis KA, Rowe CC, Macaulay SL, Darby D, Martins RN, Ames D, Masters CL, Collins S; AIBL Research Group. Alzheimer's Disease Normative Cerebrospinal Fluid Biomarkers Validated in PET Amyloid-β Characterized Subjects from the Australian Imaging, Biomarkers and Lifestyle (AIBL) study. J Alzheimers Dis. 2015;48(1):175-87. doi: 10.3233/JAD-150247.

Liao H, Xi P, Chen Q, Yi L, Zhao Y. Clinical study on acupuncture, moxibustion, acupuncture plus moxibustion at Weiwanxiashu (EX-B3) for treatment of diabetes. Zhongguo Zhen Jiu. 2007 Jul;27(7):482-4.

Lieber AL. Human aggression and the lunar synodic cycle. J Clin Psychiatry. 1978 May;39(5):385-92.

Lim AS, Yu L, Kowgier M, Schneider JA, Buchman AS, Bennett DA. Modification of the Relationship of the Apolipoprotein E ε4 Allele to the Risk of Alzheimer Disease and Neurofibrillary Tangle Density by Sleep. JAMA Neurol. 2013 Oct 21. doi: 10.1001/jamaneurol.2013.4215.

Limpeanchob N, Jaipan S, Rattanakaruna S, Phrompittayarat W, Ingkaninan K. Neuroprotective effect of Bacopa monnieri on beta-amyloid-induced cell death in primary cortical culture. J Ethnopharmacol. 2008 Oct 30;120(1):112-7.

Lin GH, Lee YJ, Choi DY, Han SB, Jung JK, Hwang BY, Moon DC, Kim Y, Lee MK, Oh KW, Jeong HS, Leem JY, Shin HK, Lee JH, Hong JT. Anti-amyloidogenic effect of thiacremonone through anti-inflamation in vitro and in vivo models. J Alzheimers Dis. 2012;29(3):659-76. doi: 10.3233/JAD-2012-111709. PubMed PMID: 22297647.

Lin PW, Chan WC, Ng BF, Lam LC. Efficacy of aromatherapy (Lavandula angustifolia) as an intervention for agitated behaviours in Chinese older persons with dementia: a cross-over randomized trial. Int J Geriatr Psychiatry. 2007 May;22(5):405-10.

Ling-Sing Seow S, Naidu M, David P, Wong KH, Sabaratnam V. Potentiation of neuritogenic activity of medicinal mushrooms in rat pheochromocytoma cells. BMC Complement Altern Med. 2013 Jul 4;13:157. doi: 10.1186/1472-6882-13-157.

Lininger S, Gaby A, Austin S, Brown D, Wright J, Duncan A. The Natural Pharmacy. New York: Three Rivers, 1999.

Lipkind M. Can the vitalistic Entelechia principle be a working instrument ? (The theory of the biological field of Alexander G.Gurvich). In: Popp F, Li K, Gu Q (eds.). Recent Advances in Biophoton Research. Singapore: World Sci Publ, 1992:469-494.

Lipkind M. Registration of spontaneous photon emission from virus-infected cell cultures: development of experimental system. Indian J Exp Biol. 2003 May;41(5):572-72.

Lipski E. Digestive Wellness. Los Angeles, CA: Keats, 2000.

Litime M, Aïssa J, Benveniste J. Antigen signaling at high dilution. FASEB Jnl. 1993;7: A602.

Litscher G. Bioengineering assessment of acupuncture, part 5: cerebral near-infrared spectroscopy. Crit Rev Biomed Eng. 2006;34(6):439-57.

Liu CH, Bu XL, Wang J, Zhang T, Xiang Y, Shen LL, Wang QH, Deng B, Wang X, Zhu C, Yao XQ, Zhang M, Zhou HD, Wang YJ. The Associations between a Capsaicin-Rich Diet and Blood Amyloid-β Levels and Cognitive Function. J Alzheimers Dis. 2016 Apr 8.

Liu CM, Kao CL, Wu HM, Li WJ, Huang CT, Li HT, Chen CY. Antioxidant and anticancer aporphine alkaloids from the leaves of Nelumbo nucifera Gaertn. cv. Rosa-plena. Molecules. 2014 Nov 3;19(11):17829-38. doi: 10.3390/molecules191117829.

Liu J, Zhang J, Shi Y, Grimsgaard S, Alraek T, Fonnebo V. Chinese red yeast rice (Monascus purpureus) for primary hyperlipidemia: a meta-analysis of randomized controlled trials. Chin Med. 2006 Nov 23;1:4.

Liu JY, Hu JH, Zhu QG, Li FQ, Wang J, Sun HJ. Effect of matrine on the expression of substance P receptor and inflammatory cytokines production in human skin keratinocytes and fibroblasts. Int Immunopharmacol. 2007 Jun;7(6):816-23.

Liu L, Zubik L, Collins FW, Marko M, Meydani M. The antiatherogenic potential of oat phenolic compounds. Atherosclerosis. 2004 Jul;175(1):39-49.

Liu P, Kong M, Liu S, Chen G, Wang P. Effect of reinforcing kidney-essence, removing phlegm, and promoting mental therapy on treating Alzheimer's disease. J Tradit Chin Med. 2013 Aug;33(4):449-54.

Liu Q, Chen X, Yang G, Min X, Deng M. Apigenin inhibits cell migration through MAPK pathways in human bladder smooth muscle cells. Biocell. 2011 Dec;35(3):71-9.

Liu SH, Lu TH, Su CC, Lay IS, Lin HY, Fang KM, Ho TJ, Chen KL, Su YC, Chiang WC, Chen YW. Lotus leaf (Nelumbo nucifera) and its active constituents prevent inflammatory responses in macrophages via JNK/NF-κB signaling pathway. Am J Chin Med. 2014;42(4):869-89. doi: 10.1142/S0192415X14500554.

Liu T, Valdez R, Yoon PW, Crocker D, Mooneshinghe R, Khoury MJ. The association between family history of asthma and the prevalence of asthma among US adults: National Health and Nutrition Examination Survey, 1999-2004. Genet Med. 2009 May;11(5):323-8.

Liu X, Beaty TH, Deindl P, Huang SK, Lau S, Sommerfeld C, Fallin MD, Kao WH, Wahn U, Nickel R. Associations between specific serum IgE response and 6 variants within the genes IL4, IL13, and IL4RA in German children: the German Multicenter Atopy Study. J Allergy Clin Immunol. 2004 Mar;113(3):489-95.

Liu X, Shibata T, Hisaka S, Osawa T. Astaxanthin inhibits reactive oxygen species-mediated cellular toxicity in dopaminergic SH-SY5Y cells via mitochondria-targeted protective mechanism. Brain Res. 2009;1254:18–27.

Liu X, Yue R, Zhang J, Shan L, Wang R, Zhang W. Neuroprotective effects of bacopaside I in ischemic brain injury. Restor Neurol Neurosci. 2012 Nov 16.

Liu XJ, Cao MA, Li WH, Shen CS, Yan SQ, Yuan CS. Alkaloids from Sophora flavescens Aition. Fitoterapia. 2010 Sep;81(6):524-7.

Liu Z, Wang Q, Cui J, Wang L, Xiong L, Wang W, Li D, Liu N, Wu Y, Mao C. Systemic Screening of Strains of the Lion's Mane Medicinal Mushroom Hericium erinaceus (Higher Basidiomycetes) and Its Protective Effects on Aβ-Triggered Neurotoxicity in PC12 Cells. Int J Med Mushrooms. 2015;17(3):219-29.

Liukkonen-Lilja H, Piepponen S. Leaching of aluminium from aluminium dishes and packages. Food Addit Contam. 1992 May-Jun;9(3):213-23.

Livanova L, Levshina I, Nozdracheva L, Elbakidze MG, Airapetiants MG. The protective action of negative air ions in acute stress in rats with different typological behavioral characteristics. Zh Vyssh Nerv Deiat Im I P Pavlova. 1998 May-Jun;48(3):554-7.

Lloyd D and Murray D. Redox rhythmicity: clocks at the core of temporal coherence. BioEssays. 2007;29(5): 465-473.

Lloyd JU. American Materia Medica, Therapeutics and Pharmacognosy. Portland, OR: Eclectic Medical Publications, 1989-1983.

Lloyd-Still JD, Powers CA, Hoffman DR, Boyd-Trull K, Lester LA, Benisek DC, Arterburn LM. Bioavailability and safety of a high dose of docosahexaenoic acid triacylglycerol of algal origin in cystic fibrosis patients: a randomized, controlled study. Nutrition. 2006 Jan;22(1):36-46.

López A, El-Naggar T, Dueñas M, Ortega T, Estrella I, Hernández T, Gómez-Serranillos MP, Palomino OM, Carretero ME. Effect of cooking and germination on phenolic composition and biological properties of dark beans (Phaseolus vulgaris L.). Food Chem. 2013 May 1;138(1):547-55.

Lopez-Garcia E, Schulze MB, Meigs JB, Manson JE, Rifai N, Stampfer MJ, Willett WC, Hu FB. Consumption of trans fatty acids is related to plasma biomarkers of inflammation and endothelial dysfunction. J Nutr. 2005 Mar;135(3):562-6.

Lopez-Garcia E, Schulze MB, Meigs JB, Manson JE, Rifai N, Stampfer MJ, Willett WC, Hu FB. Consumption of trans fatty acids is related to plasma biomarkers of inflammation and endothelial dysfunction. J Nutr. 2005 Mar;135(3):562-6.

Lorenz I, Schneider EM, Stolz P, Brack A, Strube J. Sensitive flow cytometric method to test basophil activation influenced by homeopathic histamine dilutions. Forsch Komplementarmed Klass Naturheilkd. 2003 Dec;10(6):316-24.

Lott IT, Doran E, Nguyen VQ, Tournay A, Head E, Gillen DL. Down syndrome and dementia: a randomized, controlled trial of antioxidant supplementation. Am J Med Genet A. 2011 Aug;155A(8):1939-48. doi: 10.1002/ajmg.a.34114.

REFERENCES AND BIBLIOGRAPHY

Lovejoy S, Pecknold S, Schertzer D. Stratified multifractal magnetization and surface geomagnetic fields-I. Spectral analysis and modeling. Geophysical Journal International. 2001 145(1):112-126.

Lovelock, J. Gaia: A New Look at Life on Earth. Oxford: Oxford Press, 1979.

Lovely RH. Recent studies in the behavioral toxicology of ELF electric and magnetic fields. Prog Clin Biol Res. 1988;257:327-47.

Lu J, Cui Y, Shi R. A Practical English-Chinese Library of Traditional Chinese Medicine: Chinese Acupuncture and Moxibustion. Shanghai: Publishing House of the Shanghai College of Traditional Chinese Medicine, 1988.

Lu Y, Zhang C, Bucheli P, Wei D. Citrus flavonoids in fruit and traditional Chinese medicinal food ingredients in China. Plant Foods Hum Nutr. 2006 Jun;61(2):57-65.

Lucas A, Morley R, Cole T, Lister G, Leeson-Payne C. Breast milk and subsequent intelligence quotient in children born premature. Lancet. 1992;339:261-264.

Lucas WB (ed). Regression Therapy: A Handbook for Professionals. Past-Life Therapy. Crest Park, CA: Deep Forest Press, 1993.

Luo C, Zhang Y, Ding Y, Shan Z, Chen S, Yu M, Hu FB, Liu L. Nut consumption and risk of type 2 diabetes, cardiovascular disease, and all-cause mortality: a systematic review and meta-analysis. Am J Clin Nutr. 2014 May 21. pii: ajcn.076109.

Lydic R, Schoene WC, Czeisler CA, Moore-Ede MC. Suprachiasmatic region of the human hypothalamus: homolog to the primate circadian pacemaker? Sleep. 1980;2(3):355-61.

Lykken DT, Tellegen A, DeRubeis R: Volunteer bias in twin research: the rule of two-thirds. Soc Biol 1978, 25(1): 1-9. Phillips DI: Twin studies in medical research: can they tell us whether diseases are genetically determined? Lancet 1993;341(8851): 1008-1009.

Lynch M, Walsh B. Genetics and Analysis of Quantitative Traits. Sunderland, MA: Sinauer, 1998.

Lythgoe JN. Visual pigments and environmental light. Vision Res. 1984;24(11):1539-50.

Lytle CD, Sagripanti JL. Predicted inactivation of viruses of relevance to biodefense by solar radiation. J Virol. 2005 Nov;79(22):14244-52.

Maas J, Jayson, J. K.. & Kleiber, D. A. Effects of spectral differences in illumination on fatigue. J Appl Psychol. 1974;59:524-526.

Mabey R, ed. The New Age Herbalist. New York: Simon & Schuster, 1941.

Maccabee PJ, Amassian VE, Cracco RQ, Cracco JB, Eberle L, Rudell A. Stimulation of the human nervous system using the magnetic coil. J Clin Neurophysiol. 1991 Jan;8(1):38-55.

Macdessi JS, Randell TL, Donaghue KC, Ambler GR, van Asperen PP, Mellis CM. Adrenal crises in children treated with high-dose inhaled corticosteroids for asthma. Med J Aust. 2003 Mar 3;178(5):214-6.

Macdonald TT, Monteleone G. Immunity, inflammation, and allergy in the gut. Science. 2005 Mar 25;307(5717):1920-5.

MacDougall D. The Soul: Hypothesis Concerning Soul Substance Together with Experimental Evidence of The Existence of Such Substance. J Am Soc Psych Res. 1907 May.

Machado RF, Laskowski D, Deffenderfer O, Burch T, Zheng S, Mazzone PJ, Mekhail T, Jennings C, Stoller JK, Pyle J, Duncan J, Dweik RA, Erzurum SC. Detection of lung cancer by sensor array analyses of exhaled breath. Am J Respir Crit Care Med. 2005 Jun 1;171(11):1286-91.

MacKay D. Science, Chance, and Providence. Oxford: Oxford Univ Press, 1978.

MacKay D. The Open Mind and Other Essays. Downer's Grove, IL: Inter-Varsity Press, 1988.

Maes HH, Silberg JL, Neale MC, Eaves LJ. Genetic and cultural transmission of antisocial behavior: an extended twin parent model. Twin Res Hum Genet. 2007 Feb;10(1):136-50.

Maes HH, Silberg JL, Neale MC, Eaves LJ. Genetic and cultural transmission of antisocial behavior: an extended twin parent model. Twin Res Hum Genet. 2007 Feb;10(1):136-50.

Magni P, Motta M, Martini L. Leptin: a possible link between food intake, energy expenditure, and reproductive function. Regul Pept. 2000 Aug 25;92(1-3):51-6.

Magnusson A, Stefansson JG. Prevalence of seasonal affective disorder in Iceland. Arch Gen Psychiatry. 1993 Dec;50(12):941-6.

Mahachoklertwattana P, Sudkronrayudh K, Direkwattanachai C, Choubtum L, Okascharoen C. Decreased cortisol response to insulin induced hypoglycaemia in asthmatics treated with inhaled fluticasone propionate. Arch Dis Child. 2004 Nov;89(11):1055-8.

Mainardi T, Kapoor S, Bielory L. Complementary and alternative medicine: herbs, phytochemicals and vitamins and their immunologic effects. J Allergy Clin Immunol. 2009 Feb;123(2):283-94; quiz 295-6.

Maity T, Adhikari A, Bhattacharya K, Biswas S, Debnath PK, Maharana CS. A study on evalution of antidepressant effect of imipramine adjunct with Aswagandha and Bramhi. Nepal Med Coll J. 2011 Dec;13(4):250-3.

Makomaski Illing EM, Kaiserman MJ. Mortality attributable to tobacco use in Canada and its regions, 1998. Can J Public Health. 2004;95(1):38-44.

Makrides M, Neumann M, Byard R, Simmer K, Gibson R. Fatty acid composition of brain, retina, and erythrocytes in breast- and formula-fed infants. Am J Clin Nutr. 1994;60:189-94.

Makrides M, Neumann M, Gibson R. Effect of maternal docosahexaenoic acid (DHA) supplementation on breast milk composition. Europ Jrnl of Clin Nutr. 1996;50:352-357.

Maliszewska-Cyna E, Lynch M, Oore JJ, Nagy PM, Aubert I. The benefits of exercise and metabolic interventions for the prevention and early treatment of Alzheimer's disease. Curr Alzheimer Res. 2016 Aug 19.

Mamidi P, Thakar AB. Efficacy of Ashwagandha (Withania somnifera Dunal. Linn.) in the management of psychogenic erectile dysfunction. Ayu. 2011 Jul;32(3):322-8.

Mander BA, Rao V, Lu B, Saletin JM, Lindquist JR, Ancoli-Israel S, Jagust W, Walker MP. Prefrontal atrophy, disrupted NREM slow waves and impaired hippocampal-dependent memory in aging. Nat Neurosci. 2013 Jan 27.

Mangialasche F, Solomon A, Kåreholt I, Hooshmand B, Cecchetti R, Fratiglioni L, Soininen H, Laatikainen T, Mecocci P, Kivipelto M. Serum levels of vitamin E forms and risk of cognitive impairment in a Finnish cohort of older adults. Exp Gerontol. 2013 Dec;48(12):1428-35. doi: 10.1016/j.exger.2013.09.006.

Mangialasche F, Westman E, Kivipelto M, Muehlboeck JS, Cecchetti R, Baglioni M, Tarducci R, Gobbi G, Floridi P, Soininen H, Kloszewska I, Tsolaki M, Vellas B, Spenger C, Lovestone S, Wahlund LO, Simmons A, Mecocci P; AddNeuroMed consortium. Classification and prediction of clinical diagnosis of Alzheimer's disease based on MRI and plasma measures of α-/γ-tocotrienols and γ-tocopherol. J Intern Med. 2013 Jun;273(6):602-21. doi: 10.1111/joim.12037.

Manjunath MJ, Muralidhara. Withania somnifera prophylaxis abrogates Rotenone-induced oxidative impairments and mitochondrial dysfunctions in striatum and cerebellum of mice: relevance to Parkinson's disease. Cent Nerv Syst Agents Med Chem. 2012 Oct 17.

Manral A, Meena P, Saini V, Siraj F, Shalini S, Tiwari M. DADS Analogues Ameliorated the Cognitive Impairments of Alzheimer-Like Rat Model Induced by Scopolamine. Neurotox Res. 2016 May 5.

Manson JE, et al. Estrogen plus progestin and the risk of coronary heart disease. NE J Med. 2003; 349(6):523–534.

Mansour HA, Monk TH, Nimgaonkar VL. Circadian genes and bipolar disorder. Ann Med. 2005;37(3):196-205.

Manthey JA, Bendele P. Anti-inflammatory activity of an orange peel polymethoxylated flavone, 3',4',3,5,6,7,8-heptamethoxyflavone, in the rat carrageenan/paw edema and mouse lipopolysaccharide-challenge assays. J Agric Food Chem. 2008 Oct 22;56(20):9399-403.

Manz F. Hydration and disease. J Am Coll Nutr. 2007 Oct;26(5 Suppl):535S-541S.

Manzoni P, Mostert M, Leonessa ML, Priolo C, Farina D, Monetti C, Latino MA, Gomirato G. Oral supplementation with Lactobacillus casei subspecies rhamnosus prevents enteric colonization by Candida species in preterm neonates: a randomized study. Clin Infect Dis. 2006 Jun 15;42(12):1735-42.

Marasanov SB, Matveev II. Correlation between protracted premedication and complication in cancer patients operated on during intense solar activity. Vopr Onkol. 2007;53(1):96-9.

Marcos A, Wärnberg J, Nova E, Gómez S, Alvarez A, Alvarez R, Mateos JA, Cobo JM. The effect of milk fermented by yogurt cultures plus Lactobacillus casei DN-114001 on the immune response of subjects under academic examination stress. Eur J Nutr. 2004 Dec;43(6):381-9.

Marcuard SP, Albernaz L, Khazanie PG. Omeprazole therapy causes malabsorption of cyanocobalamin (Vitamin B12). Ann Intern Med. 1994;120:211-5.

Marcucci F, Duse M, Frati F, Incorvaia C, Marseglia GL, La Rosa M. The future of sublingual immunotherapy. Int J Immunopathol Pharmacol. 2009 Oct-Dec;22(4 Suppl):31-3.

Marder K, Gu Y, Eberly S, Tanner CM, Scarmeas N, Oakes D, Shoulson I. Relationship of Mediterranean Diet and Caloric Intake to Phenoconversion in Huntington Disease. JAMA Neurol. 2013 Sep 2.

Margioris AN. Fatty acids and postprandial inflammation. Curr Opin Clin Nutr Metab Care. 2009 Mar;12(2):129-37.

Marie PJ. Optimizing bone metabolism in osteoporosis: insight into the pharmacologic profile of strontium ranelate. Osteoporos Int. 2003;14 Suppl 3:S9-12.

Marie PJ. Strontium ranelate: a physiological approach for optimizing bone formation and resorption. Bone. 2006 Feb;38(2 Suppl 1):S10-4.

Marin C, Ramirez R, Delgado-Lista J, Yubero-Serrano EM, Perez-Martinez P, Carracedo J, Garcia-Rios A, Rodriguez F, Gutierrez-Mariscal FM, Gomez P, Perez-Jimenez F, Lopez-Miranda J. Mediterranean diet reduces endothelial damage and improves the regenerative capacity of endothelium. Am J Clin Nutr. 2011 Feb;93(2):267-74.

Markesbery WR, Ehmann WD, Hossain TI, Alauddin M, Goodin DT. Instrumental neutron activation analysis of brain aluminum in Alzheimer disease and aging. Ann Neurol. 1981 Dec;10(6):511-6.

Marks C. Commissurotomy, Consciousness, and Unity of Mind. Cambridge: MIT Press, 1981.

Marks L. The Unity of the Senses: Interrelations among the Modalities. New York: Academic Press, 1978.

Martinez M. Docosahexaenoic acid therapy in docosahexaenoic acid-deficient patients with disorders of peroxisomal biogenesis. Versicherungsmedizin. 1996;31 Suppl:145-152

Martínez-Lapiscina EH, Clavero P, Toledo E, Estruch R, Salas-Salvadó J, San Julián B, Sanchez-Tainta A, Ros E, Valls-Pedret C, Martinez-Gonzalez MÁ. Mediterranean diet improves cognition: the PREDIMED-NAVARRA randomised trial. J Neurol Neurosurg Psychiatry. 2013 Dec;84(12):1318-25. doi: 10.1136/jnnp-2012-304792.

Martínez-Lapiscina EH, Clavero P, Toledo E, San Julián B, Sanchez-Tainta A, Corella D, Lamuela-Raventós RM, Martínez JA, Martinez-Gonzalez MÁ. Virgin olive oil supplementation and long-term cognition: the PREDIMED-NAVARRA randomized, trial. J Nutr Health Aging. 2013;17(6):544-52. doi: 10.1007/s12603-013-0027-6.

Martínez-Moreno M, Cerulla N, Chico G, Quintana M, Garolera M. Comparison of neuropsychological and functional outcomes in Alzheimer's disease patients with good or bad response to a cognitive stimulation treatment: a retrospective analysis. Int Psychogeriatr. 2016 Aug 9:1-13.

Martín-Moreno AM, Brera B, Spuch C, Carro E, García-García L, Delgado M, Pozo MA, Innamorato NG, Cuadrado A, de Ceballos ML. Prolonged oral cannabinoid administration prevents neuroinflammation, lowers β-amyloid levels and improves cognitive performance in Tg APP 2576 mice. J Neuroinflammation. 2012 Jan 16;9:8. doi: 10.1186/1742-2094-9-8.

278

REFERENCES AND BIBLIOGRAPHY

Martin-Venegas R, Roig-Perez S, Ferrer R, Moreno JJ. Arachidonic acid cascade and epithelial barrier function during Caco-2 cell differentiation. J Lipid Res. 2006 Apr;3.

Marwat SK, Rehman F, Khan EA, Khakwani AA, Ullah I, Khan KU, Khan IU. Useful ethnophytomedicinal recipes of angiosperms used against diabetes in South East Asian Countries (India, Pakistan & Sri Lanka). Pak J Pharm Sci. 2014 Sep;27(5):1333-58.

Mason D, Moore J, Green S, Liggett S. A gain-of-function polymorphism in a G-protein coupling domain of the human β1-adrenergic receptor. J. Biol. Chem. 1999;274:12670-12674.

Masoumi A, Goldenson B, Ghirmai S, Avagyan H, Zaghi J, Abel K, Zheng X, Espinosa-Jeffrey A, Mahanian M, Liu PT, Hewison M, Mizwickie M, Cashman J, Fiala M. 1alpha,25-dihydroxyvitamin D3 interacts with curcuminoids to stimulate amyloid-beta clearance by macrophages of Alzheimer's disease patients. J Alzheimers Dis. 2009;17(3):703-17. doi: 10.3233/JAD-2009-1080.

Mastorakos G, Pavlatou M. Exercise as a stress model and the interplay between the hypothalamus-pituitary-adrenal and the hypothalamus-pituitary-thyroid axes. Horm Metab Res. 2005 Sep;37(9):577-84.

Mattix KD, Winchester PD, Scherer LR. Incidence of abdominal wall defects is related to surface water atrazine and nitrate levels. J Pediatr Surg. 2007 Jun;42(6):947-9.

Matutinovic Z, Galic M. Relative magnetic hearing threshold. Laryngol Rhinol Otol. 1982 Jan;61(1):38-41.

Maurer HR. Bromelain: biochemistry, pharmacology and medical use. Cell Mol Life Sci. 2001 Aug;58(9):1234-45.

Mayr E. Toward a New Philosophy of Biology: Observations of an evolutionist. Boston: Belknap Press, 1988.

Mayron L, Ott J, Nations R, Mayron E. Light, radiation and academic behaviour: Initial studies on the effects of full-spectrum lighting and radiation shielding on behaviour and academic performance of school children. Acad Ther. 1974;10, 33-47.

McAnulty LS, Nieman DC, Dumke CL, Shooter LA, Henson DA, Utter AC, Milne G, McAnulty SR. Effect of blueberry ingestion on natural killer cell counts, oxidative stress, and inflammation prior to and after 2.5 h of running. Appl Physiol Nutr Metab. 2011 Dec;36(6):976-84. doi: 10.1139/h11-120.

McCauley B. 2005. Achieving Great Health. Spartan, Lansing, MI.

McConnaughey E. Sea Vegetables. Happy Camp, CA: Naturegraph, 1985.

McConnel JV, Cornwell PR, Clay M. An apparatus for conditioning Planaria. Am J Psychol. 1960 Dec;73:618-22.

McCrimmon RJ, Ryan CM, Frier BM. Diabetes and cognitive dysfunction. Lancet. 2012 Jun 16;379(9833):2291-9.

McCulloch M, Jezierski T, Broffman M, Hubbard A, Turner K, Janecki T. Diagnostic accuracy of canine scent detection in early- and late-stage lung and breast cancers. Integr Cancer Ther. 2006 Mar;5(1):30-9.

McDougall J, McDougall M. The McDougal Plan. Clinton, NJ: New Win, 1983.

McKhann G, Drachman D, Folstein M, Katzman R, Price D, Stadlan EM. Clinical diagnosis of Alzheimer's disease: report of the NINCDS-ADRDA Work Group under the auspices of Department of Health and Human Services Task Force on Alzheimer's Disease. Neurology 1984;34:939-44.

McLean CA, Cherny RA, Fraser FW, Fuller SJ, Smith MJ, Beyreuther K, et al. Soluble pool of Abeta amyloid as a determinant of severity of neurodegeneration in Alzheimer's disease. Ann Neurol 1999;46:860-6.

McNaught CE, Woodcock NP, MacFie J, Mitchell CJ. A prospective randomised study of the probiotic Lactobacillus plantarum 299V on indices of gut barrier function in elective surgical patients. Gut. 2002 Dec;51(6):827-31.

McTaggart L. The Field. New York: Quill, 2003.

Meador K, Loring D, Nichols M, Zamrini E, Rivner M, Posas H, Thompson E, Moore E. Preliminary findings of high-dose thiamine in dementia of Alzheimer's type. J Geriatr Psychiatry Neurol. 1993 Oct-Dec;6(4):222-9.

Mehta VV, Rajesh G, Rao A, Shenoy R, B H MP. Antimicrobial Efficacy of Punica granatum mesocarp, Nelumbo nucifera Leaf, Psidium guajava Leaf and Coffea Canephora Extract on Common Oral Pathogens: An In-vitro Study. J Clin Diagn Res. 2014 Jul;8(7):ZC65-8. doi: 10.7860/JCDR/2014/9122.4629.

Meier B, Shao Y, Julkunen-Tiitto R, Bettschart A, Sticher O. A chemotaxonomic survey of phenolic compounds in Swiss willow species. Planta Med. 1992;58:A698.

Meier B, Sticher O, Julkunen-Tiitto R. Pharmaceutical aspects of the use of willows in herbal remedies. Planta Med. 1988;54(6):559-560.

Meinecke FW. Sequelae and rehabilitation of spinal cord injuries. Curr Opin Neurol Neurosurg. 1991 Oct;4(5):714-9.

Melzack R, Coderre TJ, Katz J, Vaccarino AL. Central neuroplasticity and pathological pain. Ann N Y Acad Sci. 2001 Mar;933:157-74.

Melzack R, Wall PD. Pain mechanisms: a new theory. Science. 1965 Nov 19;150(699):971-9.

Melzack R. Evolution of the neuromatrix theory of pain. The prithvi raj lecture: presented at the third world congress of world institute of pain, barcelona 2004. Pain Pract. 2005 Jun;5(2):85-94.

Melzack R. Pain: past, present and future. Can J Exp Psychol. 1993 Dec;47(4):615-29.

Melzack R. Pain—an overview. Acta Anaesthesiol Scand. 1999 Oct;43(9):880-4.

Mendoza J. Circadian clocks: setting time by food. J Neuroendocrinol. 2007 Feb;19(2):127-37.

Merchant RE and Andre CA. 2001. A review of recent clinical trials of the nutritional supplement Chlorella pyrenoidosa in the treatment of fibromyalgia, hypertension, and ulcerative colitis. Altern Ther Health Med. May-Jun;7(3):79-91.

Messina M. Insights gained from 20 years of soy research. J Nutr. 2010 Dec;140(12):2289S-2295S. 2010 Oct 27.

Meyer A, Kirsch H, Domergue F, Abbadi A, Sperling P, Bauer J, Cirpus P, Zank TK, Moreau H, Roscoe TJ, Zahringer U, Heinz E. Novel fatty acid elongases and their use for the reconstitution of docosahexaenoic acid biosynthesis. J Lipid Res. 2004 Oct;45(10):1899-909.

Meyer A, Kirsch H, Domergue F, Abbadi A, Sperling P, Bauer J, Cirpus P, Zank TK, Moreau H, Roscoe TJ, Zahringer U, Heinz E. Novel fatty acid elongases and their use for the reconstitution of docosahexaenoic acid biosynthesis. J Lipid Res. 2004 Oct;45(10):1899-909.

Meyer AL, Elmadfa I, Herbacek I, Micksche M. Probiotic, as well as conventional yogurt, can enhance the stimulated production of proinflammatory cytokines. J Hum Nutr Diet. 2007 Dec;20(6):590-8.

Micha R, Wallace SK, Mozaffarian D. Red and processed meat consump-tion and risk of incident coronary heart disease, stroke, and diabetes mellitus: a systematic review and meta-analysis. Circulation. 2010 Jun 1;121(21):2271-83.

Milke Garcia Mdel P. Ghrelin: beyond hunger regulation. Rev Gastroenterol Mex. 2005 Oct-Dec;70(4):465-74.

Miller GT. Living in the Environment. Belmont, CA: Wadsworth, 1996.

Miller JD, Morin LP, Schwartz WJ, Moore RY. New insights into the mammalian circadian clock. Sleep. 1996 Oct;19(8):641-67.

Miller K. Cholesterol and In-Hospital Mortality in Elderly Patients. Am Family Phys. 2004 May.

Mills A. A replication study: Three cases of children in northern India who are said to remember a previous life," J. Sci. Explor. 1989;3(2):133-184.

Mimori Y, Katsuoka H, Nakamura S. Thiamine therapy in Alzheimer's disease. Metab Brain Dis. 1996 Mar;11(1):89-94.

Mindell E, Hopkins V. Prescription Alternatives. New Canaan, CT: Keats, 1998.

Mineev VN, Bulatova NI, Fedoseev GB. Erythrocyte insulin-reactive system and carbohydrate metabolism in bronchial asthma. Ter Arkh. 2002;74(3):14-7.

Minhas U, Minz R, Bhatnagar A. Prophylactic effect of Withania somnifera on inflammation in a non-autoimmune prone murine model of lupus. Drug Discov Ther. 2011 Aug;5(4):195-201.

Miranda H, Outeiro TF. The sour side of neurodegenerative disorders: the effects of protein glycation. J Pathol. 2010 May;221(1):13-25.

Mishkin M, Appenzeller T. The Anatomy of Memory. Sci. Am. 1987 June.

Mishkin M. Memory in monkeys severely impaired by combined but not by separate removal of amygdala and hippocampus. Nature. 1978;273: 297-298.

Mitchell AE, Hong YJ, Koh E, Barrett DM, Bryant DE, Denison RF, Kaffka S. Ten-year comparison of the influence of organic and conventional crop management practices on the content of flavonoids in tomatoes. J Agric Food Chem. 2007 Jul 25;55(15):6154-9.

Mitchell JL. Out-of-Body Experiences: A Handbook. New York: Ballantine Books, 1981.

Miu AC, Benga O. Aluminum and Alzheimer's disease: a new look. J Alzheimers Dis. 2006 Nov;10(2-3):179-201.

Miyazawa T, Nakagawa K, Kimura F, Satoh A, Miyazawa T. Erythrocytes carotenoids after astaxanthin supplementation in middle-aged and senior Japanese subjects. J Oleo Sci. 2011;60(10):495-9.

Miyazawa T, Nakagawa K, Kimura F, Satoh A, Miyazawa T. Plasma carotenoid concentrations before and after supplementation with astaxanthin in middle-aged and senior subjects. Biosci Biotechnol Biochem. 2011;75(9):1856-8.

Mizwicki MT, Menegaz D, Zhang J, Barrientos-Durán A, Tse S, Cashman JR, Griffin PR, Fiala M. Genomic and Nongenomic Signaling Induced by 1α,25(OH)2-Vitamin D3 Promotes the Recovery of Amyloid-β Phagocytosis by Alzheimer's Disease Macrophages. J Alzheimers Dis. 2011 Dec 29.

Modern Biology. Austin: Harcourt Brace, 1993.

Moeller AH, Ochman H. Factors that drive variation among gut microbial communities. Gut Microbes. 2013 Aug 9;4(5).

Mohammad MA, Molloy A, Scott J, Hussein L. Plasma cobalamin and folate and their metabolic markers methylmalonic acid and total homocysteine among Egyptian children before and after nutritional supplementation with the probiotic bacteria Lactobacillus acidophilus in yoghurt matrix. Int J Food Sci Nutr. 2006 Nov-Dec;57(7-8):470-80.

Mohammed AE, Smit I, Pawelzik E, Keutgen AJ, Horneburg B. Organically grown tomato (Lycopersicon esculentum Mill.): bioactive compounds in the fruit and infection with Phytophthora infestans. J Sci Food Agric. 2011 Dec 7.

Mohseni HK, Cowan D, Chettle DR, Milić AP, Priest N, Matysiak W, Atanackovic J, Byun SH, Prestwich WV. A Pilot Study Measuring Aluminum in Bone in Alzheimer's Disease and control Subjects Using in vivo Neutron Activation Analysis. J Alzheimers Dis. 2016 Jun 18;53(3):933-42.

Moini H, Packer L, Saris NE. Antioxidant and Prooxidant Activities of Alpha-Lipoic Acid and Dihydrolipoic Acid. Toxicol Appl Pharmacol. 2002;182(1):84-90.

Mok V, Xiong Y, Wong KK, Wong A, Schmidt R, Chu WW, Hu X, Lung Leung EY, Chen S, Chen Y, Tang WK, Chen X, Ho CL, Wong KS, Wong ST. Predictors for cognitive decline in patients with confluent white matter hyperintensities. Alzheimers Dement. 2012 Nov;8(5 Suppl):S96-S103. doi: 10.1016/j.jalz.2011.10.004.

Monarca S. Zerbini I, Simonati C, Gelatti U. Drinking water hardness and chronic degenerative diseases. Part II. Cardiovascular diseases. Ann. Ig. 2003;15:41-56.

Monji A. The neuroinflammation hypothesis of psychiatric disorders. Seishin Shinkeigaku Zasshi. 2012;114(2):124-33.

Monod J. Chance and Necessity. New York: Vintage, 1972.

Monroe R. Far Journeys. Garden City, NY: Doubleday & Co., 1985.

Monroe R. Journeys Out of the Body. Garden City, NY: Anchor Press, 1977.

Montanes P, Goldblum MC, Boller F. The naming impairment of living and nonliving items in Alzheimer's disease. J Int Neuropsychol Soc. 1995 Jan;1(1):39-48.

REFERENCES AND BIBLIOGRAPHY

Moody R. Coming Back: A Psychiatrist Explores Past-Life Journeys. New York: Bantam Books, 1991.

Moody R. Life After Life. New York: Bantam, 1975.

Moody, R. Reflections on Life After Life: More Important Discoveries In The Ongoing Investigation Of Survival Of Life After Bodily Death. New York: Bantam, 1977.

Moore KH. Conservative management for urinary incontinence. Baillieres Best Pract Res Clin Obstet Gynaecol. 2000 Apr;14(2):251-89.

Moore R. Circadian Rhythms: A Clock for the Ages. Science 1999 June 25;284(5423):2102 – 2103.

Moore RY, Speh JC. Serotonin innervation of the primate suprachiasmatic nucleus. Brain Res. 2004 Jun 4;1010(1-2):169-73.

Moore RY. Neural control of the pineal gland. Behav Brain Res. 1996;73(1-2):125-30.

Moore RY. Organization and function of a central nervous system circadian oscillator: the suprachiasmatic hypothalamic nucleus. Fed Proc. 1983 Aug;42(11):2783-9.

Morasch KC, Aaron CL, Moon JE, Gordon RK. Physiological and neurobehavioral effects of cholinesterase inhibition in healthy adults. Physiol Behav. 2015 Jan;138:165-72. doi: 10.1016/j.physbeh.2014.09.010.

Morick H. Introduction to the Philosophy of Mind: Readings from Descartes to Strawson. Glenview, Ill: Scott Foresman, 1970.

Morimoto K, Takeshita T, Nanno M, Tokudome S, Nakayama K. Modulation of natural killer cell activity by supplementation of fermented milk containing Lactobacillus casei in habitual smokers. Prev Med. 2005 May;40(5):589-94.

Mormino EC, Brandel MG, Madison CM, Rabinovici GD, Marks S, Baker SL, et al. Not quite PIB-positive, not quite PIB-negative: slight PIB elevations in elderly normal control subjects are biologically relevant. Neuroimage 2012;59:1152-60.

Morris JC, Roe CM, Grant EA, Head D, Storandt M, Goate AM, et al. Pittsburgh compound B imaging and prediction of progression from cognitive normality to symptomatic Alzheimer disease. Arch Neurol 2009;66:1469-75.

Morris MS. The role of B vitamins in preventing and treating cognitive impairment and decline. Adv Nutr. 2012 Nov 1;3(6):801-12.

Morse M. Closer to the Light. New York: Ivy Books, 1990.

Morton C. Velocity Alters Electric Field. www.amasci.com/ freenrg/ morton1.html. Accessed 2007 July.

Morton G. Hypothalamic Leptin Regulation of Energy Homeostasis and Glucose Metabolism. J Physiol. 2007 Jun 21.

Moshe M. Method and apparatus for predicting the occurrence of an earthquake by identifying electromagnetic precursors. US Patent Issued on May 28, 1996. Number 5521508.

Moss M, Cook J, Wesnes K, Duckett P. Aromas of rosemary and lavender essential oils differentially affect cognition and mood in healthy adults. Int J Neurosci. 2003 Jan;113(1):15-38.

Motoyama H. Acupuncture Meridians. Science & Medicine. 1999 July/August.

Motoyama H. Before Polarization Current and the Acupuncture Meridians. Journal of Holistic Medicine. 1986;8(1&2).

Motoyama H. Deficient/ Excessive Patterns Found in Meridian Functioning in Cases of Liver Disease. Subtle Energy & Energy Medicine. 2000; 11(2).

Motoyama H. Energetic Medicine: new science of healing: An interview with A. Jackson. www.shareintl.org/archives/health-healing/hh_adjenergetic.html. Acc. 2007 Oct.

Motoyama H. Smith, W. Harada T. Pre-Polarization Resistance of the Skin as Determined by the Single Square Voltage Pulse. Psychophysiology. 1984;21(5).

Moussaieff A, Shein NA, Tsenter J, Grigoriadis S, Simeonidou C, Alexandrovich AG, Trembovler V, Ben-Neriah Y, Schmitz ML, Fiebich BL, Munoz E, Mechoulam R, Shohami E. Incensole acetate: a novel neuroprotective agent isolated from Boswellia carterii. J Cereb Blood Flow Metab. 2008 Jul;28(7):1341-52.

Mozafar A. Enrichment of some B-vitamin in plants with application of organic fertilizers. Plant and Soil. 1994;167:305-11.

Mozafar A. Is there vitamin B12 in plants or not? A plant nutritionist's view. Veg Nutr. 1997;1/2:50-52.

Mozaffarian D, Aro A, Willett WC. Health effects of trans fatty acids: experimental and observational evidence. Eur J Clin Nutr. 2009 May;63 Suppl 2:S5-21.

Muhlack S, Lemmer W, Klotz P, Muller T, Lehmann E, Klieser E. Anxiolytic effect of rescue remedy for psychiatric patients: a double-blind, placebo-controlled, randomized trial. J Clin Psychopharmacol. 2006 Oct;26(5):541-2.

Mukaetova-Ladinska EB, Garcia-Siera F, Hurt J, Gertz HJ, Xuereb JH, Hills R, et al. Staging of cytoskeletal and beta-amyloid changes in human isocortex reveals biphasic synaptic protein response during progression of Alzheimer's disease. Am J Pathol 2000;157:623-36.

Muller H, Lindman AS, Blomfeldt A, Seljeflot I, Pedersen JI. A diet rich in coconut oil reduces diurnal postprandial variations in circulating tissue plasminogen activator antigen and fasting lipoprotein (a) compared with a diet rich in unsaturated fat in women. J Nutr. 2003 Nov;133(11):3422-7.

Müller JP, Steinegger A, Schlatter C. Contribution of aluminum from packaging materials and cooking utensils to the daily aluminum intake. Z Lebensm Unters Forsch. 1993 Oct;197(4):332-41.

Mulvihill EE, Assini JM, Lee JK, Allister EM, Sutherland BG, Koppes JB, Sawyez CG, Edwards JY, Telford DE, Charbonneau A, St-Pierre P, Marette A, Huff MW. Nobiletin attenuates VLDL overproduction, dyslipidemia, and atherosclerosis in mice with diet-induced insulin resistance. Diabetes. 2011 May;60(5):1446-57.

Mumby DG, Wood ER, Pinel J. Object-recognition memory is only mildly impaired in rats with lesions of the hippocampus and amygdala. Psychobio. 1992;20: 18-27.

281

Municino A, Nicolino A, Milanese M, Gronda E, Andreuzzi B, Oliva F, Chiarella F, Cardio-HKT Study Group. Hydrotherapy in advanced heart failure: the cardio-HKT pilot study. Monaldi Arch Chest Dis. 2006 Dec;66(4):247-54.

Munro, I. C., Harwood, M., Hlywka, J. J., Stephen, A. M., Doull, J., Flamm, W. G. & Adlercreutz, H. 2005. Soy isoflavones: a safety review. Nutr. Rev. 61:1-33. J Pediatr Gastroenterol Nutr. Nov;41(5):660-6.

Muralikrishna G, Rao MV. Cereal non-cellulosic polysaccharides: structure and function relationship—an overview. Crit Rev Food Sci Nutr. 2007;47(6):599-610.

Murchie G. The Seven Mysteries of Life. Boston: Houghton Mifflin Company, 1978.

Murphy M, Eliot K, Heuertz RM, Weiss E. Whole beetroot consumption acutely improves running performance. J Acad Nutr Diet. 2012 Apr;112(4):548-52.

Murphy R. Organon Philosophy Workbook. Blacksburg, VA: HANA, 1994.

Murray M and Pizzorno J. Encyclopedia of Natural Medicine. 2nd Edition. Roseville, CA: Prima Publishing, 1998.

Murray ME, Ferman TJ, Boeve BF, Przybelski SA, Lesnick TG, Liesinger AM, Senjem ML, Gunter JL, Preboske GM, Lowe VJ, Vemuri P, Dugger BN, Knopman DS, Smith GE, Parisi JE, Silber MH, Graff-Radford NR, Petersen RC, Jack CR Jr, Dickson DW, Kantarci K. MRI and pathology of REM sleep behavior disorder in dementia with Lewy bodies. Neurology. 2013 Oct 9.

Musaev AV, Nasrullaeva SN, Zeinalov RG. Effects of solar activity on some demographic indices and morbidity in Azerbaijan with reference to A. L. Chizhevsky's theory. Vopr Kurortol Fizioter Lech Fiz Kult. 2007 May-Jun;(3):38-42.

Muzzarelli L, Force M, Sebold M. Aromatherapy and reducing preprocedural anxiety: A controlled prospective study. Gastroenterol Nurs. 2006 Nov-Dec;29(6):466-71.

Myss C. Anatomy of the Spirit. New York: Harmony, 1996.

Mythri RB, Bharath MS. Curcumin: A Potential Neuroprotective Agent in Parkinson's Disease. Curr Pharm Des. 2012 Jan 1.

Mythri RB, Harish G, Dubey SK, Misra K, Bharath MM. Glutamoyl diester of the dietary polyphenol curcumin offers improved protection against peroxynitrite-mediated nitrosative stress and damage of brain mitochondria in vitro: implications for Parkinson's disease. Mol Cell Biochem. 2011 Jan;347(1-2):135-43.

Nadkarni AK, Nadkarni KM. Indian Materia Medica. (Vols 1 and 2). Bombay, India: Popular Pradashan, 1908, 1976.

Nagappan A, Karunanithi N, Sentrayaperumal S, Park KI, Park HS, Lee do H, Kang SR, Kim JA, Senthil K, Natesan S, Muthurajan R, Kim GS. Comparative root protein profiles of Korean ginseng (Panax ginseng) and Indian ginseng (Withania somnifera). Am J Chin Med. 2012;40(1):203-18.

Nair PK, Rodriguez S, Ramachandran R, Alamo A, Melnick SJ, Escalon E, Garcia PI Jr, Wnuk SF, Ramachandran C. Immune stimulating properties of a novel polysaccharide from the medicinal plant Tinospora cordifolia. Int Immunopharmacol. 2004 Dec 15;4(13):1645-59.

Nakajima H, Fukazawa K, Wakabayashi Y, Wakamatsu K, Imokawa G. Erratum to: Withania somnifera extract attenuates stem cell factor-stimulated pigmentation in human epidermal equivalents through interruption of ERK phosphorylation within melanocytes. J Nat Med. 2013 Jan 25.

Nakajima H, Wakabayashi Y, Wakamatsu K, Imokawa G. An Extract of Withania somnifera Attenuates Endothelin-1-stimulated Pigmentation in Human Epidermal Equivalents through the Interruption of PKC Activity Within Melanocytes. Phytother Res. 2012 Dec 3.

Nakamura K, Urayama K, Hoshino Y. Lumbar cerebrospinal fluid pulse wave rising from pulsations of both the spinal cord and the brain in humans. Spinal Cord. 1997 Nov;35(11):735-9.

Nakamura MT, Nara TY. Structure, function, and dietary regulation of delta6, delta5, and delta9 desaturases. Ann Rev Nutr. 2004;24:345-76.

Nakatani K, Yau KW. Calcium and light adaptation in retinal rods and cones. Nature. 1988 Jul 7;334(6177):69-71.

Napoli N, Thompson J, Civitelli R, Armamento-Villareal R. Effects of dietary calcium compared with calcium supplements on estrogen metabolism and bone mineral density. Am J Clin Nutr. 2007;85(5): 1428-1433.

Naruszewicz M, Daniewski M, Nowicka G, Kozlowska-Wojciechowska M. Trans-unsaturated fatty acids and acrylamide in food as potential atherosclerosis progression factors. Based on own studies. Acta Microbiol Pol. 2003;52 Suppl:75-81.

Naruszewicz M, Daniewski M, Nowicka G, Kozlowska-Wojciechowska M. Trans-unsaturated fatty acids and acrylamide in food as potential atherosclerosis progression factors. Based on own studies. Acta Microbiol Pol. 2003;52 Suppl:75-81.

Natarajan E, Grissom C. The Origin of Magnetic Field Dependent Recombination in Alkylcobalamin Radical Pairs. Photochem Photobiol. 1996;64: 286-295.

National Institutes of Health. Third Report of the National Cholesterol Education Program (NCEP) Expert Panel on Detection, Evaluation, and Treatment of High Blood Cholesterol in Adults (PDF), July 2004, The National Institutes of Heath: The National Heart, Lung, and Blood Institute.

National Toxicology Program. Final Report on Carcinogens Background Document for Formaldehyde. Rep Carcinog Backgr Doc. 2010 Jan;(10-5981):i-512.

Navarro Silvera SA, Rohan TE. Trace elements and cancer risk: a review of the epidemiologic evidence. Cancer Causes Control. 2007 Feb;18(1):7-27.

NDL, BHNRC, ARS, USDA. Oxygen Radical Absorbance Capacity (ORAC) of Selected Foods—2007. Beltsville, MD: USDA-ARS. 2007.

Neal EG, Chaffe H, Schwartz RH, Lawson MS, Edwards N, Fitzsimmons G, Whitney A, Cross JH. The ketogenic diet for the treatment of childhood epilepsy: a randomised controlled trial. Lancet Neurol. 2008;7:500–506.

REFERENCES AND BIBLIOGRAPHY

Neal EG, Chaffe H, Schwartz RH, Lawson MS, Edwards N, Fitzsimmons G, Whitney A, Cross JH. The ketogenic diet for the treatment of childhood epilepsy: a randomised controlled trial. Lancet Neurol. 2008;7:500–506.

Neeck G, Riedel W. Hormonal perturbations in fibromyalgia syndrome. Ann N Y Acad Sci. 1999;876:325-38.

Neff LM, Culiner J, Cunningham-Rundles S, Seidman C, Meehan D, Maturi J, Wittkowski KM, Levine B, Breslow JL. Algal docosahexaenoic acid affects plasma lipoprotein particle size distribution in overweight and obese adults. J Nutr. 2011 Feb;141(2):207-13.

Nelson PT, Braak H, Markesbery WR. Neuropathology and cognitive impairment in Alzheimer disease: a complex but coherent relationship. J Neuropathol Exp Neurol 2009;68:1-14.

Nestel PJ. Adulthood—prevention: Cardiovascular disease. Med J Aust. 2002 Jun 3;176(11 Suppl):S118-9.

Nestor PJ, Graham KS, Bozeat S, Simons JS, Hodges JR. Memory consolidation and the hippocampus: further evidence from studies of autobiographical memory in semantic dementia and frontal variant frontotemporal dementia. Neuropsychologia. 2002;40(6):633-54.

Newall CA, Anderson LA, Phillipson JD (eds). Herbal Medicines: A Guide for Health-Care Professionals. London: Pharmaceut Press; 1996.

Newmark T, Schulick P. Beyond Aspirin. Prescott, AZ: Holm, 2000.

Newton PE. The Effect of Sound on Plant Grwoth. JAES. 1971 Mar;19(3): 202-205.

Neyestani TR, Shariatzadeh N, Gharavi A, Kalayi A, Khalaji N. Physiological dose of lycopene suppressed oxidative stress and enhanced serum levels of immunoglobulin M in patients with Type 2 diabetes mellitus: a possible role in the prevention of long-term complications. J Endocrinol Invest. 2007 Nov;30(10):833-8.

Ngai SP, Jones AY, Hui-Chan CW, Ko FW, Hui DS. Effect of Acu-TENS on post-exercise expiratory lung volume in subjects with asthma-A randomized controlled trial. Respir Physiol Neurobiol. 2009 Jul 31;167(3):348-53. 2009 Jun 18.

Nicholls SJ, Lundman P, Harmer JA, Cutri B, Griffiths KA, Rye KA, Barter PJ, Celermajer DS. Consumption of saturated fat impairs the anti-inflammatory properties of high-density lipoproteins and endothelial function. J Am Coll Cardiol. 2006 Aug 15;48(4):715-20.

Niculescu MD, Wu R, Guo Z, da Costa KA, Zeisel SH. Diethanolamine alters proliferation and choline metabolism in mouse neural precursor cells. Toxicol Sci. 2007 Apr;96(2):321-6.

Nie L, Wise M, Peterson D, Meydani M. Mechanism by which avenanthramide-c, a polyphenol of oats, blocks cell cycle progression in vascular smooth muscle cells. Free Radic Biol Med. 2006 Sep 1;41(5):702-8.

Nie L, Wise ML, Peterson DM, Meydani M. Avenanthramide, a polyphenol from oats, inhibits vascular smooth muscle cell proliferation and enhances nitric oxide production. Atherosclerosis. 2006 Jun;186(2):260-6.

Niederau C, Göpfert E. The effect of chelidonium- and turmeric root extract on upper abdominal pain due to functional disorders of the biliary system. Results from a placebo-controlled double-blind study. Med Klin. 1999 Aug 15;94(8):425-30.

Nies LK, Cymbala AA, Kasten SL, Lamprecht DG, Olson KL. Complementary and alternative therapies for the management of dyslipidemia. Ann Pharmacother. 2006 Nov;40(11):1984-92.

Nievergelt CM, Kripke DF, Remick RA, Sadovnick AD, McElroy SL, Keck PE Jr, Kelsoe JR. Examination of the clock gene Cryptochrome 1 in bipolar disorder: mutational analysis and absence of evidence for linkage or association. Psychiatr Genet. 2005 Mar;15(1):45-52.

Niggli H. Temperature dependence of ultraweak photon emission in fibroblastic differentiation after irradiation with artificial sunlight. Indian J Exp Biol. 2003 May;41:419-423.

Nishigori C, Hattori Y, Toyokuni S. Role of reactive oxygen species in skin carcinogenesis. Antioxid Redox Signal. 2004 Jun;6(3):561-70.

Noone EJ, Roche HM, Nugent AP, Gibney MJ. The effect of dietary supplementation using isomeric blends of conjugated linoleic acid on lipid metabolism in healthy human subjects. Br J Nutr. 2002 Sep;88(3):243-51.

Noorbakhsh R, Mortazavi SA, Sankian M, Shahidi F, Assarehzadegan MA, Varasteh A. Cloning, expression, characterization, and computational approach for cross-reactivity prediction of manganese superoxide dismutase allergen from pistachio nut. Allergol Int. 2010 Sep;59(3):295-304.

North J. The Fontana History of Astronomy and Cosmology. London: Fontana Press, 1994.

O'Brien J, Okereke O, Devore E, Rosner B, Breteler M, Grodstein F. Long-term intake of nuts in relation to cognitive function in older women. J Nutr Health Aging. 2014;18(5):496-502. doi: 10.1007/s12603-014-0014-6.

O'Connor J., Bensky D. (ed). Shanghai College of Traditional Chinese Medicine: Acupuncture: A Comprehensive Text. Seattle: Eastland Press, 1981.

O'Donnell MJ, Yusuf S, Mente A, Gao P, Mann JF, Teo K, McQueen M, Sleight P, Sharma AM, Dans A, Probstfield J, Schmieder RE. Urinary sodium and potassium excretion and risk of cardiovascular events. JAMA. 2011 Nov 23;306(20):2229-38. doi: 10.1001/jama.2011.1729.

O'Dwyer JJ. College Physics. Pacific Grove, CA: Brooks/Cole, 1990.

O'Neil CE, Nicklas TA, Rampersaud GC, Fulgoni VL 3rd. One hundred percent orange juice consumption is associated with better diet quality, improved nutrient adequacy, and no increased risk for overweight/obesity in children. Nutr Res. 2011 Sep;31(9):673-82.

O'Brien SJ, Shannon JE, Gail MH. A molecular approach to the identification and individualization of human and animal cells in culture: isozyme and allozyme genetic signatures. In Vitro. 1980 Feb;16(2):119-35.

O'Connell OF, Ryan L, O'Brien N. Xanthophyll carotenoids are more bioaccessible from fruits than dark green vegetables. Nutr Res. 2007;27(5):258-264.

O'Connor J., Bensky D. (ed). Shanghai College of Traditional Chinese Medicine: Acupuncture: A Comprehensive Text. Seattle: Eastland Press, 1981.

Oehme FW (ed.). Toxicity of heavy metals in the environment. Part 1. New York: M.Dekker, 1979.

Oh CK, Lücker PW, Wetzelsberger N, Kuhlmann F. The determination of magnesium, calcium, sodium and potassium in assorted foods with special attention to the loss of electrolytes after various forms of food preparations. Mag.-Bull. 1986;8:297-302.

Oh CK, Lücker PW, Wetzelsberger N, Kuhlmann F. The determination of magnesium, calcium, sodium and potassium in assorted foods with special attention to the loss of electrolytes after various forms of food preparations. Mag.-Bull. 1986;8:297-302.

Ohara T, Doi Y, Ninomiya T, Hirakawa Y, Hata J, Iwaki T, Kanba S, Kiyohara Y. Glucose tolerance status and risk of dementia in the community: The Hisayama Study. Neurology. 2011 Sep 20;77(12):1126-34.

Okamura H. Clock genes in cell clocks: roles, actions, and mysteries. J Biol Rhythms. 2004 Oct;19(5):388-99.

Okayama Y, Begishvili TB, Church MK. Comparison of mechanisms of IL-3 induced histamine release and IL-3 priming effect on human basophils. Clin Exp Allergy. 1993 Nov;23(11):901-10.

Okazaki Y, Isobe T, Iwata Y, Matsukawa T, Matsuda F, Miyagawa H, Ishihara A, Nishioka T, Iwamura H. Metabolism of avenanthramide phytoalexins in oats. Plant J. 2004 Aug;39(4):560-72.

Okello A, Koivunen J, Edison P, Archer HA, Turkheimer FE, Någren K, et al. Conversion of amyloid positive and negative MCI to AD over 3 years: an 11C-PIB PET study. Neurology 2009;73:754-60.

Olde Rikkert MG, Verhey FR, Blesa R, von Arnim CA, Bongers A, Harrison J, Sijben J, Scarpini E, Vandewoude MF, Vellas B, Witkamp R, Kamphuis PJ, Scheltens P. Tolerability and safety of Souvenaid in patients with mild Alzheimer's disease: results of multi-center, 24-week, open-label extension study. J Alzheimers Dis. 2015;44(2):471-80. doi: 10.3233/JAD-141305.

Ole D. Rughede, On the Theory and Physics of the Aether. Progress in Physics. 2006; (1).

O'Leary KD, Rosenbaum A, Hughes PC. Fluorescent lighting: a purported source of hyperactive behavior. J Abnorm Child Psychol. 1978 Sep;6(3):285-9.

Olney JW, Farber NB, Spitznagel E, Robins LN. Increasing brain tumor rates: is there a link to aspartame? J Neuropathol Exp Neurol. 1996;55:1115-23.

Olney JW. Excitotoxins in foods. Neurotoxicology. 1994;15:535-44.

Onder G, Landi F, Volpato S, Fellin R, Carbonin P, Gambassi G, Bernabei R. Serum cholesterol levels and in-hospital mortality in the elderly. Am J Med. 2003 Sept;115:265-71

One Hundred Million Americans See Medical Mistakes Directly Touching Them as Patients, Friends, Relatives. National Patient Safety Foundation. Press Release. 1997 Oct 9. http://npsf.org/pr/pressrel/ finalsur.htm. Acc. 2007 Mar.

Oosterga M, ten Vaarwerk IA, DeJongste MJ, Staal MJ. Spinal cord stimulation in refractory angina pectoris—clinical results and mechanisms. Z Kardiol. 1997;86 Suppl 1:107-13.

Ostrander S, Schroeder L, Ostrander N. Super-Learning. New York: Delta, 1979.

Otani S. Memory trace in prefrontal cortex: theory for the cognitive switch. Biol Rev Camb Philos Soc. 2002 Nov;77(4):563-77.

Otsu A, Chinami M, Morgenthale S, Kaneko Y, Fujita D, Shirakawa T. Correlations for number of sunspots, unemployment rate, and suicide mortality in Japan. Percept Mot Skills. 2006 Apr;102(2):603-8.

Ott J. Color and Light: Their Effects on Plants, Animals, and People (Series of seven articles in seven issues). Internl J Biosoc Res. 1985-1991.

Ott J. Health and Light: The Effects of Natural and Artificial Light on Man and Other Living Things. Self published, 1973,

Otto SJ, van Houwelingen AC, Hornstra G. The effect of supplementation with docosahexaenoic and arachidonic acid derived from single cell oils on plasma and erythrocyte fatty acids of pregnant women in the second trimester. Prost Leuk Essent Fatty Acids. 2000 Nov;63(5):323-8.

Ou CC, Tsao SM, Lin MC, Yin MC. Protective action on human LDL against oxidation and glycation by four organosulfur compounds derived from garlic. Lipids. 2003 Mar;38(3):219-24.

Ozawa M, Ninomiya T, Ohara T, Doi Y, Uchida K, Shirota T, Yonemoto K, Kitazono T, Kiyohara Y. Dietary patterns and risk of dementia in an elderly Japanese population: the Hisayama Study. Am J Clin Nutr. 2013 May;97(5):1076-82. doi: 10.3945/ajcn.112.045575.

Packard CC. Pocket Guide to Ayurvedic Healing. Freedom, CA: Crossing Press, 1996.

Palo-Bengtsson L, Ekman SL. Emotional response to social dancing and walks in persons with dementia. Am J Alzheimers Dis Other Demen. 2002 May-Jun;17(3):149-53.

Palo-Bengtsson L, Ekman SL. Social dancing in the care of persons with dementia in a nursing home setting: a phenomenological study. Sch Inq Nurs Pract. 1997 Spring;11(2):101-18; discussion 119-23.

Palo-Bengtsson L, Winblad B, Ekman SL. Social dancing: a way to support intellectual, emotional and motor functions in persons with dementia. J Psychiatr Ment Health Nurs. 1998 Dec;5(6):545-54.

Pan A, Chen M, Chowdhury R, Wu JH, Sun Q, Campos H, Mozaffarian D, Hu FB. α-Linolenic acid and risk of cardiovascular disease: a systematic review and meta-analysis. Am J Clin Nutr. 2012 Oct 17.

Pan A, Sun Q, Bernstein AM, Manson JE, Willett WC, Hu FB. Changes in red meat consumption and subsequent risk of type 2 diabetes mellitus: three cohorts of US men and women. JAMA Intern Med. 2013 Jul 22;173(14):1328-35. doi: 10.1001/jamainternmed.2013.6633.

Pan A, Sun Q, Bernstein AM, Schulze MB, Manson JE, Stampfer MJ, Willett WC, Hu FB. Red meat consumption and mortality: results from 2 prospective cohort studies. Arch Intern Med. 2012 Apr 9;172(7):555-63. doi: 10.1001/archinternmed.2011.2287.

REFERENCES AND BIBLIOGRAPHY

Pan A, Sun Q, Bernstein AM, Schulze MB, Manson JE, Willett WC, Hu FB. Red meat consumption and risk of type 2 diabetes: 3 cohorts of US adults and an updated meta-analysis. Am J Clin Nutr. 2011 Oct;94(4):1088-96.

Pandit S, Chang KW, Jeon JG. Effects of Withania somnifera on the growth and virulence properties of Streptococcus mutans and Streptococcus sobrinus at sub-MIC levels. Anaerobe. 2013 Feb;19:1-8.

Panghal S, Mallapur SS, Kumar M, Ram V, Singh BK. Antiinflammatory Activity of Piper longum Fruit Oil. Indian J Pharm Sci. 2009 Jul;71(4):454-6.

Pardini M, Serrati C, Guida S, Mattei C, Abate L, Massucco D, Sassos D, Amore M, Krueger F, Cocito L, Emberti Gialloreti L. Souvenaid reduces behavioral deficits and improves social cognition skills in frontotemporal dementia: a proof-of-concept study. Neurodegener Dis. 2015;15(1):58-62. doi: 10.1159/000369811.

Park AE, Fernandez JJ, Schmedders K, Cohen MS. The Fibonacci sequence: relationship to the human hand. J Hand Surg. 2003 Jan;28(1):157-60.

Park BJ, Tsunetsugu Y, Kasetani T, Kagawa T, Miyazaki Y. The physiological effects of Shinrin-yoku (taking in the forest atmosphere or forest bathing): evidence from field experiments in 24 forests across Japan. Environ Health Prev Med. 2010 Jan;15(1):18-26.

Parra MD, Martínez de Morentin BE, Cobo JM, Mateos A, Martínez JA. Daily ingestion of fermented milk containing Lactobacillus casei DN114001 improves innate-defense capacity in healthy middle-aged people. J Physiol Biochem. 2004 Jun;60(2):85-91.

Partonen T, Haukka J, Nevanlinna H, Lonnqvist J. Analysis of the seasonal pattern in suicide. J Affect Disord. 2004 Aug;81(2):133-9.

Patocka J. Anti-inflammatory triterpenoids from mysterious mushroom Ganoderma lucidum and their potential possibility in modern medicine. Acta Medica (Hradec Kralove). 1999;42(4):123-5

Patwardhan B, Gautam M. Botanical immunodrugs: scope and opportunities. Drug Discov Today. 2005 Apr 1;10(7):495-502.

Pavlin M, Repič M, Vianello R, Mavri J. The Chemistry of Neurodegeneration: Kinetic Data and Their Implications. Mol Neurobiol. 2016 Jul;53(5):3400-15. doi: 10.1007/s12035-015-9284-1. Epub 2015 Jun 18.

Pedrosa MC, Golner BB, Goldin BR, Barakat S, Dallal GE, Russell RM. Survival of yogurt-containing organisms and Lactobacillus gasseri (ADH) and their effect on bacterial enzyme activity in the gastrointestinal tract of healthy and hypochlorhydric elderly subjects. Am J Clin Nutr. 1995 Feb;61(2):353-9.

Pehowich DJ, Gomes AV, Barnes JA. Fatty acid composition and possible health effects of coconut constituents. West Indian Med J. 2000 Jun;49(2):128-33.

Pelsser LM, Frankena K, Toorman J, Savelkoul HF, Dubois AE, Pereira RR, Haagen TA, Rommelse NN, Buitelaar JK. Effects of a restricted elimination diet on the behaviour of children with attention-deficit hyperactivity disorder (INCA study): a randomised controlled trial. Lancet. 2011 Feb 5;377(9764):494-503.

Pendell D. Plant Powers, Poisons, and Herbcraft. San Francisco: Mercury House, 1995.

Peng Y, Hu Y, Xu S, Feng N, Wang L, Wang X. L-3-n-butylphthalide regulates amyloid precursor protein processing by PKC and MAPK pathways in SK-N-SH cells over-expressing wild type human APP695. Neurosci Lett. 2011 Jan 7;487(2):211-6.

Peng Y, Hu Y, Xu S, Li P, Li J, Lu L, Yang H, Feng N, Wang L, Wang X. L-3-n-butylphthalide Reduces Tau Phosphorylation and Improves Cognitive Deficits in AβPP/PS1-Alzheimer's Transgenic Mice. J Alzheimers Dis. 2012 Jan 10.

Peng Y, Sun J, Hon S, Nylander AN, Xia W, Feng Y, Wang X, Lemere CA. L-3-n-butylphthalide improves cognitive impairment and reduces amyloid-beta in a transgenic model of Alzheimer's disease. J Neurosci. 2010 Jun 16;30(24):8180-9.

Peng Y, Yang X, Zhang Y. 2005. Microbial fibrinolytic enzymes: an overview of source, production, properties, and thrombolytic activity in vivo. Appl Microbiol Biotechnol. Nov;69(2):126-32.

Pengelly A, Snow J, Mills SY, Scholey A, Wesnes K, Butler LR. Short-term study on the effects of rosemary on cognitive function in an elderly population. J Med Food. 2012 Jan;15(1):10-7. doi: 10.1089/jmf.2011.0005.

Penn RD, Hagins WA. Kinetics of the photocurrent of retinal rods. Biophys J. 1972 Aug;12(8):1073-94.

Penn RD, Hagins WA. Signal transmission along retinal rods and the origin of the electroretinographic a-wave. Nature. 1969 Jul 12;223(5202):201-4.

Penson RT, Kyriakou H, Zuckerman D, Chabner BA, Lynch TJ Jr. Teams: communication in multidisciplinary care. Oncologist. 2006 May;11(5):520-6.

Perez-Galvez A, Martin HD, Sies H, Stahl W. Incorporation of carotenoids from paprika oleoresin into human chylomicrons. Br J Nutr. 2003 Jun;89(6):787-93.

Perez-Galvez A, Martin HD, Sies H, Stahl W. Incorporation of carotenoids from paprika oleoresin into human chylomicrons. Br J Nutr. 2003 Jun;89(6):787-93.

Perez-Pena R. Secrets of the Mummy's Medicine Chest. NY Times. 2005 Sept 10.

Perl DP, Moalem S. Aluminum and Alzheimer's disease, a personal perspective after 25 years. J Alzheimers Dis. 2006;9(3 Suppl):291-300.

Peroxisomes from pepper fruits (Capsicum annuum L.): purification, characterisation and antioxidant activity. J Plant Physiol. 2003 Dec;160(12):1507-16.

Perreau-Lenz S, Kalsbeek A, Van Der Vliet J, Pevet P, Buijs RM. In vivo evidence for a controlled offset of melatonin synthesis at dawn by the suprachiasmatic nucleus in the rat. Neuroscience. 2005;130(3):797-803.

Perrin RJ, Fagan AM, Holtzman DM. Multimodal techniques for diagnosis and prognosis of Alzheimer's disease. Nature 2009;461:916-22.

Perry G, Phelix CF, Nunomura A, Colom LV, Castellani RJ, Petersen RB, Lee HG, Zhu X. Untangling the vascular web from Alzheimer disease and oxidative stress. Can J Neurol Sci. 2012 Jan;39(1):4.

Perry J. A Dialogue on Personal Identity and Immortality. Indianapolis, IN: Hackett, 1978.

Perry J. Personal Identity. Berkeley: University of California Press, 1975.

Persinger M.A. Psi phenomena and temporal lobe activity: The geomagnetic factor. In L.A. Henkel & R.E. Berger (Eds.), Research in parapsychology. (121- 156). Metuchen, NJ: Scarecrow Press, 1989.

Persinger M.A., Krippner S. Dream ESP experiments and geomagnetic activity. Journal of the American Society of Psychical Research. 1989;83:101- 106.

Persson R, Orbaek P, Kecklund G, Akerstedt T. Impact of an 84-hour workweek on biomarkers for stress, metabolic processes and diurnal rhythm. Scand J Work Environ Health. 2006 Oct;32(5):349-58.

Persson R, Orbaek P, Kecklund G, Akerstedt T. Impact of an 84-hour workweek on biomarkers for stress, metabolic processes and diurnal rhythm. Scand J Work Environ Health. 2006 Oct;32(5):349-58.

Pert C. Molecules of Emotion. New York: Scribner, 1997.

Peter JJ, Beecher GR, Bhagwat SA, Dwyer JT, Gebhardt SE, Haytowitz DB, Holden JM. Flavanones in grapefruit, lemons, and limes: A compilation and review of the data from the analytical literature. Jrnl Food Comp and Anal. 2006;19:S74-S80.

Petersen RC, Smith GE, Waring SC, Ivnik RJ, Tangalos EG, Kokmen E. Mild cognitive impairment: clinical characterization and outcome. Arch Neurol 1999;56:303-8.

Petersen RC. Alzheimer's disease: progress in prediction. Lancet Neurol 2010;9:4-5.

Peth-Nui T, Wattanathorn J, Muchimapura S, Tong-Un T, Piyavhatkul N, Rangseekajee P, Ingkaninan K, Vittaya-Areekul S. Effects of 12-Week Bacopa monnieri Consumption on Attention, Cognitive Processing, Working Memory, and Functions of Both cholinergic and Monoaminergic Systems in Healthy Elderly Volunteers. Evid Based Complement Alternat Med. 2012;2012:606424.

Petiot JF, Sainte-Laudy J, Benveniste J. Interpretation of results on a human basophil degranulation test. Ann Biol Clin (Paris). 1981;39(6):355-9.

Pfundstein B, El Desouky SK, Hull WE, Haubner R, Erben G, Owen RW. Polyphenolic compounds in the fruits of Egyptian medicinal plants (Terminalia bellerica, Terminalia chebula and Terminalia horrida): characterization, quantitation and determination of antioxidant capacities. Phytochemistry. 2010 Jul;71(10):1132-48.

Phan CW, David P, Naidu M, Wong KH, Sabaratnam V. Therapeutic potential of culinary-medicinal mushrooms for the management of neurodegenerative diseases: diversity, metabolite, and mechanism. Crit Rev Biotechnol. 2015;35(3):355-68. doi: 10.3109/07388551.2014.887649.

Phillips M, Cataneo RN, Cummin AR, Gagliardi AJ, Gleeson K, Greenberg J, Maxfield RA, Rom WN. Detection of lung cancer with volatile markers in the breath. Chest. 2003 Jun;123(6):2115-23.

Physicians' Desk Reference. Montvale, NJ: Thomson, 2003.

Pieterse Z, Jerling JC, Oosthuizen W, Kruger HS, Hanekom SM, Smuts CM, Schutte AE. Substitution of high monounsaturated fatty acid avocado for mixed dietary fats during an energy-restricted diet: effects on weight loss, serum lipids, fibrinogen, and vascular function. Nutrition. 2005 Jan;21(1):67-75

Pietrzik K, Bailey L, Shane B. Folic acid and L-5-methyltetrahydrofolate: comparison of clinical pharmacokinetics and pharmacodynamics. Clin Pharmacokinet. 2010 Aug;49(8):535-48.

Piggins HD. Human clock genes. Ann Med. 2002;34(5):394-400.

Piluso LG, Moffatt-Smith C. Disinfection using ultraviolet radiation as an antimicrobial agent: a review and synthesis of mechanisms and concerns. PDA J Pharm Sci Technol. 2006 Jan-Feb;60(1):1-16.

Pimentel D. Environmental and Economic Costs of the Application of Pesticides Primarily in the United States. Environment, Development and Sustainability. 2005. 7: 229-252.

Ping Liu, Mingwang Kong, Shihe Yuan, Junfeng Liu, and Ping Wang, "History and Experience: A Survey of Traditional Chinese Medicine Treatment for Alzheimer's Disease," Evidence-Based Complementary and Alternative Medicine, vol. 2014, Article ID 642128, 5 pages, 2014. doi:10.1155/2014/642128

Piolino P, Desgranges B, Belliard S, Matuszewski V, Lalevee C, De la Sayette V, Eustache F. Autobiographical memory and autonoetic consciousness: triple dissociation in neurodegenerative diseases. Brain. 2003 Oct;126(Pt 10):2203-19.

Piper PW. Yeast superoxide dismutase mutants reveal a pro-oxidant action of weak organic acid food preservatives. Free Radic Biol Med. 1999 Dec;27(11-12):1219-27.

Pitt-Rivers R, Trotter WR. The Thyroid Gland. London: Butterworth Publisher, 1954.

Plaut T, Jones T. Asthma Guide for People of All Ages. Amherst MA: Pedipress, 1999.

Plohmann B, Bader G, Hiller K, Franz G. Immunomodulatory and antitumoral effects of triterpenoid saponins. Pharmazie. 1997 Dec;52(12):953-7.

Plotkin H. Darwin Machines and the Nature of Knowledge: Concerning adaptations, instinct and the evolution of intelligence. New York: Penguin, 1994.

Plotnikoff G, Quigley J. Prevalence of Severe Hypovitaminosis D in Patients With Persistent, Nonspecific Musculoskeletal Pain. Mayo Clin Proc. 2003;78:1463-1470.

Poblocka-Olech L, Krauze-Baranowska M. SPE-HPTLC of procyanidins from the barks of different species and clones of Salix. J Pharm Biomed Anal. 2008 Nov 4;48(3):965-8.

Poitevin B, Davenas E, Benveniste J. In vitro immunological degranulation of human basophils is modulated by lung histamine and Apis mellifica. Br J Clin Pharmacol. 1988 Apr;25(4):439-44.

Polkinghorne J. Science and Providence. Boston: Shambhala Publications, 1989.

Pongratz W, Endler PC, Poitevin B, Kartnig T. Effect of extremely diluted plant hormone on cell culture, Proc. 1995 AAAS Ann. Meeting, Atlanta, 1995.

Ponsonby AL, McMichael A, van der Mei I. Ultraviolet radiation and autoimmune disease: insights from epidemiological research. Toxicology. 2002 Dec 27;181-182:71-8.

REFERENCES AND BIBLIOGRAPHY

Pool R. Is there an EMF-Cancer connection? Science. 1990;249: 1096-1098.

Pope SK, Shue VM, Beck C. Will a healthy lifestyle help prevent Alzheimer's disease? Annu Rev Public Health. 2003;24:111-32.

Popp F, Chang J. Mechanism of interaction between electromagnetic fields and living organisms. Science in China. 2000 Series C;43(5):507-518.

Popp F, Chang J, Herzog A, Yan Z, Yan Y. Evidence of non-classical (squeezed) light in biological systems. Physics Lett. 2002;293:98-102.

Popp F, Yan Y. Delayed luminescence of biological systems in terms of coherent states. Phys.Lett. 2000;293:91-97.

Popp F. Molecular Aspects of Carcinogenesis. In Deutsch E, Moser K, Rainer H, Stacher A (eds.). Molecular Base of Malignancy. Stuttgart: G.Thieme, 1976:47-55.

Popp F. Properties of biophotons and their theoretical implications. Indian J Exper Biology. 2003 May;41:391-402.

Popper KR, Eccles, JC. The Self and Its Brain. London: Routledge, 1983.

Postlethwait EM. Scavenger receptors clear the air. J Clin Invest. 2007 Mar;117(3):601-4.

Poulos LM, Toelle BG, Marks GB. The burden of asthma in children: an Australian perspective. Paediatr Respir Rev. 2005 Mar;6(1):20-7.

Power MC, Adar SD, Yanosky JD, Weuve J. Exposure to air pollution as a potential contributor to cognitive function, cognitive decline, brain imaging, and dementia: A systematic review of epidemiologic research. Neurotoxicology. 2016 Jun 18. pii: S0161-813X(16)30105-X.

Prabu PC, Panchapakesan S, Raj CD. Acute and Sub-Acute Oral Toxicity Assessment of the Hydroalcoholic Extract of Withania somnifera Roots in Wistar Rats. Phytother Res. 2012 Sep 21.

Prescott J. Alienation of Affection. Psych Today. 1979 Dec.

Prescott J. The Origins of Human Love and Violence. Pre- and Perinatal Psych J. 1996;10(3):143-188.

Pribram K. Brain and perception: holonomy and structure in figural processing. Hillsdale, N. J.: Lawrence Erlbaum Assoc., 1991.

Pronina TS. Circadian and infradian rhythms of testosterone and aldosterone excretion in children. Probl Endokrinol. 1992 Sep-Oct;38(5):38-42.

Protheroe WM, Captiotti ER, Newsom GH. Exploring the Universe. Columbus, OH: Merrill, 1989,

Provalova NV, Suslov NI, Skurikhin EG, Dygaï AM. Local mechanisms of the regulatory action of Scutellaria baicalensis and ginseng extracts on the erythropoiesis after paradoxical sleep deprivation. Eksp Klin Farmakol. 2006 Sep-Oct;69(5):31-5.

Prucksunand C, Indrasukhsri B, Leethochawalit M, Hungspreugs K. Phase II clinical trial on effect of the long turmeric (Curcuma longa Linn) on healing of peptic ulcer. Southeast Asian J Trop Med Public Health. 2001 Mar;32(1):208-15.

Puthoff H, Targ R, May E. Experimental Psi Research: Implication for Physics. AAAS Proceedings of the 1979 Symposium on the Role of Consciousness in the Physical World. 1981.

Puthoff H, Targ R. A Perceptual Channel for Information Transfer Over Kilometer distances: Historical Perspective and Recent Research. Proc. IEEE. 1976;64(3):329-254.

Qu Z, Mossine VV, Cui J, Sun GY, Gu Z. Protective Effects of AGE and Its Components on Neuroinflammation and Neurodegeneration. Neuromolecular Med. 2016 Sep;18(3):474-82. doi: 10.1007/s12017-016-8410-1.

Quinn J, Suh J, Moore MM, Kaye J, Frei B. Antioxidants in Alzheimer's disease-vitamin C delivery to a demanding brain. J Alzheimers Dis. 2003 Aug;5(4):309-13.

Radin D. The Conscious Universe. San Francisco: HarperEdge, 1997.

Rafii MS, Walsh S, Little JT, Behan K, Reynolds B, Ward C, Jin S, Thomas R, Aisen PS; Alzheimer's Disease Cooperative Study. A phase II trial of huperzine A in mild to moderate Alzheimer disease. Neurology. 2011 Apr 19;76(16):1389-94. doi: 10.1212/WNL.0b013e318216eb7b.

Raha S, Lee HJ, Yumnam S, Hong GE, Saralamma VV, Ha YL, Kim JO, Kim YS, Heo JD, Lee SJ, Eun HK, Kim GS. Vitamin D(2) suppresses amyloid-β 25-35 induced microglial activation in BV2 cells by blocking the NF-κB inflammatory signaling pathway. Life Sci. 2016 Jul 28. pii: S0024-3205(16)30454-4. doi: 10.1016/j.lfs.2016.07.017.

Rahman K. Garlic and aging: new insights into an old remedy. Ageing Res Rev. 2003 Jan;2(1):39-56.

Rahman MM, Bhattacharya A, Fernandes G. Docosahexaenoic acid is more potent inhibitor of osteoclast differentiation in RAW 264.7 cells than eicosapentaenoic acid. J Cell Physiol. 2008 Jan;214(1):201-9.

Raiten DJ, Talbot JM, Fisher KD, eds. Life Sciences Research Office Report. Executive summary from the report. Analysis of adverse reactions to monosodium glutamate (MSG). J Nutr. 1995;125 (suppl).:2892-906.

Raloff J. Ill Winds. Science News: 2001;160(14):218.

Ramachandran C, Quirin KW, Escalon E, Melnick SJ. Improved neuroprotective effects by combining Bacopa monnieri and Rosmarinus officinalis supercritical CO2 extracts. J Evid Based Complementary Altern Med. 2014 Apr;19(2):119-27. doi: 10.1177/2156587214524577.

Ranilla LG, Genovese MI, Lajolo FM. Polyphenols and antioxidant capacity of seed coat and cotyledon from Brazilian and Peruvian bean cultivars (Phaseolus vulgaris L.). J Agric Food Chem. 2007 Jan 10;55(1):90-8.

Ranjbaran Z, Keefer L, Stepanski E, Farhadi A, Keshavarzian A. The relevance of sleep abnormalities to chronic inflammatory conditions. Inflamm Res. 2007 Feb;56(2):51-7.

Rapley G. Keeping mothers and babies together—breastfeeding and bonding. RCM Midwives. 2002 Oct;5(10):332-4.

Rappoport J. Both sides of the pharmaceutical death coin. Townsend Letter for Doctors and Patients. 2006 Oct.

Rastogi M, Ojha R, Prabu PC, Devi DP, Agrawal A, Dubey GP. Amelioration of age associated neuroinflammation on long term bacosides treatment. Neurochem Res 2012;37: 869–874.

287

Rauma A. Antioxidant status in vegetarians versus omnivores. Nutrition. 2003;16(2): 111-119.

Raut AA, Rege NN, Tadvi FM, Solanki PV, Kene KR, Shirolkar SG, Pandey SN, Vaidya RA, Vaidya AB. Exploratory study to evaluate tolerability, safety, and activity of Ashwagandha (Withania somnifera) in healthy volunteers. J Ayurveda Integr Med. 2012 Jul;3(3):111-4.

Rawlings M. Beyond Death's Door. New York: Bantam, 1979.

Razdan S, Bhat WW, Rana S, Dhar N, Lattoo SK, Dhar RS, Vishwakarma RA. Molecular characterization and promoter analysis of squalene epoxidase gene from Withania somnifera (L.) Dunal. Mol Biol Rep. 2013 Feb;40(2):905-16.

Reddy KP, Shahani KM, Kulkarni SM. B-complex vitamins in cultured and acidified yogurt. J Dairy Sci. 1976 Feb;59(2):191-5.

Reger D, Goode S, Mercer E. Chemistry: Principles & Practice. Fort Worth, TX: Harcourt Brace, 1993.

Reger MA, Henderson ST, Hale C, Cholerton B, Baker LD, Watson GS, Hyde K, Chapman D, Craft S. Effects of beta-hydroxybutyrate on cognition in memory-impaired adults. Neurobiol Aging. 2004;25:311–314.

Regis E. Virus Ground Zero. New York: Pocket, 1996.

Reiffenberger DH, Amundson LH. Fibromyalgia syndrome: a review. Am Fam Physician. 1996;53:1698-704.

Reilly T, Taylor M, McSharry C, Aitchison T. Is homoeopathy a placebo response? Controlled trial of homoeopathic potency, with pollen in hayfever as model. Lancet. 1986;II: 881-886.

Reiter RJ, Garcia JJ, Pie J. Oxidative toxicity in models of neurodegeneration: responses to melatonin. Restor Neurol Neurosci. 1998 Jun;12(2-3):135-42.

Reiter RJ, Tan DX, Manchester LC, Qi W. Biochemical reactivity of melatonin with reactive oxygen and nitrogen species: a review of the evidence. Cell Biochem Biophys. 2001;34(2):237-56.

Reitz C. Dyslipidemia and the risk of Alzheimer's disease. Curr Atheroscler Rep. 2013 Mar;15(3):307. doi: 10.1007/s11883-012-0307-3

Remington R, Bechtel C, Larsen D, Samar A, Doshanjh L, Fishman P, Luo Y, Smyers K, Page R, Morrell C, Shea TB. A Phase II Randomized Clinical Trial of a Nutritional Formulation for Cognition and Mood in Alzheimer's Disease. J Alzheimers Dis. 2015;45(2):395-405. doi: 10.3233/JAD-142499.

Remington R, Chan A, Paskavitz J, Shea TB. Efficacy of a vitamin/nutriceutical formulation for moderate-stage to later-stage Alzheimer's disease: a placebo-controlled pilot study. Am J Alzheimers Dis Other Demen. 2009 Feb-Mar;24(1):27-33. doi: 10.1177/1533317508325094.

Renaud S, Lanzmann-Petithory D. Dietary fats and coronary heart disease pathogenesis. Curr Atheroscler Rep. 2002;4(6):419-24.

Renault S, De Lucca AJ, Boue S, Bland JM, Vigo CB, Selitrennikoff CP. CAY-1, a novel antifungal compound from cayenne pepper. Med Mycol. 2003 Feb;41(1):75-81.

Resnick SM, Sojkova J, Zhou Y, An Y, Ye W, Holt DP, et al. Longitudinal cognitive decline is associated with fibrillar amyloid-beta measured by [11C]PiB. Neurology 2010;74:807-15.

Retallack D. The Sound of Music and Plants. Marina Del Rey, CA: Devorss, 1973.

Reuland DJ, Khademi S, Castle CJ, Irwin DC, McCord JM, Miller BF, Hamilton KL. Upregulation of phase II enzymes through phytochemical activation of Nrf2 protects cardiomyocytes against oxidant stress. Free Radic Biol Med. 2012 Nov 30;56C:102-111.

Reyna-Villasmil N, Bermúdez-Pirela V, Mengual-Moreno E, Arias N, Cano-Ponce C, Leal-Gonzalez E, Souki A, Inglett GE, Israili ZH, Hernández-Hernández R, Valasco M, Arraiz N. Oat-derived beta-glucan significantly improves HDLC and diminishes LDLC and non-HDL cholesterol in overweight individuals with mild hypercholesterolemia. Am J Ther. 2007 Mar-Apr;14(2):203-12.

Richards R. Darwin and the Emergence of Evolutionary Theories of Mind and Behavior. Chicago: Univ Chicago Press, 1987.

Rietbrock N, Hamel M, Hempel B, Mitrovic V, Schmidt T, Wolf GK. Actions of standardized extracts of Crataegus berries on exercise tolerance and quality of life in patients with congestive heart failure. Arzneimittelforschung. 2001 Oct;51(10):793-8.

Rinaldi P, Polidori MC, Metastasio A, Mariani E, Mattioli P, Cherubini A, Catani M, Cecchetti R, Senin U, Mecocci P. Plasma antioxidants are similarly depleted in mild cognitive impairment and in Alzheimer's disease. Neurobiol Aging. 2003 Nov;24(7):915-9.

Rindos D. The Origins of Agriculture: An evolutionary perspective. Burlington, MA: Academic Press, 1984.

Ring K. Life at Death: A Scientific Investigation of the Near-Death Experience. New York: Quill, 1982.

Rinne JO, Brooks DJ, Rossor MN, Fox NC, Bullock R, Klunk WE, et al. 11C-PiB PET assessment of change in fibrillar amyloid-beta load in patients with Alzheimer's disease treated with bapineuzumab: a phase 2, double-blind, placebo-controlled, ascending-dose study. Lancet Neurol 2010;9:363-72.

Riso P, Martini D, Møller P, Loft S, Bonacina G, Moro M, Porrini M. DNA damage and repair activity after broccoli intake in young healthy smokers. Mutagenesis. 2010 Nov;25(6):595-602. doi: 10.1093/mutage/geq045.

Riso P, Vendrame S, Del Bo' C, Martini D, Martinetti A, Seregni E, Visioli F, Parolini M, Porrini M. Effect of 10-day broccoli consumption on inflammatory status of young healthy smokers. Int J Food Sci Nutr. 2013 Sep 2.

Rizos EC, Ntzani EE, Bika E, Kostapanos MS, Elisaf MS. Association between omega-3 fatty acid supplementation and risk of major cardiovascular disease events: a systematic review and meta-analysis. JAMA. 2012 Sep 12;308(10):1024-33.

Roach M. Stiff: The Curious Lives of Human Cadavers. New York: W.W. Norton, 2003.

Robbins KS, Shin EC, Shewfelt RL, Eitenmiller RR, Pegg RB. Update on the Healthful Lipid Constituents of Commercially Important Tree Nuts. J Agric Food Chem. 2011 Oct 27.

Robert AM, Groult N, Six C, Robert L. The effect of procyanidolic oligomers on mesenchymal cells in culture II—Attachment of elastic fibers to the cells. Pathol Biol. 1990 Jun;38(6):601-7.

Robert AM, Robert L, Renard G. Protection of cornea against proteolytic damage. Experimental study of procyanidolic oligomers (PCO) on bovine cornea. J Fr Ophtalmol. 2002 Apr;25(4):351-5.

Robert AM, Tixier JM, Robert L, Legeais JM, Renard G. Effect of procyanidolic oligomers on the permeability of the blood-brain barrier. Pathol Biol. 2001 May;49(4):298-304.

Roberts JE. Light and immunomodulation. Ann N Y Acad Sci. 2000;917:435-45.

Roberts RO, Knopman DS, Cha RH, Mielke MM, Pankratz VS, Boeve BF, Kantarci K, Geda YE, Jack CR, Petersen RC, Lowe VJ. Diabetes and elevated hemoglobin A1c levels are associated with brain hypometabolism but not amyloid accumulation. J. Nucl. Med. 2014 55:759–764. doi:10.2967/jnumed.113.132647

Robilliard DL, Archer SN, Arendt J, Lockley SW, Hack LM, English J, Leger D, Smits MG, Williams A, Skene DJ, Von Schantz M. The 3111 Clock gene polymorphism is not associated with sleep and circadian rhythmicity in phenotypically characterized human subjects. J Sleep Res. 2002 Dec;11(4):305-12.

Rodale R. Our Next Frontier. Emmaus, PA: Rodale, 1981.

Rodermel SR, Smith-Sonneborn J. Age-correlated changes in expression of micronuclear damage and repair in Paramecium tetraurelia. Genetics. 1977 Oct;87(2):259-74.

Rodgers JT, Puigserver P. Fasting-dependent glucose and lipid metabolic response through hepatic sirtuin 1. Proc Natl Acad Sci USA. 2007 Jul 31;104(31):12861-6.

Rodriguez-Fragoso L, Reyes-Esparza J, Burchiel SW, Herrera-Ruiz D, Torres E. Risks and benefits of commonly used herbal medicines in Mexico. Toxicol Appl Pharmacol. 2008 Feb 15;227(1):125-35.

Rohrmann S, Zoller D, Hermann S, Linseisen J. Intake of heterocyclic aromatic amines from meat in the European Prospective Investigation into Cancer and Nutrition (EPIC)-Heidelberg cohort. Br J Nutr. 2007 Dec;98(6):1112-5.

Romaguera D, Ängquist L, Du H, Jakobsen MU, Forouhi NG, Halkjær J, Feskens EJ, van der A DL, Masala G, Steffen A, Palli D, Wareham NJ, Overvad K, Tjønneland A, Boeing H, Riboli E, Sorensen TI. Food composition of the diet in relation to changes in waist circumference adjusted for body mass index. PLoS One. 2011;6(8):e23384. doi: 10.1371/journal.pone.0023384.

Rondeau V, Commenges D, Jacqmin-Gadda H, Dartigues JF. Relation between aluminum concentrations in drinking water and Alzheimer's disease: an 8-year follow-up study. Am J Epidemiol. 2000 Jul 1;152(1):59-66.

Rondina R 2nd, Olsen RK, McQuiggan DA, Fatima Z, Li L, Oziel E, Meltzer JA, Ryan JD. Age-related changes to oscillatory dynamics in hippocampal and neocortical networks. Neurobiol Learn Mem. 2015 Dec 9. pii: S1074-7427(15)00226-9. doi: 10.1016/j.nlm.2015.11.017.

Ros E, Mataix J. Fatty acid composition of nuts—implications for cardiovascular health. Br J Nutr. 2006 Nov;96 Suppl 2:S29-35.

Rosenfeldt V, Benfeldt E, Nielsen SD, Michaelsen KF, Jeppesen DL, Valerius NH, Paerregaard A. Effect of probiotic Lactobacillus strains in children with atopic dermatitis. J Allergy Clin Immunol. 2003 Feb;111(2):389-95.

Rosenlund M, Picciotto S, Forastiere F, Stafoggia M, Perucci CA. Traffic-related air pollution in relation to incidence and prognosis of coronary heart disease. Epidemiology. 2008 Jan;19(1):121-8.

Rosenthal N, Blehar M (Eds.). Seasonal affective disorders and phototherapy. New York: Guildford Press, 1989.

Rossouw JE, Prentice RL, Manson JE, Wu L, Barad D, Barnabei VM, Ko M, LaCroix AZ, Margolis KL, Stefanick ML. Postmenopausal hormone therapy and risk of cardiovascular disease by age and years since menopause. JAMA. 2007 Apr 4;297(13):1465-77.

Rousseaux C, Thuru X, Gelot A, Barnich N, Neut C, Dubuquoy L, Dubuquoy C, Merour E, Geboes K, Chamaillard M, Ouwehand A, Leyer G, Carcano D, Colombel JF, Ardid D, Desreumaux P. Lactobacillus acidophilus modulates intestinal pain and induces opioid and cannabinoid receptors. Nat Med. 2007 Jan;13(1):35-7

Routasalo P, Isola A. The right to touch and be touched. Nurs Ethics. 1996 Jun;3(2):165-76.

Rowe CC, Ellis KA, Rimajova M, Bourgeat P, Pike KE, Jones G, et al. Amyloid imaging results from the Australian Imaging, Biomarkers and Lifestyle (AIBL) study of aging. Neurobiol Aging 2010;31:1275-83.

Rowland AS, Baird DD, Long S, Wegienka G, Harlow SD, Alavanja M, Sandler DP. Influence of medical conditions and lifestyle factors on the menstrual cycle. Epidemiology. 2002 Nov;13(6):668-74.

Roy M, Kirschbaum C, Steptoe A. Intraindividual variation in recent stress exposure as a moderator of cortisol and testosterone levels. Ann Behav Med. 2003 Dec;26(3):194-200.

Roybal K, Theobold D, Graham A, DiNieri JA, Russo SJ, Krishnan V, Chakravarty S, Peevey J, Oehrlein N, Birnbaum S, Vitaterna MH, Orsulak P, Takahashi JS, Nestler EJ, Carlezon WA Jr, McClung CA. Mania-like behavior induced by disruption of CLOCK. Proc Natl Acad Sci USA. 2007 Apr 10;104(15):6406-11.

Royer RJ, Schmidt CL. Evaluation of venotropic drugs by venous gas plethysmography. A study of procyanidolic oligomers Sem Hop. 1981 Dec 18-25;57(47-48):2009-13.

Rozycki VR, Baigorria CM, Freyre MR, Bernard CM, Zannier MS, Charpentier M. Nutrient content in vegetable species from the Argentine Chaco. Arch Latinoam Nutr. 1997 Sep;47(3):265-70.

Rubenowitz E, Molin I, Axelsson G, Rylander R. (2000) Magnesium in drinking water in relation to morbidity and mortality from acute myocardial infarction. Epidemiology. 2000;11:416-421.

Rubin E and Farber J. Pathology 3rd Edition. Lippincott-Raven, Philadelphia, PA, 1999.

Russ MJ, Clark WC, Cross LW, Kemperman I, Kakuma T, Harrison K. Pain and self-injury in borderline patients: sensory decision theory, coping strategies, and locus of control. Psychiatry Res. 1996 Jun 26;63(1):57-65.

Russ T, Murianni L, Icaza G, Slachevsky A, Starr J. Geographical Variation in Dementia Mortality in Italy, New Zealand, and Chile: The Impact of Latitude, Vitamin D, and Air Pollution. Dement Geriatr Cogn Disord. 2016 Aug 19;42(1-2):31-41.

Russek LG, Schwartz GE. Narrative descriptions of parental love and caring predict health status in midlife: a 35-year follow-up of the Harvard Mastery of Stress Study. Altern Ther Health Med. 1996 Nov;2(6):55-62.

Russell IJ. Advances in fibromyalgia: possible role for central neurochemicals. Am J Med Sci. 1998;315:377-84.

Russell RM, Golner BB, Krasinski SD, Sadowski JA, Suter PM, Braun CL. Effect of antacid and H2 receptor antagonists on the intestinal absorption of folic acid. J Lab Clin Med. 1988;112:458-63.

Russo PA, Halliday GM. Inhibition of nitric oxide and reactive oxygen species production improves the ability of a sunscreen to protect from sunburn, immunosuppression and photocarcinogenesis. Br J Dermatol. 2006 Aug;155(2):408-15.

Saarijarvi S, Lauerma H, Helenius H, Saarilehto S. Seasonal affective disorders among rural Finns and Lapps. Acta Psychiatr Scand. 1999 Feb;99(2):95-101.

Sabia S, Elbaz A, Dugravot A, Head J, Shipley M, Hagger-Johnson G, Kivimaki M, Singh-Manoux A. Impact of Smoking on Cognitive Decline in Early Old Age: The Whitehall II Cohort Study. Arch Gen Psychiatry. 2012 Feb 6.

Sabia S, Elbaz A, Dugravot A, Head J, Shipley M, Hagger-Johnson G, Kivimaki M, Singh-Manoux A. Impact of smoking on cognitive decline in early old age: the Whitehall II cohort study. Arch Gen Psychiatry. 2012 Jun;69(6):627-35.

Sabir F, Mishra S, Sangwan RS, Jadaun JS, Sangwan NS. Qualitative and quantitative variations in withanolides and expression of some pathway genes during different stages of morphogenesis in Withania somnifera Dunal. Protoplasma. 2012 Aug 10.

Sabom M. Light and Death: One Doctor's Fascinating Account of Near Death Experiences. Grand Rapids, MI: Zondervan Publishing, 1998.

Sabom M. Recollections of Death: A Medical Investigation. New York: Harper and Row, 1982.

Sacks O. The Man Who Mistook his Wife for a Hat and Other Clinical Tales. New York: Simon & Schuster, 1998.

Sahlin C, Pettersson FE, Nilsson LN, Lannfelt L, Johansson AS. Docosahexaenoic acid stimulates non-amyloidogenic APP processing resulting in reduced Abeta levels in cellular models of Alzheimer's disease. Eur J Neurosci. 2007 Aug;26(4):882-9.

Saini N, Mathur R, Agrawal SS. Qualitative and quantitative assessment of four marketed formulations of brahmi. Indian J Pharm Sci. 2012 Jan;74(1):24-8.

Sainte-Laudy J, Belon P. Analysis of immunosuppressive activity of serial dilutions of histamine on human basophil activation by flow cytometry. Inflam Rsrch. 1996 Suppl. 1: S33-S34.

Sakae N, Liu CC, Shinohara M, Frisch-Daiello J, Ma L, Yamazaki Y, Tachibana M, Younkin L, Kurti A, Carrasquillo MM, Zou F, Sevlever D, Bisceglio G, Gan M, Fol R, Knight P, Wang M, Han X, Fryer JD, Fitzgerald ML, Ohyagi Y, Younkin SG, Bu G, Kanekiyo T. ABCA7 Deficiency Accelerates Amyloid-β Generation and Alzheimer's Neuronal Pathology. J Neurosci. 2016 Mar 30;36(13):3848-59. doi: 10.1523/JNEUROSCI.3757-15.2016

Sakugawa H, Cape JN. Harmful effects of atmospheric nitrous acid on the physiological status of

Salem N, Wegher B, Mena P, Uauy R. Arachidonic and docosahexaenoic acids are biosynthesized from their 18-carbon precursors in human infants. Proc Natl Acad Sci. 1996;93:49-54.

Salem N, Wegher B, Mena P, Uauy R. Arachidonic and docosahexaenoic acids are biosynthesized from their 18-carbon precursors in human infants. Proc Natl Acad Sci. 1996;93:49-54.

Salloway S, Sperling R, Keren R, Porsteinsson AP, van Dyck CH, Tariot PN, Gilman S, Arnold D, Abushakra S, Hernandez C, Crans G, Liang E, Quinn G, Bairu M, Pastrak A, Cedarbaum JM; ELND005-AD201 Investigators. A phase 2 randomized trial of ELND005, scyllo-inositol, in mild to moderate Alzheimer disease. Neurology. 2011 Sep 27;77(13):1253-62. doi: 10.1212/WNL.0b013e3182309fa5.

Salminen S, Isolauri E, Salminen E. Clinical uses of probiotics for stabilizing the gut mucosal barrier: successful strains and future challenges. Antonie Van Leeuwenhoek. 1996 Oct;70(2-4):347-58.

Salom IL, Silvis SE, Doscherholmen A. Effect of cimetidine on the absorption of vitamin B12. Scand J Gastroenterol. 1982;17:129-31.

Samberkar S, Gandhi S, Naidu M, Wong KH, Raman J, Sabaratnam V. Lion's Mane, Hericium erinaceus and Tiger Milk, Lignosus rhinocerotis (Higher Basidiomycetes) Medicinal Mushrooms Stimulate Neurite Outgrowth in Dissociated Cells of Brain, Spinal Cord, and Retina: An In Vitro Study. Int J Med Mushrooms. 2015;17(11):1047-54.

Samieri C, Okereke OI, E Devore E, Grodstein F. Long-term adherence to the Mediterranean diet is associated with overall cognitive status, but not cognitive decline, in women. J Nutr. 2013 Apr;143(4):493-9. doi: 10.3945/jn.112.169896.

Sandberg AS. The effect of food processing on phytate hydrolysis and availability of iron and zinc. Adv Exp Med Biol. 1991;289:499-508.

Sanders R. Slow brain waves play key role in coordinating complex activity. UC Berkeley News. 2006 Sep 14.

Sano M, Ernesto C, Thomas RG, Klauber MR, Schafer K, Grundman M, Woodbury P, Growdon J, Cotman CW, Pfeiffer E, Schneider LS, Thal LJ. A controlled trial of selegiline, alpha-tocopherol, or both as treatment for Alzheimer's disease. The Alzheimer's Disease Cooperative Study. N Engl J Med. 1997 Apr 24;336(17):1216-22.

REFERENCES AND BIBLIOGRAPHY

Santos-Lozano A, Pareja-Galeano H, Sanchis-Gomar F, Quindós-Rubial M, Fiuza-Luces C, Cristi-Montero C, Emanuele E, Garatachea N, Lucia A. Physical Activity and Alzheimer Disease: A Protective Association. Mayo Clin Proc. 2016 Aug;91(8):999-1020. doi: 10.1016/j.mayocp.2016.04.024.

Sarah Janssen S, Solomon G, Schettler T. Chemical Contaminants and Human Disease: A Summary of Evidence. The Collaborative on Health and the Environment. 2006. http://www.healthandenvironment.org. Acc. 2007 Jul.

Saran, S., Gopalan, S. and Krishna, T. P. Use of fermented foods to combat stunting and failure to thrive. Nutrition. 2002;8:393-396.

Sarkar S, Mishra BR, Praharaj SK, Nizamie SH. Add-on effect of Brahmi in the management of schizophrenia. J Ayurveda Integr Med. 2012 Oct;3(4):223-5.

Sarveiya V, Risk S, Benson HA. Liquid chromatographic assay for common sunscreen agents: application to in vivo assessment of skin penetration and systemic absorption in human volunteers. J Chromatogr B Analyt Technol Biomed Life Sci. 2004 Apr 25;803(2):225-31.

Sato TK, Yamada RG, Ukai H, Baggs JE, Miraglia LJ, Kobayashi TJ, Welsh DK, Kay SA, Ueda HR, Hogenesch JB. Feedback repression is required for mammalian circadian clock function. Nat Genet. 2006 Mar;38(3):312-9.

Satoh A, Tsuji S, Okada Y, Murakami N, Urami M, Nakagawa K, Ishikura M, Katagiri M, Koga Y, Shirasawa T. Preliminary Clinical Evalua-tion of Toxicity and Efficacy of A New Astaxanthin-rich Haematococcus pluvialis Extract. J Clin Biochem Nutr. 2009 May;44(3):280-4.

Satoh A, Tsuji S, Okada Y, Murakami N, Urami M, Nakagawa K, Ishikura M, Katagiri M, Koga Y, Shirasawa T. Preliminary Clinical Evaluation of Toxicity and Efficacy of A New Astaxanthin-rich Haematococcus pluvialis Extract. J Clin Biochem Nutr. 2009 May;44(3):280-4.

Satoh K, Abe-Dohmae S, Yokoyama S, St George-Hyslop P, Fraser PE. ATP-binding cassette transporter A7 (ABCA7) loss of function alters Alzheimer amyloid processing. J Biol Chem. 2015 Oct 2;290(40):24152-65. doi: 10.1074/jbc.M115.655076.

Sattler C, Toro P, Schönknecht P, Schröder J. Cognitive activity, education and socioeconomic status as preventive factors for mild cognitive impairment and Alzheimer's disease. Psychiatry Res. 2012 Mar 30;196(1):90-5. doi: 10.1016/j.psychres.2011.11.012.

Satyanarayana S, Sushruta K, Sarma GS, Srinivas N, Subba Raju GV. Antioxidant activity of the aqueous extracts of spicy food additives—evaluation and comparison with ascorbic acid in in-vitro systems. J Herb Pharmacother. 2004;4(2):1-10.

Sauvant M, Pepin D. Drinking water and cardiovascular disease. Food Chem Toxicol. 2002;40:1311-1325.

Scarmeas N, Luchsinger JA, Mayeux R, Stern Y. Mediterranean diet and Alzheimer disease mortality. Neurology. 2007 Sep 11;69(11):1084-93.

Scarmeas N, Luchsinger JA, Schupf N, Brickman AM, Cosentino S, Tang MX, Stern Y. Physical activity, diet, and risk of Alzheimer disease. JAMA. 2009 Aug 12;302(6):627-37.

Scarmeas N, Stern Y, Mayeux R, Luchsinger JA. Mediterranean diet, Alzheimer disease, and vascular mediation. Arch Neurol. 2006 Dec;63(12):1709-17.

Scarmeas N, Stern Y, Tang MX, Mayeux R, Luchsinger JA. Mediterranean diet and risk for Alzheimer's disease. Ann Neurol. 2006 Jun;59(6):912-21.

Schauenberg P, Paris F. Guide to Medicinal Plants. New Canaan, CT: Keats Publ, 1977.

Schauss AG, Wu X, Prior RL, Ou B, Huang D, Owens J, Agarwal A, Jensen GS, Hart AN, Shanbrom E. Antioxidant capacity and other bioactivities of the freeze-dried Amazonian palm berry, Euterpe oleraceae mart. (acai). J Agric Food Chem. 2006 Nov 1;54(22):8604-10.

Scheiber, M. D., J. H. Liu, et al. 2001. Dietary inclusion of whole soy foods results in significant reductions in clinical risk factors for osteoporosis and cardiovascular disease in normal postmenopausal women. Menopause 8(5): 384-92.

Scheinin NM, Aalto S, Koikkalainen J, Lötjönen J, Karrasch M, Kemppainen N, et al. Follow-up of [11C]PIB uptake and brain volume in patients with Alzheimer disease and controls. Neurology 2009;73:1186-92.

Schempp H, Weiser D, Elstner EF. Biochemical model reactions indicative of inflammatory processes. Activities of extracts from Fraxinus excelsior and Populus tremula. Arzneimittelforschung. 2000 Apr;50(4):362-72.

Schenk BE, Festen HP, Kuipers EJ, Klinkenberg-Knol EC, Meuwissen SG. Effect of short-and long-term treatment with omeprazole on the absorption and serum levels of cobalamin. Aliment Pharmacol Ther. 1996;10:541-5.

Schirber M. Earth as a Giant Pinball Machine. LiveScience. 2004; 19 Nov 19. http://www.livescience.com/ environ-ment/041119_earth_layers.html. Acc. 2006 Nov.

Schlebusch KP, Maric-Oehler W, Popp FA. Biophotonics in the infrared spectral range reveal acupuncture meridian structure of the body. J Altern Complement Med. 2005 Feb;11(1):171-3.

Schlumpf M, Cotton B, Conscience M, Haller V, Steinmann B, Lichtensteiger W. In vitro and in vivo estrogenicity of UV screens. Environ Health Perspect. 2001 Mar;109(3):239-44.

Schmid B, Kötter I, Heide L. Pharmacokinetics of salicin after oral administration of a standardised willow bark extract. Eur J Clin Pharmacol. 2001 Aug;57(5):387-91.

Schmidt H, Quantum processes predicted? New Sci. 1969 Oct 16.

Schmitt B, Frölich L. Creative therapy options for patients with dementia—a systematic review. Fortschr Neurol Psychiatr. 2007 Dec;75(12):699-707.

Schoeninger MJ, Murray S, Bunn HT, Marlett JA. Composition of tubers used by Hadza foragers of Tanzania. J Food Compost Anal. 2001;14:15—25.

Schonberger B. Bladder dysfunction and surgery in the small pelvis. Therapeutic possibilities. Urologe A. 2003 Dec;42(12):1569-75.

Schottner M, Gansser D, Spiteller G. Lignans from the roots of Urtica dioica and their metabolites bind to human sex hormone binding globulin (SHBG). Planta Med. 1997;65:529-532.

Schulick P. Ginger: Common Spice & Wonder Drug. Brattleboro, VT: Herbal Free Perss, 1996.

Schulman G. A nexus of progression of chronic kidney disease: charcoal, tryptophan and profibrotic cytokines. Blood Purif. 2006;24(1):143-8.

Schulz T, Zarse K, Voigt A, Urban N, Birringer M, Ristow M. Glucose Restriction Extends Caenorhabditis elegans Life Span by Inducing Mitochondrial Respiration and Increasing Oxidative Stress. Cell Metabolism. 2007 Oct 3;6:280-293.

Schulz V, Hansel R, Tyler VE. Rational Phytotherapy. Berlin: Springer-Verlag; 1998.

Schulze MB, Manson JE, Willett WC, Hu FB. Processed meat intake and incidence of Type 2 diabetes in younger and middle-aged women. Diabetologia. 2003 Nov;46(11):1465-73.

Schumacher P. Biophysical Therapy Of Allergies. Stuttgart: Thieme, 2005.

Schwartz GG, Skinner HG. Vitamin D status and cancer: new insights. Curr Opin Clin Nutr Metab Care. 2007 Jan;10(1):6-11.

Schwartz S, De Mattei R, Brame E, Spottiswoode S. Infrared spectra alteration in water proximate to the palms of therapeutic practitioners. In: Wiener D, Nelson R (Eds.): Research in parapsychology 1986. Metuchen, NJ: Scarecrow Press, 1987:24-29.

Schwellenbach IJ, Olson KL. McConnell KJ, Stolepart RS, Nash JD, Merenich JA. The triglyceride-lowering effects of a modest dose of docosahexaenoic acid alone versus in combination with low dose eicosapentaenoic acid in patients with coronary artery disease and elevated triglycerides. J Am Coll Nutr. 2006;25(6):480-485.

Schwellenbach IJ, Olson KL. McConnell KJ, Stolepart RS, Nash JD, Merenich JA. The triglyceride-lowering effects of a modest dose of docosahexaenoic acid alone versus in combination with low dose eicosapentaenoic acid in patients with coronary artery disease and elevated triglycerides. J Am Coll Nutr. 2006;25(6):480-485.

Scoville WB, Milner B. Loss of recent memory after bilateral hippocampal lesions. J Neurol Neurosurg Psychiatry. 1957;20:11-21.

Sehgal N, Gupta A, Valli RK, Joshi SD, Mills JT, Hamel E, Khanna P, Jain SC, Thakur SS, Ravindranath V. Withania somnifera reverses Alzheimer's disease pathology by enhancing low-density lipoprotein receptor-related protein in liver. Proc Natl Acad Sci U S A. 2012 Feb 28;109(9):3510-5.

Semenza C. Retrieval pathways for common and proper names. Cortex. 2006 Aug;42(6):884-91.

Senekowitsch F, Endler PC, Pongratz W, Smith CW. Hormone effects by CD record /replay. FASEB J. 1995:A12025.

Senior F. Fallout. New York Magazine. Fall: 2003.

Şenol FS, Yilmaz G, Şener B, Koyuncu M, Orhan I. Preliminary screening of acetylcholinesterase inhibitory and antioxidant activities of Anatolian Heptaptera species. Pharm Biol. 2010 Mar;48(3):337-41. doi: 10.3109/13880200903133837.

Seo JS, Yun JH, Baek IS, Leem YH, Kang HW, Cho HK, Lyu YS, Son HJ, Han PL. Oriental medicine Jang-wonhwan reduces Abeta(1-42) level and beta-amyloid deposition in the brain of Tg-APPswe/PS1dE9 mouse model of Alzheimer disease. J Ethnopharmacol. 2010 Mar 2;128(1):206-12. doi: 10.1016/j.jep.2010.01.014

Seo K, Jung S, Park M, Song Y, Choung S. Effects of leucocyanidines on activities of metabolizing enzymes and antioxidant enzymes. Biol Pharm Bull. 2001 May;24(5):592-3.

Serra-Valls A. Electromagnetic Industrion and the Conservation of Momentum in the Spiral Paradox. Cornell University Library. http://arxiv.org/ftp/physics/papers/0012/0012009.pdf. Acc. 2007 Jul.

Serway R. Physicis For Scientists & Engineers. Philadelphia: Harcourt Brace, 1992.

Shaffer D. Developmental Psychology: Theory, Research and Applications. Monterey, CA: Brooks/Cole, 1985.

Shafik A. Role of warm-water bath in anorectal conditions. The "thermosphincteric reflex". J Clin Gastroenterol. 1993 Jun;16(4):304-8.

Shankar R. My Music, My Life. New York: Simon & Schuster, 1968.

Shao ZQ. Comparison of the efficacy of four cholinesterase inhibitors in combination with memantine for the treatment of Alzheimer's disease. Int J Clin Exp Med. 2015 Feb 15;8(2):2944-8.

Sharma DR, Wani WY, Sunkaria A, Kandimalla RJ, Sharma RK, Verma D, Bal A, Gill KD. Quercetin attenuates neuronal death against aluminum-induced neurodegeneration in the rat hippocampus. Neuroscience. 2016 Jun 2;324:163-76. doi: 10.1016/j.neuroscience.2016.02.055.

Sharma V, Sharma S, Pracheta. Protective effect of Withania somnifera roots extract on hematoserological profiles against lead nitrate-induced toxicity in mice. Indian J Biochem Biophys. 2012 Dec;49(6):458-62.

Sharp KC. After the Light. New York: William Morrow & Co., 1995.

Shay CM, Van Horn L, Stamler J, Dyer AR, Brown IJ, Chan Q, Miura K, Zhao L, Okuda N, Daviglus ML, Elliott P; INTERMAP Research Group. Food and nutrient intakes and their associations with lower BMI in middle-aged US adults: the International Study of Macro-/Micronutrients and Blood Pressure (INTERMAP). Am J Clin Nutr. 2012 Sep;96(3):483-91.

Shearman LP, Zylka MJ, Weaver DR, Kolakowski LF Jr, Reppert SM. Two period homologs: circadian expression and photic regulation in the suprachiasmatic nuclei. Neuron. 1997 Dec;19(6):1261-9.

Shen YF, Goddard G. The short-term effects of acupuncture on myofascial pain patients after clenching. Pain Pract. 2007 Sep;7(3):256-64.

Shenoy S, Chaskar U, Sandhu JS, Paadhi MM. Effects of eight-week supplementation of Ashwagandha on cardio-respiratory endurance in elite Indian cyclists. J Ayurveda Integr Med. 2012 Oct;3(4):209-14.

Shevelev IA, Kostelianetz NB, Kamenkovich VM, Sharaev GA. EEG alpha-wave in the visual cortex: check of the hypothesis of the scanning process. Int J Psychophysiol. 1991 Aug;11(2):195-201.

REFERENCES AND BIBLIOGRAPHY

Shi GX, Liu CZ, Wang LP, Guan LP, Li SQ. Biomarkers of oxidative stress in vascular dementia patients. Can J Neurol Sci. 2012 Jan;39(1):65-8.

Shiino A, Watanabe T, Shirakashi Y, Kotani E, Yoshimura M, Morikawa S, Inubushi T, Akiguchi I. The profile of hippocampal metabolites differs between Alzheimer's disease and subcortical ischemic vascular dementia, as measured by proton magnetic resonance spectroscopy. J Cereb Blood Flow Metab. 2012 May;32(5):805-15. doi: 10.1038/jcbfm.2012.9.

Shimabukuro M, Higa M, Kinjo R, Yamakawa K, Tanaka H, Kozuka C, Yabiku K, Taira SI, Sata M, Masuzaki H. Effects of the brown rice diet on visceral obesity and endothelial function: the BRAVO study. Br J Nutr. 2013 Aug 12:1-11.

Shinto L, Quinn J, Montine T, Dodge HH, Woodward W, Baldauf-Wagner S, Waichunas D, Bumgarner L, Bourdette D, Silbert L, Kaye J. A randomized placebo-controlled pilot trial of omega-3 fatty acids and alpha lipoic acid in Alzheimer's disease. J Alzheimers Dis. 2014;38(1):111-20. doi: 10.3233/JAD-130722.

Shishehbor F, Behroo L, Ghafouriyan Broujerdnia M, Namjoyan F, Latifi SM. Quercetin effectively quells peanut-induced anaphylactic reactions in the peanut sensitized rats. Iran J Allergy Asthma Immunol. 2010 Mar;9(1):27-34.

Shivpuri DN, Menon MP, Parkash D. Preliminary studies in Tylophora indica in the treatment of asthma and allergic rhinitis. J Assoc Physicians India. 1968 Jan;16(1):9-15.

Shivpuri DN, Menon MP, Prakash D. A crossover double-blind study on Tylophora indica in the treatment of asthma and allergic rhinitis. J Allergy. 1969 Mar;43(3):145-50.

Shivpuri DN, Singhal SC, Parkash D. Treatment of asthma with an alcoholic extract of Tylophora indica: a crossover, double-blind study. Ann Allergy. 1972; 30:407-12.

Shu-huai Xing, Chun-xiao Zhu, Rui Zhang, and Li An. Huperzine A in the Treatment of Alzheimer's Disease and Vascular Dementia: A Meta-Analysis. Evidence-Based Complementary and Alternative Medicine, vol. 2014, Article ID 363985, 10 pages, 2014. doi:10.1155/2014/363985

Shukla K, Dikshit P, Shukla R, Gambhir JK. The aqueous extract of Withania coagulans fruit partially reverses nicotinamide/streptozotocin-induced diabetes mellitus in rats. J Med Food. 2012 Aug;15(8):718-25.

Shukla K, Dikshit P, Tyagi MK, Shukla R, Gambhir JK. Ameliorative effect of Withania coagulans on dyslipidemia and oxidative stress in nicotinamide-streptozotocin induced diabetes mellitus. Food Chem Toxicol. 2012 Oct;50(10):3595-9.

Shupak NM, Prato FS, Thomas AW. Human exposure to a specific pulsed magnetic field: effects on thermal sensory and pain thresholds. Neurosci Lett. 2004 Jun 10;363(2):157-62.

Shutov AA, Panasiuk Ila. Efficacy of rehabilitation of patients with chronic primary low back pain at the spa Klyuchi using balneopelotherapy and transcranial electrostimulation. Vopr Kurortol Fizioter Lech Fiz Kult. 2007 Mar-Apr;(2):16-8.

Sicher F, Targ E, Moore D, Smith H. A Randomized Double-Blind Study of the Effect of Distant Healing in a Population With Advanced AIDS. Western Journal of Medicine. 1998;169 Dec::356-363.

Siegfried J. Electrostimulation and neurosurgical measures in cancer pain. Recent Results Cancer Res. 1988;108:28-32.

Silveri MM, Dikan J, Ross AJ, Jensen JE, Kamiya T, Kawada Y, Renshaw PF, Yurgelun-Todd DA. Citicoline enhances frontal lobe bioenergetics as measured by phosphorus magnetic resonance spectroscopy. NMR Biomed. 2008 Nov;21(10):1066-75.

Simpson G. The Major Features of Evolution. New York: Columbia Univ Press, 1953.

Sin DD, Man J, Sharpe H, Gan WQ, Man SF. Pharmacological management to reduce exacerbations in adults with asthma: a systematic review and meta-analysis. JAMA. 2004 Jul 21;292(3):367-76.

Singer P, Shapiro H, Theilla M, Anbar R, Singer J, Cohen J. Anti-inflammatory properties of omega-3 fatty acids in critical illness: novel mechanisms and an integrative perspective. Intensive Care Med. 2008 Sep;34(9):1580-92.

Singh AB, Singh N, Akanksha, Jayendra, Maurya R, Srivastava AK. Coagulanolide modulates hepatic glucose metabolism in C57BL/KsJ-db/db mice. Hum Exp Toxicol. 2012 Oct;31(10):1056-65. : 10.1177/0960327112438289.

Singh S, Khajuria A, Taneja SC, Johri RK, Singh J, Qazi GN. Boswellic acids: A leukotriene inhibitor also effective through topical application in inflammatory disorders. Phytomedicine. 2008 Jun;15(6-7):400-7.

Singh-Manoux A, Czernichow S, Elbaz A, Dugravot A, Sabia S, Hagger-Johnson G, Kaffashian S, Zins M, Brunner EJ, Nabi H, Kivimaki M. Obesity phenotypes in midlife and cognition in early old age: The Whitehall II cohort study. Neuro. 2012; 79 (8): 755.

Sinha R, Cross AJ, Graubard BI, Leitzmann MF, Schatzkin A. Meat in-take and mortality: a prospective study of over half a million people. Arch Intern Med. 2009 Mar 23;169(6):562-71.

Sivanandhan G, Arun M, Mayavan S, Rajesh M, Jeyaraj M, Dev GK, Manickavasagam M, Selvaraj N, Ganapathi A. Optimization of elicitation conditions with methyl jasmonate and salicylic acid to improve the productivity of withanolides in the adventitious root culture of Withania somnifera (L.) Dunal. Appl Biochem Biotechnol. 2012 Oct;168(3):681-96.

Sivanandhan G, Kapil Dev G, Jeyaraj M, Rajesh M, Muthuselvam M, Selvaraj N, Manickavasagam M, Ganapathi A. A promising approach on biomass accumulation and withanolides production in cell suspension culture of Withania somnifera (L.) Dunal. Protoplasma. 2012 Dec 18.

Sivanandhan G, Rajesh M, Arun M, Jeyaraj M, Dev GK, Manickavasagam M, Selvaraj N, Ganapathi A. Optimization of carbon source for hairy root growth and withaferin A and withanone production in Withania somnifera. Nat Prod Commun. 2012 Oct;7(10):1271-2.

293

Skoczylas A, Wiecek A. Ghrelin, a new hormone involved not only in the regulation of appetite. Wiad Lek. 2006;59(9-10):697-701.

Skwerer RG, Jacobsen FM, Duncan CC, Kelly KA, Sack DA, Tamarkin L, Gaist PA, Kasper S, Rosenthal NE. Neurobiology of Seasonal Affective Disorder and Phototherapy. J Biolog Rhyth. 1988;3(2):135-154.

Sloan F and Gelband (ed). Cancer Control Opportunities in Low- and Middle-Income Countries. Committee on Cancer Control in Low- and Middle-Income Countries. 2007.

Smith AD, Smith SM, de Jager CA, Whitbread P, Johnston C, Agacinski G, Oulhaj A, Bradley KM, Jacoby R, Refsum H. Homocysteine-lowering by B vitamins slows the rate of accelerated brain atrophy in mild cognitive impairment: a randomized controlled trial. PLoS One. 2010 Sep 8;5(9):e12244. doi: 10.1371/journal.pone.0012244.

Smith CW. Coherence in living biological systems. Neural Network World. 1994:4(3):379-388.

Smith MJ. "Effect of Magnetic Fields on Enzyme Reactivity" in Barnothy M.(ed.), Biological Effects of Magnetic Fields. New York: Plenum Press, 1969.

Smith MJ. The Influence on Enzyme Growth By the 'Laying on of Hands: Dimensions of Healing. Los Altos, California: Academy of Parapsychology and Medicine, 1973.

Smith S, Sullivan K. Examining the influence of biological and psychological factors on cognitive performance in chronic fatigue syndrome: a randomized, double-blind, placebo-controlled, crossover study. Int J Behav Med. 2003;10(2):162-73.

Smith T. Homeopathic Medicine: A Doctor's Guide. Rochester, VT: Healing Arts, 1989.

Smith-Sonneborn J. Age-correlated effects of caffeine on non-irradiated and UV-irradiated Paramecium Aurelia. J Gerontol. 1974 May;29(3):256-60.

Smith-Sonneborn J. DNA repair and longevity assurance in Paramecium tetraurelia. Science. 1979 Mar 16;203(4385):1115-7.

Snyder K. Researchers Produce Firsts with Bursts of Light: Team generates most energetic terahertz pulses yet, observes useful optical phenomena. Press Release: Brookhaven National Laboratory. 2007 July 24.

Sofic E, Denisova N, Youdim K, Vatrenjak-Velagic V, De Filippo C, Mehmedagic A, Causevic A, Cao G, Joseph JA, Prior RL. Antioxidant and pro-oxidant capacity of catecholamines and related compounds. Effects of hydrogen peroxide on glutathione and sphingomyelinase activity in pheochromocytoma PC12 cells: potential relevance to age-related diseases. J Neural Transm. 2001;108(5):541-57.

Sojkova J, Driscoll I, Iacono D, Zhou Y, Codispoti K-E, Kraut MA, et al. In vivo fibrillar beta-amyloid detected using [11C]PiB positron emission tomography and neuropathologic assessment in older adults. Arch Neurol 2011a;68:232-40.

Sojkova J, Zhou Y, An Y, Kraut MA, Ferrucci L, Wong DF, et al. Longitudinal patterns of β-amyloid deposition in nondemented older adults. Arch Neurol 2011b;68:644-9.

Solá R, Fitó M, Estruch R, Salas-Salvadó J, Corella D, de La Torre R, Muñoz MA, López-Sabater Mdel C, Martínez-González MA, Arós F, Ruiz-Gutierrez V, Fiol M, Casals E, Wärnberg J, Buil-Cosiales P, Ros E, Konstantinidou V, Lapetra J, Serra-Majem L, Covas MI. Effect of a traditional Mediterranean diet on apolipoproteins B, A-I, and their ratio: a randomized, controlled trial. Atherosclerosis. 2011 Sep;218(1):174-80.

Soleo L, Colosio C, Alinovi R, Guarneri D, Russo A, Lovreglio P, Vimercati L, Birindelli S, Cortesi I, Flore C, Carta P, Colombi A, Parrinello G, Ambrosi L. Immunologic effects of exposure to low levels of inorganic mercury. Med Lav. 2002 May-Jun;93(3):225-32.

Soler M, Chandra S, Ruiz D, Davidson E, Hendrickson D, Christou G. A third isolated oxidation state for the Mn12 family of singl molecule magnets. ChemComm; 2000; Nov 22.

Solfrizzi V, Frisardi V, Seripa D, Logroscino G, Imbimbo BP, D'Onofrio G, Addante F, Sancarlo D, Cascavilla L, Pilotto A, Panza F. Mediterranean diet in predementia and dementia syndromes. Curr Alzheimer Res. 2011 Aug;8(5):520-42.

Solfrizzi V, Frisardi V, Seripa D, Logroscino G, Imbimbo BP, D'Onofrio G, Addante F, Sancarlo D, Cascavilla L, Pilotto A, Panza F. Mediterranean diet in predementia and dementia syndromes. Curr Alzheimer Res. 2011 Aug;8(5):520-42.

Solfrizzi V, Panza F, Frisardi V, Seripa D, Logroscino G, Imbimbo BP, Pilotto A. Diet and Alzheimer's disease risk factors or prevention: the current evidence. Expert Rev Neurother. 2011 May;11(5):677-708.

Soman S, Korah PK, Jayanarayanan S, Mathew J, Paulose CS. Oxidative stress induced NMDA receptor alteration leads to spatial memory deficits in temporal lobe epilepsy: ameliorative effects of Withania somnifera and Withanolide A. Neurochem Res. 2012 Sep;37(9):1915-27.

Sompamit K, Kukongviriyapan U, Nakmareong S, Pannangpetch P, Kukongviriyapan V. Curcumin improves vascular function and alleviates oxidative stress in non-lethal lipopolysaccharide-induced endotoxaemia in mice. Eur J Pharmacol. 2009 Aug 15;616(1-3):192-9.

Song JX, Sze SC, Ng TB, Lee CK, Leung GP, Shaw PC, Tong Y, Zhang YB. Anti-Parkinsonian drug discovery from herbal medicines: What have we got from neurotoxic models? J Ethnopharmacol. 2011 Dec 29.

Soni MG, Carabin IG, Burdock GA. Safety assessment of esters of p-hydroxybenzoic acid (parabens). Food Chem Toxicol. 2005 Jul;43(7):985-1015.

Sorelle JA, Itoh T, Peng H, Kanak MA, Sugimoto K, Matsumoto S, Levy MF, Lawrence MC, Naziruddin B. Withaferin A inhibits pro-inflammatory cytokine-induced damage to islets in culture and following transplantation. Diabetologia. 2013 Jan 15.

Soul Has Weight, Physician Thinks. The New York Times. 1907 March 11:5.

REFERENCES AND BIBLIOGRAPHY

Southgate, D. Nature and variability of human food consumption. Philosophical Transactions of the Royal Society of London. 1991;B(334): 281-288.

Spanagel R, Rosenwasser AM, Schumann G, Sarkar DK. Alcohol consumption and the body's biological clock. Alcohol Clin Exp Res. 2005 Aug;29(8):1550-7.

Speed Of Light May Not Be Constant, Physicist Suggests. Science Daily. 1999 Oct 6. www.sciencedaily.com/releases/1999/10/991005114024.htm. Acc. 2007 Jun.

Spence A. Basic Human Anatomy. Menlo Park, CA: Benjamin/Commings, 1986.

Sperling RA, Aisen PS, Beckett LA, Bennett DA, Craft S, Fagan AM, et al. Toward defining the preclinical stages of Alzheimer's disease: recommendations from the National Institute on Aging-Alzheimer's Association workgroups on diagnostic guidelines for Alzheimer's disease. Alzheimers Dement 2011a;7:280-92.

Sperling RA, Jack CR Jr., Aisen PS. Testing the right target and right drug at the right stage. Sci Transl Med 2011b;3:111cm33.

Spetner L. Not By Chance! -Shattering The Modern Theory of Evolution. New York: The Judaica Press, 1997.

Spillane M. Good Vibrations, A Sound 'Diet' for Plants. The Growing Edge. 1991 Spring.

Spiller G. The Super Pyramid. New York: HRS Press, 1993.

Spira AP, Gamaldo AA, An Y, Wu MN, Simonsick EM, Bilgel M, Zhou Y, Wong DF, Ferrucci L, Resnick SM. Self-reported Sleep and β-Amyloid Deposition in Community-Dwelling Older Adults. JAMA Neurol. 2013 Oct 21. doi:10.1001/jamaneurol.2013.4258.

Spira AP, Yager C, Brandt J, Smith GS, Zhou Y, Mathur A, Kumar A, Brašić JR, Wong DF, Wu MN. Objectively Measured Sleep and β-amyloid Burden in Older Adults: A Pilot Study. SAGE Open Med. 2014 Aug 12;2. doi: 10.1177/2050312114546520.

Squire LR, Zola-Morgan S. The medial temporal lobe memory system. Science. 1991;253(5026):1380-1386.

St Hilaire MA, Klerman EB, Khalsa SB, Wright KP Jr, Czeisler CA, Kronauer RE. Addition of a non-photic component to a light-based mathematical model of the human circadian pacemaker. J Theor Biol. 2007 Aug 21;247(4):583-99.

Stabler SP, Allen RH. Vitamin B12 Deficiency as a Worldwide Problem. Annual Review of Nutrition. Vol. 24: 299-326. July 2004.

Stachowska E, Dolegowska B, Chlubek D, Wesolowska T, Ciechanowski K, Gutowski P, Szumilowicz H, Turowski R. Dietary trans fatty acids and composition of human atheromatous plaques. Eur J Nutr. 2004 Oct;43(5):313-8.

Stachowska E, Dolegowska B, Chlubek D, Wesolowska T, Ciechanowski K, Gutowski P, Szumilowicz H, Turowski R. Dietary trans fatty acids and composition of human atheromatous plaques. Eur J Nutr. 2004 Oct;43(5):313-8.

Stahler C. 1994. How many vegetarians are there?" Veget Jnl. 1994: July/August.

Stamets P. Mycelium Running. Berkeley, CA: Ten Speed Press, 2005.

Stampfer MJ, Willett WC, Colditz GA, Rosner B, Speizer FE, Hennekens CH. A prospective study of postmenopausal estrogen therapy and coronary heart disease. N Engl J Med. 1985 Oct 24;313(17):1044-9.

Stanford, C. B. The hunting ecology of wild chimpanzees: Implications for the evolutionary ecology of Pliocene hominids. American Anthropologist. 1996;98: 96-113.

Stanley M, Macauley SL, Holtzman DM. Changes in insulin and insulin signaling in Alzheimer's disease: cause or consequence? J Exp Med. 2016 Jul 25;213(8):1375-85. doi: 10.1084/jem.20160493.

State Pharmacopoeia Commission of The People's Republic of China. Pharmacopoeia of the People's Republic of China. Beijing: Chemical Industry Press; 2005.

Steck B. Effects of optical radiation on man. Light Resch Techn. 1982;14:130-141.

Steele JW, Brautigam H, Short JA, Sowa A, Shi M, Yadav A, Weaver CM, Westaway D, Fraser PE, St George-Hyslop PH, Gandy S, Hof PR, Dickstein DL. Early fear memory defects are associated with altered synaptic plasticity and molecular architecture in the TgCRND8 Alzheimer's disease mouse model. J Comp Neurol. 2014 Jul 1;522(10):2319-35. doi: 10.1002/cne.23536.

Steenhuysen J. New theory of Alzheimer's explains drug failures. Reuters Life. Wed May 12, 2010.

Stein MS, Scherer SC, Ladd KS, Harrison LC. A randomized controlled trial of high-dose vitamin D2 followed by intranasal insulin in Alzheimer's disease. J Alzheimers Dis. 2011;26(3):477-84. doi: 10.3233/JAD-2011-110149.

Steinberg S, Stefansson H, Jonsson T, Johannsdottir H, Ingason A, Helgason H, Sulem P, Magnusson OT, Gudjonsson SA, Unnsteinsdottir U, Kong A, Helisalmi S, Soininen H, Lah JJ; DemGene, Aarsland D, Fladby T, Ulstein ID, Djurovic S, Sando SB, White LR, Knudsen GP, Westlye LT, Selbæk G, Giegling I, Hampel H, Hiltunen M, Levey AI, Andreassen OA, Rujescu D, Jonsson PV, Bjornsson S, Snaedal J, Stefansson K. Loss-of-function variants in ABCA7 confer risk of Alzheimer's disease. Nat Genet. 2015 May;47(5):445-7. doi: 10.1038/ng.3246.

Steinberg S, Stefansson H, Jonsson T, Johannsdottir H, Ingason A, Helgason H, et al. (May 2015). "Loss-of-function variants in ABCA7 confer risk of Alzheimer's disease". Nature Genetics. 47 (5): 445–7. doi:10.1038/ng.3246

Steiner R. Agriculture. Kimberton, PA: Bio-Dynamic Farming, 1924-1993.

Stengler M. The Natural Physician's Healing Therapies. Stamford, CT: Bottom Line Books, 2008.

Stojanovic MP, Abdi S. Spinal cord stimulation. Pain Physician. 2002 Apr;5(2):156-66.

Stough C, Downey LA, Lloyd J, Silber B, Redman S, Hutchison C, Wesnes K, Nathan PJ.Examining the nootropic effects of a special extract of Bacopa monniera on human cognitive functioning: 90 day double-blind placebo-controlled randomized trial. Phytother Res. 2008 Dec;22(12):1629-34. doi: 10.1002/ptr.2537.

Stough C, Lloyd J, Clarke J, Downey LA, Hutchison CW, Rodgers T, Nathan PJ. The chronic effects of an extract of Bacopa monniera (Brahmi) on cognitive function in healthy human subjects. Psychopharmacology (Berl). 2001 Aug;156(4):481-4.

Stoupel E, Babyev E, Mustafa F, Abramson E, Israelevich P, Sulkes J. Acute myocardial infarction occurrence: Environmental links - Baku 2003-2005 data. Med Sci Monit. 2007 Aug;13(8):BR175-179.

Stoupel E, Kalediene R, Petrauskiene J, Gaizauskiene A, Israelevich P, Abramson E, Sulkes J. Monthly number of newborns and environmental physical activity. Medicina Kaunas. 2006;42(3):238-41.

Stoupel E, Monselise Y, Lahav J. Changes in autoimmune markers of the anti-cardiolipin syndrome on days of extreme geomamagnetic activity. J Basic Clin Physiol Pharmacol. 2006;17(4):269-78.

Stoupel EG, Frimer H, Appelman Z, Ben-Neriah Z, Dar H, Fejgin MD, Gershoni-Baruch R, Manor E, Barkai G, Shalev S, Gelman-Kohan Z, Reish O, Lev D, Davidov B, Goldman B, Shohat M. Chromosome aberration and environmental physical activity: Down syndrome and solar and cosmic ray activity, Israel, 1990-2000. Int J Biometeorol. 2005 Sep;50(1):1-5.

Strange BA, Dolan RJ. Anterior medial temporal lobe in human cognition: memory for fear and the unexpected. Cognit Neuropsychiatry. 2006 May;11(3):198-218.

Streitberger K, Ezzo J, Schneider A. Acupuncture for nausea and vomiting: an update of clinical and experimental studies. Auton Neurosci. 2006 Oct 30;129(1-2):107-17.

Strickland KC, Krupenko NI, Krupenko SA. Molecular mechanisms underlying the potentially adverse effects of folate. Clin Chem Lab Med. 2012 Dec 12:1-10.

Stuerenburg HJ, Ganzer S, Müller-Thomsen T. Plasma beta carotene in Alzheimer's disease. Association with cerebrospinal fluid beta-amyloid 1-40, (Abeta40), beta-amyloid 1-42 (Abeta42) and total Tau. Neuro Endocrinol Lett. 2005 Dec;26(6):696-8.

Stull AJ, Cash KC, Johnson WD, Champagne CM, Cefalu WT. Bioactives in blueberries improve insulin sensitivity in obese, insulin-resistant men and women. J Nutr. 2010 Oct;140(10):1764-8. doi: 10.3945/jn.110.125336.

Sugimoto Y, Nishimura K, Itoh A, Tanahashi T, Nakajima H, Oshiro H, Sun S, Toda T, Yamada J. Serotonergic mechanisms are involved in antidepressant-like effects of bisbenzylisoquinolines liensinine and its analogs isolated from the embryo of Nelumbo nucifera Gaertner seeds in mice. J Pharm Pharmacol. 2015 Aug 5. doi: 10.1111/jphp.12473.

Sulman FG, Levy D, Lunkan L, Pfeifer Y, Tal E. New methods in the treatment of weather sensitivity. Fortschr Med. 1977 Mar 17;95(11):746-52.

Sulman FG. Migraine and headache due to weather and allied causes and its specific treatment. Ups J Med Sci Suppl. 1980;31:41-4.

Sumiyoshi M, Sakanaka M, Kimura Y. Effects of Red Ginseng extract on allergic reactions to food in Balb/c mice. J Ethnopharmacol. 2010 Aug 14.

Sun Y, Lu CJ, Chien KL, Chen ST, Chen RC. Efficacy of multivitamin supplementation containing vitamins B6 and B12 and folic acid as adjunctive treatment with a cholinesterase inhibitor in Alzheimer's disease: a 26-week, randomized, double-blind, placebo-controlled study in Taiwanese patients. Clin Ther. 2007 Oct;29(10):2204-14.

Sung JH, Lee JO, Son JK, Park NS, Kim MR, Kim JG, Moon DC. Cytotoxic constituents from Solidago virga-aurea var. gigantea MIQ. Arch Pharm Res. 1999 Dec;22(6):633-7.

Suppes P, Han B, Epelboim J, Lu ZL. Invariance of brain-wave representations of simple visual images and their names. Proc Natl Acad Sci Psych-BS. 1999;96(25):14658-14663.

Sur R, Nigam A, Grote D, Liebel F, Southall MD. Avenanthramides, polyphenols from oats, exhibit anti-inflammatory and anti-itch activity. Arch Dermatol Res. 2008 May .

Suzuki R, Rylander-Rudqvist T, Ye W, Saji S, Adlercreutz H, Wolk A. Dietary fiber intake and risk of postmenopausal breast cancer defined by estrogen and progesterone receptor status—a prospective cohort study among Swedish women. Int J Cancer. 2008 Jan 15;122(2):403-12.

Suzuki R, Ye W, Rylander-Rudqvist T, Saji S, Colditz GA, Wolk A. Alcohol and postmenopausal breast cancer risk defined by estrogen and progesterone receptor status: a prospective cohort study. J Natl Cancer Inst. 2005 Nov 2;97(21):1601-8.

Suzuki Y, Kondo K, Ichise H, Tsukamoto Y, Urano T, Umemura K. Dietary supplementation with fermented soybeans suppresses intimal thickening. Nutrition. 2003 Mar;19(3):261-4.

Svedberg MM, Rahman O, Hall H. Preclinical studies of potential amyloid binding PET/SPECT ligands in Alzheimer's disease. Nucl Med Biol. 2012 Jan 4.

Szyf M, McGowan P, Meaney MJ. The social environment and the epigenome. Environ Mol Mutagen. 2008 Jan;49(1):46-60.

Tahmasbi AM, Mirakzehi MT, Hosseini SJ, Agah MJ, Fard MK. The effects of phytase and root hydroalcoholic extract of Withania somnifera on productive performance and bone mineralisation of laying hens in the late phase of production. Br Poult Sci. 2012;53(2):204-14.

Tajadini H, Saifadini R, Choopani R, Mehrabani M, Kamalinejad M, Haghdoost AA. Herbal medicine Davaie Loban in mild to moderate Alzheimer's disease: A 12-week randomized double-blind placebo-controlled clinical trial. Complement Ther Med. 2015 Dec;23(6):767-72. doi: 10.1016/j.ctim.2015.06.009.

Takata Y, Shu XO, Gao YT, Li H, Zhang X, Gao J, Cai H, Yang G, Xiang YB, Zheng W. Red meat and poultry intakes and risk of total and cause-specific mortality: results from cohort studies of Chinese adults in Shanghai. PLoS One. 2013;8(2):e56963. doi: 10.1371/journal.pone.0056963.

Talairach J, Tournoux P. Co-planar stereotaxic atlas of the human brain. New York: Thieme; 1988.

Tan DX, Manchester LC, Reiter RJ, Qi WB, Karbownik M, Calvo JR. Significance of melatonin in antioxidative defense system: reactions and products. Biol Signals Recept. 2000 May-Aug;9(3-4):137-59.

Tanagho EA. Principles and indications of electrostimulation of the urinary bladder. Urologe A. 1990 Jul;29(4):185-90.

Tang G, Serfaty-Lacrosniere C, Camilo ME, Russell RM. Gastric acidity influences the blood response to a beta-carotene dose in humans. Am J Clin Nutr. 1996;64:622-6.

Taoka S, Padmakumar R, Grissom C, Banerjee R. Magnetic Field Effects on Coenzyme B-12 Dependent Enzymes: Validation of Ethanolamine Ammonia Lyase Results and Extension to Human Methylmalonyl CoA Mutase. Bioelectromagnetics. 1997;18: 506-513.

Tapiero H, Ba GN, Couvreur P, Tew KD. Polyunsaturated fatty acids (PUFA) and eicosanoids in human health and pathologies. Biomed Pharmacother. 2002 Jul;56(5):215-22.

Tapola N, Karvonen H, Niskanen L, Mikola M, Sarkkinen E. Glycemic responses of oat bran products in type 2 diabetic patients. Nutr Metab Cardiovasc Dis. 2005 Aug;15(4):255-61.

Tapsell LC, Hemphill I, Cobiac L, Patch CS, Sullivan DR, Fenech M, Roodenrys S, Keogh JB, Clifton PM, Williams PG, Fazio VA, Inge KE. Health benefits of herbs and spices: the past, the present, the future. Med J Aust. 2006 Aug 21;185(4 Suppl):S4-24.

Taraban M, Leshina T, Anderson M, Grissom C. Magnetic Field Dependence and the Role of electron spin in Heme Enzymes: Horseradish Peroxidase. J. Am. Chem. Soc. 1997;119: 5768-5769.

Targ R, Katra J, Brown D, Wiegand W. Viewing the future: A pilot study with an error-detecting protocol. J Sci Expl. 9:3:367-380, 1995.

Targ R, Puthoff H. Information transfer under conditions of sensory shielding. Nature. 1975;251:602-607.

Tassone F, Broglio F, Gianotti L, Arvat E, Ghigo E, Maccario M. Ghrelin and other gastrointestinal peptides involved in the control of food intake. Mini Rev Med Chem. 2007 Jan;7(1):47-53.

Tauchert M. Efficacy and safety of crataegus extract WS 1442 in comparison with placebo in patients with chronic stable New York Heart Association class-III heart failure. Am Heart J. 2002 May;143(5):910-5.

Taussig SJ, Batkin S. Bromelain, the enzyme complex of pineapple (Ananas comosus) and its clinical application. An update. J Ethnopharmacol. 1988 Feb-Mar;22(2):191-203.

Taussig SJ, Batkin S. Bromelain, the enzyme complex of pineapple (Ananas comosus) and its clinical application. An update. J Ethnopharmacol. 1988 Feb-Mar;22(2):191-203.

Taylor A. Soul Traveler: A Guide to Out-of-Body Experiences and the Wonders Beyond. New York: Penguin, 2000.

Taylor RB, Lindquist N, Kubanek J, Hay ME. Intraspecific variation in palatability and defensive chemistry of brown seaweeds: effects on herbivore fitness. Oecologia. 2003 Aug;136(3):412-23.

Teitelbaum J. From Fatigue to Fantastic. New York: Avery, 2001.

Termanini B, Gibril F, Sutliff VE, Yu F, Venzon DJ, Jensen RT. Effect of long-term gastric acid suppressive therapy on serum vitamin B12 levels in patients with Zollinger-Ellison syndrome. Am J Med. 1998 May;104(5):422-30.

Tevini M, ed. UV-B Radiation and Ozone Depletion: Effects on humans, animals, plants, microorganisms and materials. Boca Raton: Lewis Pub, 1993.

Thakur CP, Sharma D. Full moon and crime. Br Med J. 1984 December 22; 289(6460): 1789-1791.

Thampithak A, Jaisin Y, Meesarapee B, Chongthammakun S, Piyachaturawat P, Govitrapong P, Supavilai P, Sanvarinda Y. Transcriptional regulation of iNOS and COX-2 by a novel compound from Curcuma comosa in lipopolysaccharide-induced microglial activation. Neurosci Lett. 2009 Sep 22;462(2):171-5.

Thaut MH. The future of music in therapy and medicine. Ann N Y Acad Sci. 2005 Dec;1060:303-8.

The Mystery of Smell. Howard Hughes Medical Instit. http://www.hhmi.org/senses/d110.html. Acc. 2007 Jul.

The Timechart Company. Timetables of Medicine. New York: Black Dog & Leventhal, 2000.

Theofilopoulos AN, Kono DH. The genes of systemic autoimmunity. Proc Assoc Am Physicians. 1999;111(3): 228-240.

Theuwissen E, Mensink RP. Water-soluble dietary fibers and cardiovascular disease. Physiol Behav. 2008 May 23;94(2):285-92.

Thie J. Touch for Health. Marina del Rey, CA: Devorss Publications, 1973-1994.

Thomas B, Lloyd-Jones DM, Thadhani RI, Shaw AC, Deraska DJ, Kitch BT, Vamvakas EC, Dick IM, Prince RL, Finkelstein JS. Hypovitaminosis D in medical inpatients. N Engl J Med. 1998 Mar 19;338(12):777-83

Thomas, R.G., Gebhardt, S.E. 2008. Nutritive value of pomegranate fruit and juice. Maryland Dietetic Association Annual Meeting, USDA-ARS. 2008 April 11.

Thomas-Anterion C, Jacquin K, Laurent B. Differential mechanisms of impairment of remote memory in Alzheimer's and frontotemporal dementia. Dement Geriatr Cogn Disord. 2000 Mar-Apr;11(2):100-6.

Thompson D. On Growth and Form. Cambridge: Cambridge University Press, 1992.

Thorogood M, Mann J, Appleby P, McPherson K. Risk of death from cancer and ischaemic heart disease in meat and non-meat eaters. BMJ. 1994 June 25;308:1667-1670.

Threlkeld DS, ed. Central Nervous System Drugs, Analeptics, Caffeine. Facts and Comparisons Drug Information. St. Louis, MO: Facts and Comparisons. 1998 Feb: 230-d.

Threlkeld DS, ed. Gastrointestinal Drugs, Proton Pump Inhibitors. Facts and Comparisons Drug Information. St. Louis, MO: Facts and Comparisons. 1998 Apr: 305r.

Tian FS, Zhang HR, Li WD, Qiao P, Duan HB, Jia CX. Study on acupuncture treatment of diabetic neurogenic bladder. Zhongguo Zhen Jiu. 2007 Jul;27(7):485-7.

Tian, Jinzhou, et al. P4-302: Effect of GETO extract on expression of ChAT and NGF in the brain with AD model. Alzheimer's and Dementia 2.3 (2006): S605-S606.

Tierra L. The Herbs of Life. Freedom, CA: Crossing Press, 1992.

Tierra M. The Way of Herbs. New York: Pocket Books, 1990.

Tieu K, Perier C, Caspersen C, Teismann P, Wu DC, Yan SD, Naini A, Vila M, Jackson-Lewis V, Ramasamy R, Przedborski S. D-beta-hydroxybutyrate rescues mitochondrial respiration and mitigates features of Parkinson disease. J Clin Invest. 2003;112:892–901.

Tieu K, Perier C, Caspersen C, Teismann P, Wu DC, Yan SD, Naini A, Vila M, Jackson-Lewis V, Ramasamy R, Przedborski S. D-beta-hydroxybutyrate rescues mitochondrial respiration and mitigates features of Parkinson disease. J Clin Invest. 2003;112:892–901.

Timofeev I, Steriade M. Low-frequency rhythms in the thalamus of intact-cortex and decorticated cats. J Neurophysiol. 1996 Dec;76(6):4152-68.

Ting W, Schultz K, Cac NN, Peterson M, Walling HW. Tanning bed exposure increases the risk of malignant melanoma. Int J Dermatol. 2007 Dec;46(12):1253-7.

Tiraboschi P, Hansen LA, Thal LJ, Corey-Bloom J. The importance of neuritic plaques and tangles to the development and evolution of AD. Neurology 2004;62:1984-9.

Tisserand R. The Art of Aromatherapy. New York: Inner Traditions, 1979.

Tiwari M. Ayurveda: A Life of Balance. Rochester, VT: Healing Arts, 1995.

Todd GR, Acerini CL, Ross-Russell R, Zahra S, Warner JT, McCance D. Survey of adrenal crisis associated with inhaled corticosteroids in the United Kingdom. Arch Dis Child. 2002 Dec;87(6):457-61.

Tompkins, P, Bird C. The Secret Life of Plants. New York: Harper & Row, 1973.

Tonkal AM, Morsy TA. An update review on Commiphora molmol and related species. J Egypt Soc Parasitol. 2008 Dec;38(3):763-96.

Toomer G. "Ptolemy". The Dictionary of Scientific Biography. New York: Gale Cengage, 1970.

Topçu G, Erenler R, Cakmak O, Johansson CB, Celik C, Chai HB, Pezzuto JM. Diterpenes from the berries of Juniperus excelsa. Phytochemistry. 1999 Apr;50(7):1195-9.

Trapp GA, Miner GD, Zimmerman RL, Mastri AR, Heston LL. Aluminum levels in brain in Alzheimer's disease. Biol Psychiatry. 1978 Dec;13(6):709-18.

Tresserra-Rimbau A, Medina-Remón A, Pérez-Jiménez J, Martínez-González MA, Covas MI, Corella D, Salas-Salvadó J, Gómez-Gracia E, Lapetra J, Arós F, Fiol M, Ros E, Serra-Majem L, Pintó X, Muñoz MA, Saez GT, Ruiz-Gutiérrez V, Warnberg J, Estruch R, Lamuela-Raventós RM. Dietary intake and major food sources of polyphenols in a Spanish population at high cardiovascular risk: The PREDIMED study. Nutr Metab Cardiovasc Dis. 2013 Jan 16. doi:pii: S0939-4753(12)00245-1. 10.1016/j.numecd.2012.10.008.

Triglia A, La Malfa G, Musumeci F, Leonardi C, Scordino A. Delayed luminescence as an indicator of tomato fruit quality. J Food Sci. 1998;63:512-515.

Trivedi B. Magnetic Map" Found to Guide Animal Migration. Natl Geogr Today. 2001 Oct 12.

Trovato A, Siracusa R, Di Paola R, Scuto M, Fronte V, Koverech G, Luca M, Serra A, Toscano MA, Petralia A, Cuzzocrea S, Calabrese V. Redox modulation of cellular stress response and lipoxin A4 expression by Coriolus versicolor in rat brain: Relevance to Alzheimer's disease pathogenesis. Neurotoxicology. 2016 Mar;53:350-8. doi: 10.1016/j.neuro.2015.09.012.

Tsinkalovsky O, Smaaland R, Rosenlund B, Sothern RB, Hirt A, Steine S, Badiee A, Abrahamsen JF, Eiken HG, Laerum OD. Circadian variations in clock gene expression of human bone marrow CD34+ cells. J Biol Rhythms. 2007 Apr;22(2):140-50.

Tsong T. Deciphering the language of cells. Trends in Biochem Sci. 1989;14: 89-92.

Tsuei JJ, Lam Jr. F, Zhao Z. Studies in Bioenergetic Correlations-Bioenergetic Regulatory Measurement Instruments and Devices. Am J Acupunct. 1988;16:345-9.

Tsuei JJ, Lehman CW, Lam F, Jr, Zhu D. A food allergy study utilizing the EAV acupuncture technique. Am J Acupunct. 1984;12:105-16.

Tubek S. Role of trace elements in primary arterial hypertension: is mineral water style or prophylaxis? Biol Trace Elem Res. 2006 Winter;114(1-3):1-5.

Tucker J. Life Before Life: A Scientific Investigation of Children's Memories of Previous Lives. New York: St. Martin's Press, 2005.

Tweed K. Study: Conceiving in Summer Lowers Baby's Future Test Scores. Fox News. 2007 May 9, 2007. (Study done by: Winchester P. 2007. Pediatric Academic Societies annual meeting.)

Tzourio-Mazoyer N, Landeau B, Papathanassiou D, Crivello F, Etard O, Delcroix N, et al. Automated anatomical labeling of activations in SPM using a macroscopic anatomical parcellation of the MNI MRI single-subject brain. Neuroimage 2002;15:273-89. Villemagne VL, Fodero-Tavoletti MT, Pike KE, Cappai R, Masters CL, Rowe CC. The ART of loss: Abeta imaging in the evaluation of Alzheimer's disease and other dementias. Mol Neurobiol 2008;38:1-15.

U.S. Food and Drug Administration Guidance for Industry Botanical Drug Products. CfDEaR. 2000

Udermann H, Fischer G. Studies on the influence of positive or negative small ions on the catechol amine content in the brain of the mouse following shorttime or prolonged exposure. Zentralbl Bakteriol Mikrobiol Hyg. 1982 Apr;176(1):72-8.

Uezu A, Kanak DJ, Bradshaw TW, Soderblom EJ, Catavero CM, Burette AC, Weinberg RJ, Soderling SH. Identification of an elaborate complex mediating postsynaptic inhibition. Science. 2016 Sep 9;353(6304):1123-9. doi: 10.1126/science.aag0821.

Ulett G. Electroacupuncture: mechanisms and clinical application. Biological Psychiatry. 1998;44(2):129-138.

Ullman D. Controlled clinical trials evaluating the homeopathic treatment of people with human immunodeficiency virus or acquired immune deficiency syndrome. J Altern Complement Med. 2003 Feb;9(1):133-41.

Ullman D. Discovering Homeopathy. Berkeley, CA: North Atlantic, 1991.

298

REFERENCES AND BIBLIOGRAPHY

Um HJ, Min KJ, Kim DE, Kwon TK. Withaferin A inhibits JAK/STAT3 signaling and induces apoptosis of human renal carcinoma Caki cells. Biochem Biophys Res Commun. 2012 Oct 12;427(1):24-9.

Unconventional But Effective Therapy for Alzheimer's Treatment: Dr. Mary T. Newport. http://www.youtube.com/watch?v=Dvh3JhsrQ0w.

Unger RH. Leptin physiology: a second look. Regul Pept. 2000 Aug 25;92(1-3):87-95.

Upadhyay BN, Gupta V. A clinical study on the effect of Rishyagandha (Withania coagulans) in the management of Prameha (Type II Diabetes Mellitus). Ayu. 2011 Oct;32(4):507-11.

USDA National Nutrient Database for Standard Reference, Release 21. NDB 09209. Accessed 10/21/2008.

Vakil JR, Shahani KM. Carbohydrate metabolism of lactic acid cultures. V. Lactobionate and gluconate metabolism of Streptococcus lactis UN. J Dairy Sci. 1969 Dec;52(12):1928-34.

Valgimigli L, Sapone A, Canistro D, Broccoli M, Gatta L, Soleti A, Paolini M. Oxidative stress and aging: a non-invasive EPR investigation in human volunteers. Aging Clin Exp Res. 2014 Jul 31.

Vallance A. Can biological activity be maintained at ultra-high dilution? An overview of homeopathy, evidence, and Bayesian philosophy. J Altern Complement Med. 1998 Spring;4(1):49-76.

van Beelen VA, Roeleveld J, Mooibroek H, Sijtsma L, Bino RJ, Bosch D, Rietjens IM, Alink GM. A comparative study on the effect of algal and fish oil on viability and cell proliferation of Caco-2 cells. Food Chem Toxicol. 2007 May;45(5):716-24.

Van Cauter E, Leproult R, Plat L. Age-related changes in slow wave sleep and REM sleep and relationship with growth hormone and cortisol levels in healthy men. JAMA. 2000 Aug 16;284(7):861-8.

van Dam RM, Willett WC, Rimm EB, Stampfer MJ, Hu FB. Dietary fat and meat intake in relation to risk of type 2 diabetes in men. Diabetes Care. 2002 Mar;25(3):417-24.

van den Berg H, Dagnelie P, van Staveren W. Vitamin B12 and seaweed. Lancet. 1988;1:242-3.

van den Eeden SK, Koepsell TD, Longstreth WT, van Belle G, Daling JR, McKnight B. Aspartame ingestion and headache: a randomized crossover trial. Neurology. 1994;44:1787-93.

van Dyck CH, Lyness JM, Rohrbaugh RM, Siegal AP. Cognitive and psychiatric effects of vitamin B12 replacement in dementia with low serum B12 levels: a nursing home study. Int Psychogeriatr. 2009 Feb;21(1):138-47. doi: 10.1017/S1041610208007904.

Van Maele-Fabry G, Hoet P, Vilain F, Lison D. Occupational exposure to pesticides and Parkinson's disease: a systematic review and meta-analysis of cohort studies. Environ Int. 2012 Oct 1;46:30-43.

Van Wijk R, Wiegant FAC. Cultured mammalian cells in homeopathy research: the similia principle in self-recovery. Utrecht: University Utrecht Publ, 1994.

van Woudenbergh GJ, Kuijsten A, Tigcheler B, Sijbrands EJ, van Rooij FJ, Hofman A, Witteman JC, Feskens EJ. Meat Consumption and Its Association With C-Reactive Protein and Incident Type 2 Diabetes: The Rotterdam Study. Diabetes Care. 2012 May 17.

Vandenbroucke JP. Should you eat meat, or are you confounded by methodological debate? BMJ. 1994 Jun 25;308(6945):1671.

Vaquero JM, Gallego MC. Sunspot numbers can detect pandemic influenza A: the use of different sunspot numbers. Med Hypotheses. 2007;68(5):1189-90.

Vargha-Khadem F, Polkey CE. A review of cognitive outcome after hemidecortication in humans. Adv Exp Med Biol. 1992;325:137-51.

Varraso R, Jiang R, Barr RG, Willett WC, Camargo CA Jr. Prospective study of cured meats consumption and risk of chronic obstructive pulmonary disease in men. Am J Epidemiol. 2007 Dec 15;166(12):1438-45. 2007 Sep 4. 17785711; .

Vassallo N, Scerri C. Mediterranean Diet and Dementia of the Alzheimer Type. Curr Aging Sci. 2012 Sep 27.

Vauthier JM, Lluch A, Lecomte E, Artur Y, Herbeth B. Family resemblance in energy and macronutrient intakes: the Stanislas Family Study. Int J Epidemiol. 1996 Oct;25(5):1030-7.

Velusami CC, Agarwal A, Mookambeswaran V. Effect of Nelumbo nucifera Petal Extracts on Lipase, Adipogenesis, Adipolysis, and Central Receptors of Obesity. Evid Based Complement Alternat Med. 2013;2013:145925. doi: 10.1155/2013/145925.

Venkatesan N, Punithavathi D, Babu M. Protection from acute and chronic lung diseases by curcumin. Adv Exp Med Biol. 2007;595:379-405.

Vescelius E. Music and Health. New York: Goodyear Book Shop, 1918.

Vetvicka V, Vetvickova J. Immune enhancing effects of WB365, a novel combination of Ashwagandha (Withania somnifera) and Maitake (Grifola frondosa) extracts. N Am J Med Sci. 2011 Jul;3(7):320-4.

Vickers A. Botanical medicines for the treatment of cancer: rationale, overview of current data, and methodological considerations for phase I and II trials. Cancer Invest. 2002;20(7-8):1069-79.

Vickers AJ, Kuo J, Cassileth BR. Unconventional anticancer agents: a systematic review of clinical trials. J Clin Oncol. 2006 Jan 1;24(1):136-40.

Vidgren HM, Agren JJ, Schwab U, Rissanen T, Hanninen O, Uusitupa MI. Incorporation of n-3 fatty acids into plasma lipid fractions, and erythrocyte membranes and platelets during dietary supplementation with fish, fish oil, and docosahexaenoic acid-rich oil among healthy young men. Lipids. 1997 Jul;32(7):697-705.

Vidgren HM, Agren JJ, Schwab U, Rissanen T, Hanninen O, Uusitupa MI. Incorporation of n-3 fatty acids into plasma lipid fractions, and erythrocyte membranes and platelets during dietary supplementation with fish, fish oil, and docosahexaenoic acid-rich oil among healthy young men. Lipids. 1997 Jul;32(7):697-705.

Vierling-Claassen D, Siekmeier P, Stufflebeam S, Kopell N. Modeling GABA alterations in schizophrenia: a link between impaired inhibition and altered gamma and beta range auditory entrainment. J Neurophysiol. 2008 May;99(5):2656-71.

299

Vigny P, Duquesne M. On the fluorescence properties of nucleotides and polynucleotides at room temperature. In. Birks J (ed.). Excited states of biological molecules. London-NY: J Wiley, 1976:167-177.

Villemagne VL, McLean CA, Reardon K, Boyd A, Lewis V, Klug G, et al. 11C-PiB PET studies in typical sporadic Creutzfeldt-Jakob disease. J Neurol Neurosurg Psychiatr 2009;80:998-1001.

Villemagne VL, Pike KE, Chételat G, Ellis KA, Mulligan RS, Bourgeat P, et al. Longitudinal assessment of amyloid-β and cognition in aging and Alzheimer disease. Ann Neurol 2011;69:181-92.

Viswanathan A, Raj S, Greenberg SM, Stampfer M, Campbell S, Hyman BT, Irizarry MC. Plasma Abeta, homocysteine, and cognition: the Vitamin Intervention for Stroke Prevention (VISP) trial. Neurology. 2009 Jan 20;72(3):268-72. doi: 10.1212/01.wnl.0000339486.63862.db.

Volkmann H, Dannberg G, Kuhnert H, Heinke M. Therapeutic value of trans-esophageal electrostimulation in tachycardic arrhythmias. Z Kardiol. 1991 Jun;80(6):382-8.

Voll R. The phenomenon of medicine testing in elecroacupuncture according to Voll. Am J Acupunct. 1980;8:97-104.

Voll R. Twenty years of electroacupuncture diagnosis in Germany: a progressive report. Am J Acupunct. 1975;3:7-17.

Volman JJ, Ramakers JD, Plat J. Dietary modulation of immune function by beta-glucans. Physiol Behav. 2008 May 23;94(2):276-84.

von Arnim CA, Herbolsheimer F, Nikolaus T, Peter R, Biesalski HK, Ludolph AC, Riepe M, Nagel G; ActiFE Ulm Study Group. Dietary antioxidants and dementia in a population-based case-control study among older people in South Germany. J Alzheimers Dis. 2012;31(4):717-24. doi: 10.3233/JAD-2012-120634.

von Schantz M, Archer SN. Clocks, genes and sleep. J R Soc Med. 2003 Oct;96(10):486-9.

Vuksan V, Whitham D, Sievenpiper JL, Jenkins AL, Rogovik AL, Bazinet RP, Vidgen E, Hanna A. Supplementation of conventional therapy with the novel grain Salba (Salvia hispanica L.) improves major and emerging cardiovascular risk factors in type 2 diabetes: results of a randomized controlled trial. Diabetes Care. 2007 Nov;30(11):2804-10.

Vyas P, Chandola HM, Ghanchi F, Ranthem S. Clinical evaluation of Rasayana compound as an adjuvant in the management of tuberculosis with anti-Koch's treatment. Ayu. 2012 Jan;33(1):38-43.

Vyasadeva S. Srimad Bhagavatam. Approx rec 4000 BCE.

Wachiuli M, Koyama M, Utsuyama M, Bittman BB, Kitagawa M, Hirokawa K. Recreational music-making modulates natural killer cell activity, cytokines, and mood states in corporate employees. Med Sci Monit. 2007 Feb;13(2):CR57-70.

Wade N. From Ants to Ethics: A Biologist Dreams of Unity of Knowledge. Scientist at Work, Edward O. Wilson. New York Times. 1998 May 12.

Walker AF, Marakis G, Morris AP, Robinson PA. Promising hypotensive effect of hawthorn extract: a randomized double-blind pilot study of mild, essential hypertension. Phytother Res. 2002 Feb;16(1):48-54.

Walker M. The Power of Color. Gujarat, India: Jain Publ., 2002.

Wang H, Zhai F. Program and Policy Options for Preventing Obesity in China. Obes Rev. 2013 Sep 9.

Wang LC, Wang SE, Wang JJ, Tsai TY, Lin CH, Pan TM, Lee CL. In vitro and in vivo comparisons of the effects of the fruiting body and mycelium of Antrodia camphorata against amyloid β-protein-induced neurotoxicity and memory impairment. Appl Microbiol Biotechnol. 2012 Jun;94(6):1505-19. doi: 10.1007/s00253-012-3941-3.

Wang MS, Boddapati S, Emadi S, Sierks MR. Curcumin reduces alpha-synuclein induced cytotoxicity in Parkinson's disease cell model. BMC Neurosci. 2010 Apr 30;11:57.Bezaitis A. Gatz Updates Alzheimer's Findings. Psychologist discusses her research on dementia in Swedish twins at a USC Davis School gathering. USC Dorn News. September 1, 2007

Wang MX, Liu YL, Yang Y, Zhang DM, Kong LD. Nuciferine restores potassium oxonate-induced hyperuricemia and kidney inflammation in mice. Eur J Pharmacol. 2015 Jan 15;747:59-70. doi: 10.1016/j.ejphar.2014.11.035.

Wang MY, Peng L, Weidenbacher-Hoper V, Deng S, Anderson G, West BJ. Noni juice improves serum lipid profiles and other risk markers in cigarette smokers. ScientificWorldJournal. 2012;2012:594657. doi: 10.1100/2012/594657.

Wang R, Jiang C, Lei Z, Yin K. The role of different therapeutic courses in treating 47 cases of rheumatoid arthritis with acupuncture. J Tradit Chin Med. 2007 Jun;27(2):103-5.

Wang XY, Shi X, He L. Effect of electroacupuncture on gastrointestinal dynamics in acute pancreatitis patients and its mechanism. Zhen Ci Yan Jiu. 2007;32(3):199-202.

Wang YM, Huan GX. Utilization of Classical Formulas. Beijing, China: Chinese Medicine and Pharmacology Publishing Co, 1998.

Waser M, et al. PARSIFAL Study team. Inverse association of farm milk consumption with asthma and allergy in rural and suburban populations across Europe. Clin Exp Allergy. 2007 May;37(5):661-70.

Waterman E, Lockwood B. Active components and clinical applications of olive oil. Altern Med Rev. 2007 Dec;12(4):331-42.

Watkins BA, Hannon K, Ferruzzi M, Li Y. Dietary PUFA and flavonoids as deterrents for environmental pollutants. J Nutr Biochem. 2007 Mar;18(3):196-205.

Watnick S. Pregnancy and contraceptive counseling of women with chronic kidney disease and kidney transplants. Adv Chronic Kidney Dis. 2007 Apr;14(2):126-31.

Watson L. Beyond Supernature. New York: Bantam, 1987.

Watson L. Supernature. New York: Bantam, 1973.

Watson R. Preedy VR. Botanical Medicine in Clinical Practice. Oxfordshire: CABI, 2008.

Wauters M, Considine RV, Van Gaal LF. Human leptin: from an adipocyte hormone to an endocrine mediator. Eur J Endocrinol. 2000 Sep;143(3):293-311.

Wayne R. Chemistry of the Atmospheres. Oxford Press, 1991.

WB Saunders; 1982, Fishman HC. Notalgia paresthetica. J Am Acad Dermatol. 1986;15:1304-1305

Weatherley-Jones E, Thompson E, Thomas K. The placebo-controlled trial as a test of complementary and alternative medicine: observations from research experience of individualised homeopathic treatment. Homeopathy. 2004 Oct;93(4):186-9.

Weaver J, Astumian R. The response of living cells to very weak electric fields: the thermal noise limit. Science. 1990;247: 459-462.

Wee K, Rogers T, Altan BS, Hackney SA, Hamm C. Engineering and medical applications of diatoms. J Nanosci Nanotechnol. 2005 Jan;5(1):88-91.

Wegrowski J, Robert AM, Moczar M. The effect of procyanidolic oligomers on the composition of normal and hypercholesterolemic rabbit aortas. Biochem Pharmacol. 1984 Nov 1;33(21):3491-7.

Wei A, Shibamoto T. Antioxidant activities and volatile constituents of various essential oils. J Agric Food Chem. 2007 Mar 7;55(5):1737-42.

Weikl A, Assmus KD, Neukum-Schmidt A, Schmitz J, Zapfe G, Noh HS, Siegrist J. Crataegus Special Extract WS 1442. Assessment of objective effectiveness in patients with heart failure (NYHA II). Fortschr Med. 1996 Aug 30;114(24):291-6.

Weil, A. 2004. Dr. Andrew Weil's Self Healing. September, page 6

Weinberger P, Measures M. The effect of two audible sound frequencies on the germination and growth of a spring and winter wheat. Can. J. Bot. 1968;46(9):1151-1158.

Weiner MA. Secrets of Fijian Medicine. Berkeley, CA: Univ. of Calif., 1969.

Weiner MW, Aisen PS, Jack CR Jr., Jagust WJ, Trojanowski JQ, Shaw L., et al. The Alzheimer's disease neuroimaging initiative: progress report and future plans. Alzheimers Dement 2010;6:202-11.e7.

Weinert D, Waterhouse J. The circadian rhythm of core temperature: effects of physical activity and aging. Physiol Behav. 2007 Feb 28;90(2-3):246-56.

Weiss RF. Herbal Medicine. Gothenburg, Sweden: Beaconsfield, 1988.

Weller A, Weller L. Menstrual synchrony between mothers and daughters and between roommates. Physiol Behav. 1993 May;53(5):943-9.

Weller L, Weller A, Roizman S. Human menstrual synchrony in families and among close friends: examining the importance of mutual exposure. J Comp Psychol. 1999 Sep;113(3):261-8.

Welsh D, Yoo SH, Liu A, Takahashi J, Kay S. Bioluminescence Imaging of Individual Fibroblasts Reveals Persistent, Independently Phased Circadian Rhythms of Clock Gene Expression. Current Biology. 2004;14:2289-2295.

Wen YD, Zhu YZ. The Pharmacological Effects of S-Propargyl-Cysteine, a Novel Endogenous H2S-Producing Compound. Handb Exp Pharmacol. 2015;230:325-36. doi: 10.1007/978-3-319-18144-8_16.

Werbach M. Nutritional Influences on Illness. Tarzana, CA: Third Line Press, 1996.

West P. Surf Your Biowaves. London: Quantum, 1999.

West R. Risk of death in meat and non-meat eaters. BMJ. 1994 Oct 8;309(6959):955.

Westman M, Eden D. Effects of a respite from work on burnout: vacation relief and fade-out. J Appl Psychol. 1997 Aug;82(4):516-27.

Wetterberg L. Light and biological rhythms. J Intern Med. 1994 Jan;235(1):5-19.

Wheeler FJ. The Bach Remedies Repertory. New Canaan, CN: Keats, 1997.

Wheeler JG, Bogle ML, Shema SJ, Shirrell MA, Stine KC, Pittler AJ, Burks AW, Helm RM. Impact of dietary yogurt on immune function. Am J Med Sci. 1997 Feb;313(2):120-3.

White AR, Rampes H, Ernst E. Acupuncture for smoking cessation. Cochrane Database Syst Rev. 2002;(2):CD000009.

White J, Krippner S (eds). Future Science: Life Energies & the Physics of Paranormal Phenomena. Garden City: Anchor, 1977.

White LB, Foster S. The Herbal Drugstore. Emmaus, PA: Rodale, 2000.

White S. The Unity of the Self. Cambridge: MIT Press, 1991.

Whiten, A. and E. M. Widdowson (eds.). Foraging Strategies and Natural Diet of Monkeys, Apes and Humans. Oxford: Clarendon Press, 1991.

Whitfield KE, King G, Moller S, Edwards CL, Nelson T, Vandenbergh D. Concordance rates for smoking among African-American twins. J Natl Med Assoc. 2007 Mar;99(3):213-7.

Whittaker E. History of the Theories of Aether and Electricity. New York: Nelson LTD, 1953.

Whitton J. Life Between Life. New York: Warner, 1986.

WHO. Guidelines for Drinking-water Quality. 2nd ed, vol. 2. Geneva: World Health Organization, 1996.

WHO. How trace elements in water contribute to health. WHO Chronicle. 1978;32:382-385.

Widmer W. Determination of naringin and neohesperidin in orange juice by liquid chromatography with UV detection to detect the presence of grapefruit juice: Collaborative Study. J AOAC Int. 2000 Sep-Oct;83(5):1155-65.

Wilke M, Holland SK, Altaye M, Gaser C. Template-O-Matic: a toolbox for creating customized pediatric templates. Neuroimage 2008;41:903-13.

Wilkinson SM, Love SB, Westcombe AM, Gambles MA, Burgess CC, Cargill A, Young T, Maher EJ, Ramirez AJ. Effectiveness of aromatherapy massage in the management of anxiety and depression in patients with cancer: a multicenter randomized controlled trial. J Clin Oncol. 2007 Feb 10;25(5):532-9.

Willard T, Jones K. Reishi Mushroom: Herb of Spiritual Potency and Medical Wonder. Issaquah, Washington: Sylvan Press, 1990.

Willard T. Edible and Medicinal Plants of the Rocky Mountains and Neighbouring Territories. Calgary: 1992.

Willemsen LE, Koetsier MA, Balvers M, Beermann C, Stahl B, van Tol EA. Polyunsaturated fatty acids support epithelial barrier integrity and reduce IL-4 mediated permeability in vitro. Eur J Nutr. 2008 Jun;47(4):183-91.

Williams A. Electron microscopic changes associated with water absorption in the jejunum. Gut. 1963;4:1-7.

Williams G. Natural Selection: Domains, levels, and challenges. Oxford: Oxford Univ Press, 1992.

Williams LJ, et al. Status of Folic Acid Fortification in the United States. Pediatrics 2005; 116; 580-586.

Wilson L. Nutritional Balancing and Hair Mineral Analysis. Prescott, AZ: LD Wilson, 1998.

Wilson RS, Barnes LL, Aggarwal NT, Boyle PA, Hebert LE, Mendes de Leon CF, Evans DA. Cognitive activity and the cognitive morbidity of Alzheimer disease. Neurology. 2010 Sep 14;75(11):990-6. doi: 10.1212/WNL.0b013e3181f25b5e.

Wilson RS, Scherr PA, Schneider JA, Tang Y, Bennett DA. Relation of cognitive activity to risk of developing Alzheimer disease. Neurology. 2007 Nov 13;69(20):1911-20.

Winchester AM. Biology and its Relation to Mankind. New York: Van Nostrand Reinhold, 1969.

Winfree AT. The Timing of Biological Clocks. New York: Scientific American, 1987.

Winneke G. Developmental aspects of environmental neurotoxicology: lessons from lead and polychlorinated biphenyls. J Neurol Sci. 2011 Sep 15;308(1-2):9-15. doi: 10.1016/j.jns.2011.05.020.

Winstead DK, Schwartz BD, Bertrand WE. Biorhythms: fact or superstition? Am J Psychiatry. 1981 Sep;138(9):1188-92.

Wise M, Doehlert D, McMullen M. Association of Avenanthramide Concentration in Oat (Avena sativa L.) Grain with Crown Rust Incidence and Genetic Resistance. Cereal Chem. 85(5):639-641.

Wiseman H. Vitamin D is a membrane antioxidant. Ability to inhibit iron-dependent lipid peroxidation in liposomes compared to cholesterol, ergosterol and tamoxifen and relevance to anticancer action. FEBS Lett. 1993 Jul 12;326(1-3):285-8.

Wittenberg JS. The Rebellious Body. New York: Insight, 1996.

Wixted JT. A Theory About Why We Forget What We Once Knew. CurrDir Psychol Sci. 2005;14(1):6-9.

Wolf, M. Beyond the Point Particle - A Wave Structure for the Electron. Galilean Electrodynamics. 1995 Oct;6(5): 83-91.

Wolverton BC. How to Grow Fresh Air: 50 House Plants that Purify Your Home or Office. New York: Penguin, 1997.

Woo JY, Gu W, Kim KA, Jang SE, Han MJ, Kim DH. Lactobacillus pentosus var. plantarum C29 ameliorates memory impairment and inflammaging in a D-galactose-induced accelerated aging mouse model. Anaerobe. 2014 Jun;27:22-6. doi: 10.1016/j.anaerobe.2014.03.003.

Wood M. The Book of Herbal Wisdom. Berkeley, CA: North Atlantic, 1997.

World Cancer Research Fund, American Institute for Cancer Research. Food, Nutrition and the Prevention of Cancer: A Global Perspective. 1997: 509.

Worwood VA. The Complete Book of Essential Oils & Aromatherapy. San Rafael, CA: New World, 1991.

Wright ML. Melatonin, diel rhythms, and metamorphosis in anuran amphibians. Gen Comp Endocrinol. 2002 May;126(3):251-4.

Wu ZC, Yu JT, Li Y, Tan L. Clusterin in Alzheimer's disease. Adv Clin Chem. 2012;56:155-73.

Würsch P, Pi-Sunyer FX. The role of viscous soluble fiber in the metabolic control of diabetes. A review with special emphasis on cereals rich in beta-glucan. Diabetes Care. 1997 Nov;20(11):1774-80.

Wyart C, Webster WW, Chen JH, Wilson SR, McClary A, Khan RM, Sobel N. Smelling a single component of male sweat alters levels of cortisol in women. J Neurosci. 2007 Feb 7;27(6):1261-5.

Wyka J. [Nutritional factors in prevention of Alzheimer's disease]. Rocz Panstw Zakl Hig. 2012;63(2):135-40.

Wylie LJ, Mohr M, Krustrup P, Jackman SR, Ermıdis G, Kelly J, Black MI, Bailey SJ, Vanhatalo A, Jones AM. Dietary nitrate supplementation improves team sport-specific intense intermittent exercise performance. Eur J Appl Physiol. 2013 Feb 1.

Xiao D, Srivastava SK, Lew KL, Zeng Y, Hershberger P, Johnson CS, Trump DL, Singh SV. Allyl isothiocyanate, a constituent of cruciferous vegetables, inhibits proliferation of human prostate cancer cells by causing G2/M arrest and inducing apoptosis. Carcinogenesis. 2003 May;24(5):891-7.

Xu Y, Jin-zhou T, and Shu-li S. Changes of brain myelin sheath structure and myelin basic protein content induced by amyloid β peptide (Aβ) and effect of GETO on these changes. Chinese Journal of Rehabilitation Theory & Practice 12 (2005): 004.

Xu Y, Tian JZ, Sheng SL. [Effect of GETO on expression of protein in postsynaptic dense zone of Alzheimer's disease model rats]. Zhongguo Zhong Xi Yi Jie He Za Zhi. 2006 Jan;26(1):54-7.

Yadav H, Jain S, Sinha PR. Antidiabetic effect of probiotic dahi containing Lactobacillus acidophilus and Lactobacillus casei in high fructose fed rats. Nutrition. 2007 Jan;23(1):62-8.

Yadav RK, Ray RB, Vempati R, Bijlani RL. Effect of a comprehensive yoga-based lifestyle modification program on lipid peroxidation. Indian J Physiol Pharmacol. 2005 Jul-Sep;49(3):358-62.

Yadav VS, Mishra KP, Singh DP, Mehrotra S, Singh VK. Immunomodulatory effects of curcumin. Immunopharmacol Immunotoxicol. 2005;27(3):485-97.

Yakoot M, Salem A, Helmy S. Effect of Memo®, a natural formula combination, on Mini-Mental State Examination scores in patients with mild cognitive impairment. Clin Interv Aging. 2013;8:975-81. doi: 10.2147/CIA.S44777.

Yamaoka Y. Solid cell nest (SCN) of the human thyroid gland. Acta Pathol Jpn. 1973 Aug;23(3):493-506.

Yan MZ, Chang Q, Zhong Y, Xiao BX, Feng L, Cao FR, Pan RL, Zhang ZS, Liao YH, Liu XM. Lotus Leaf Alkaloid Extract Displays Sedative-Hypnotic and Anxiolytic Effects through GABAA Receptor. J Agric Food Chem. 2015 Oct 28;63(42):9277-85. doi: 10.1021/acs.jafc.5b04141.

Yan YF, Wei YY, Chen YH, Chen MM. Effect of acupuncture on rehabilitation training of child's autism. Zhongguo Zhen Jiu. 2007 Jul;27(7):503-5.

Yang H, Wang Y, Cheryan VT, Wu W, Cui CQ, Polin LA, Pass HI, Dou QP, Rishi AK, Wali A. Withaferin a inhibits the proteasome activity in mesothelioma in vitro and in vivo. PLoS One. 2012;7(8):e41214

Yang HQ, Xie SS, Hu XL, Chen L, Li H. Appearance of human meridian-like structure and acupoints and its time correlation by infrared thermal imaging. Am J Chin Med. 2007;35(2):231-40.

Yao Y, Sang W, Zhou M, Ren G. Phenolic composition and antioxidant activities of 11 celery cultivars. J Food Sci. 2010 Jan-Feb;75(1):C9-13.

Ye Q, Huang B, Zhang X, Zhu Y, Chen X. Astaxanthin protects against MPP+-induced oxidative stress in PC12 cells via the HO-1/NOX2 axis. BMC Neurosci. 2012 Dec 29;13:156. doi: 10.1186/1471-2202-13-156.

Ye Q, Huang B, Zhang X, Zhu Y, Chen X. Astaxanthin protects against MPP+-induced oxidative stress in PC12 cells via the HO-1/NOX2 axis. BMC Neurosci. 2012 Dec 29;13:156. doi: 10.1186/1471-2202-13-156.

Yeager S. The Doctor's Book of Food Remedies. Emmaus, PA: Rodale Press, 1998.

Yeh CC, Lin CC, Wang SD, Chen YS, Su BH, Kao ST. Protective and anti-inflammatory effect of a traditional Chinese medicine, Xia-Bai-San, by modulating lung local cytokine in a murine model of acute lung injury. Int Immunopharmacol. 2006 Sep;6(9):1506-14.

Yeh CT, Yen GC. Effect of vegetables on human phenolsulfotransferases in relation to their antioxidant activity and total phenolics. Free Radic Res. 2005 Aug;39(8):893-904.

Yeung JW. A hypothesis: Sunspot cycles may detect pandemic influenza A in 1700-2000 A.D. Med Hypotheses. 2006;67(5):1016-22.

Yokoi S, Ikeya M, Yagi T, Nagai K. Mouse circadian rhythm before the Kobe earthquake in 1995. Bioelectromagnetics. 2003 May;24(4):289-91.

Yoo DH, Kim DH. Lactobacillus pentosus var. plantarum C29 increases the protective effect of soybean against scopolamine-induced memory impairment in mice. Int J Food Sci Nutr. 2015;66(8):912-8. doi: 10.3109/09637486.2015.1064865.

Yoshioka M, Doucet E, Drapeau V, Dionne I, Tremblay A. Combined effects of red pepper and caffeine consumption on 24 h energy balance in subjects given free access to foods. Br J Nutr. 2001 Feb;85(2):203-11.

You JS, Lee YJ, Kim KS, Kim SH, Chang KJ. Ethanol extract of lotus (Nelumbo nucifera) root exhibits an anti-adipogenic effect in human pre-adipocytes and anti-obesity and anti-oxidant effects in rats fed a high-fat diet. Nutr Res. 2014 Mar;34(3):258-67. doi: 10.1016/j.nutres.2014.01.003.

Yu L, Lin SM, Zhou RQ, Tang WJ, Huang PX, Dong Y, Wang J, Yu ZH, Chen JL, Wei L, Xing SL, Cao HJ, Zhao HB. Chinese herbal medicine for patients with mild to moderate Alzheimer disease based on syndrome differentiation: a randomized controlled trial. Zhong Xi Yi Jie He Xue Bao. 2012 Jul;10(7):766-76.

Yu XM, Zhu GM, Chen YL, Fang M, Chen YN. Systematic assessment of acupuncture for treatment of herpes zoster in domestic clinical studies. Zhongguo Zhen Jiu. 2007 Jul;27(7):536-40.

Yuan L, Gu X, Yin Z, Kang W. Antioxidant activities in vitro and hepatoprotective effects of Nelumbo nucifera leaves in vivo. Afr J Tradit Complement Altern Med. 2014 Apr 3;11(3):85-91.

Yuan SY, Lun X, Liu DS, Qin Z, Chen WT. Acupoint-injection of BCG polysaccharide nuclear acid for treatment of condyloma acuminatum and its immunoregulatory action on the patient. Zhongguo Zhen Jiu. 2007 Jun;27(6):407-11.

Yun CH, Estrada A, Van Kessel A, Gajadhar A, Redmond M, Laarveld B. Immunomodulatory effects of oat beta-glucan administered intragastrically or parenterally on mice infected with Eimeria vermiformis. Microbiol Immunol. 1998;42(6):457-65.

Yun HM, Jin P, Park KR, Hwang J, Jeong HS, Kim EC, Jung JK, Oh KW, Hwang BY, Han SB, Hong JT. Thiacremonone Potentiates Anti-Oxidant Effects to Improve Memory Dysfunction in an APP/PS1 Transgenic Mice Model. Mol Neurobiol. 2016 May;53(4):2409-20. doi: 10.1007/s12035-015-9208-0.

Zaets VN, Karpov PA, Smertenko PS, Blium IaB. Molecular mechanisms of the repair of UV-induced DNA damages in plants. Tsitol Genet. 2006 Sep-Oct;40(5):40-68. Review.

Zago W, Buttini M, Comery TA, Nishioka C, Gardai SJ, Seubert P, Games D, Bard F, Schenk D, Kinney GG. Neutralization of soluble, synaptotoxic amyloid β species by antibodies is epitope specific. J Neurosci. 2012 Feb 22;32(8):2696-702. doi: 10.1523/JNEUROSCI.1676-11.2012.

Zamora JL. Chemical and microbiologic characteristics and toxicity of povidone-iodine solutions. Am J Surg. 1986 Mar;151(3):400-6.

Zand J, Lanza F, Garg HK, Bryan NS. All-natural nitrite and nitrate containing dietary supplement promotes nitric oxide production and reduces triglycerides in humans. Nutr Res. 2011 Apr;31(4):262-9.

Zarate G, Gonzalez S, Chaia AP. Assessing survival of dairy propionibacteria in gastrointestinal conditions and adherence to intestinal epithelia. Centro de Referencia para Lactobacilos-CONICET. Tucuman, Argentina: Humana Press. 2004.

Zarnowski R, Suzuki Y, Yamaguchi I, Pietr SJ. Alkylresorcinols in barley Hordeum vulgare L. distichon) grains. Z Naturforsch. 2002 Jan-Feb;57(1-2):57-62.

Zarnowski R, Suzuki Y. 5-n-Alkylresorcinols from grains of winter barley (Hordeum vulgare L.). Z Naturforsch. 2004 May-Jun;59(5-6):315-7.

Zeiger RS, Heller S. The development and prediction of atopy in high-risk children: follow-up at age seven years in a prospective randomized study of combined maternal and infant food allergen avoidance. J Allergy Clin Immunol. 1995 Jun;95(6):1179-90.

Zeliger HI. Exposure to lipophilic chemicals as a cause of neurological impairments, neurodevelopmental disorders and neurodegenerative diseases. Interdiscip Toxicol. 2013 Sep;6(3):103-110.

Zhan S, Ho SC. 2005. Meta-analysis of the effects of soy protein containing isoflavones on the lipid profile. Am J Clin Nutr. Feb;81(2):397-408.

Zhang C, Popp, F., Bischof, M.(eds.). Electromagnetic standing waves as background of acupuncture system. Current Development in Biophysics - the Stage from an Ugly Duckling to a Beautiful Swan. Hangzhou: Hangzhou University Press, 1996.

Zhang J, Sun C, Yan Y, Chen Q, Luo F, Zhu X, Li X, Chen K. Purification of naringin and neohesperidin from Huyou (Citrus changshanensis) fruit and their effects on glucose consumption in human HepG2 cells. Food Chem. 2012 Dec 1;135(3):1471-8.

Zhang QH, Zhang I, Shang LX, Shao CL, Wu YX. Studies on the chemical constituents of flowers of Prunus mume. Zhong Yao Cai. 2008 Nov;31(11):1666-8.

Zhang X, Shu XO, Xiang YB, Yang G, Li H, Gao J, Cai H, Gao YT, Zheng W. Cruciferous vegetable consumption is associated with a reduced risk of total and cardiovascular disease mortality. Am J Clin Nutr. 2011 Jul;94(1):240-6.

Zhao QF, Yu JT, Tan MS, Tan L. ABCA7 in Alzheimer's Disease. Mol Neurobiol. 2015;51(3):1008-16. doi: 10.1007/s12035-014-8759-9.

Zhao X, Shen J, Chang KJ, Kim SH. Analysis of fatty acids and phytosterols in ethanol extracts of Nelumbo nucifera seeds and rhizomes by GC-MS. J Agric Food Chem. 2013 Jul 17;61(28):6841-7. doi: 10.1021/jf401710h.

Zhao XL, Wang ZM, Ma XJ, Jing WG, Liu A. [Chemical constituents from leaves of Nelumbo nucifera]. Zhongguo Zhong Yao Za Zhi. 2013 Mar;38(5):703-8.

Zheng X, Gessel MM, Wisniewski ML, Viswanathan K, Wright DL, Bahr BA, Bowers MT. Z-Phe-Ala-diazomethylketone (PADK) disrupts and remodels early oligomers states of the Alzheimer disease Beta-amyloid42 protein. J Biol Chem. 2012 Feb 24;287(9):6084-8.

Zheng X, Gessel MM, Wisniewski ML, Viswanathan K, Wright DL, Bahr BA, Bowers MT. Z-Phe-Ala-diazomethylketone (PADK) disrupts and remodels early oligomer states of the Alzheimer disease Aβ42 protein. J Biol Chem. 2012 Feb 24;287(9):6084-8.

Zielińska-Przyjemska M, Olejnik A, Kostrzewa A, Łuczak M, Jagodziński PP, Baer-Dubowska W. The beetroot component betanin modulates ROS production, DNA damage and apoptosis in human polymorphonuclear neutrophils. Phytother Res. 2012 Jun;26(6):845-52.

Zimecki M. The lunar cycle: effects on human and animal behavior and physiology. Postepy Hig Med Dosw. 2006;60:1-7.

Zizza, C. The nutrient content of the Italian food supply 1961-1992. Euro J Clin Nutr. 1997;51: 259-265.

Zou C, Montagna E, Shi Y, Peters F, Blazquez-Llorca L, Shi S, Filser S, Dorostkar MM, Herms J. Intraneuronal APP and extracellular Aβ independently cause dendritic spine pathology in transgenic mouse models of Alzheimer's disease. Acta Neuropathol. 2015 Jun;129(6):909-20. doi: 10.1007/s00401-015-1421-4.

Zou Z, Li F, Buck L. Odor maps in the olfactory cortex. Proc Natl Acad of Sci. 2005;102(May 24):7724-7729.

Zschäbitz S, Cheng TY, Neuhouser ML, Zheng Y, Ray RM, Miller JW, Song X, Maneval DR, Beresford SA, Lane D, Shikany JM, Ulrich CM. B vitamin intakes and incidence of colorectal cancer: results from the Women's Health Initiative Observational Study cohort. Am J Clin Nutr. 2012 Dec 19.

Index

*(Foods and nutrients too numerous to index—
refer to ebook for better search ability)*

Made in the USA
Monee, IL
06 July 2024

61356803R00185